Perspectives in
Behavioral Medicine

STRESS AND
DISEASE PROCESSES

Perspectives in Behavioral Medicine
Sponsored by the Academy of Behavioral Medicine Research

Perspectives in
Behavioral Medicine

STRESS AND
DISEASE PROCESSES

Edited by

Neil Schneiderman
Department of Psychology
University of Miami

Philip McCabe
Department of Psychology
University of Miami

Andrew Baum
F. Edward Hébert School of Medicine
Uniformed Services University of the Health Sciences

LEA
1992
LAWRENCE ERLBAUM ASSOCIATES, PUBLISHERS
Hillsdale, New Jersey   Hove and London

Lawrence Erlbaum Associates, Inc., Publishers
365 Broadway
Hillsdale, New Jersey 07642

Library of Congress Cataloging-in-Publication Data

Stress and disease processes / edited by Neil Schneiderman, Philip
  McCabe, Andrew Baum.
      p.   cm. — (Perspectives in behavioral medicine)
  Includes bibliographical references and indexes.
  ISBN 0–8058–1161–3
  1. Stress (Physiology) 2. Stress (Psychology)
3. Psychoneuroimmunology. I. Schneiderman, Neil. II. McCabe,
Philip M. III. Baum, Andrew. IV. Series.
  [DNLM: 1. Immune System—physiology.   2. Psychoneuroimmunology.
3. Stress, Psychological—immunology.   QZ 160 S9142]
QP82.2.S8S84   1992
616.07′9—dc20
DNLM/DLC
for Library of Congress   92–859
                                                           CIP

Printed in the United States of America
10 9 8 7 6 5 4 3 2 1

CONTENTS

PREFACE

As we have learned more about the relationships between stress and illness, we have been able to clearly delineate pathways by which stress may interfere with health maintenance and contribute directly to disease etiology and progression. Sympathetic nervous system arousal that drives many of the biological sequelae of stress appears to affect atherosclerosis, hypertension-related blood pressure changes, and a host of other pathogenic processes important in behaviorally-mediated disease. Although much of the research in behavioral medicine has focused on stress-related physiological changes and heart disease, there are rapidly growing research efforts addressing immune and endocrine changes and their effects on infectious disease, AIDS, diabetes, and other diseases.

A second pathway by which stress may alter health is less direct. We know that stress affects behavior in ways that can affect health. For example, it is widely believed that stress increases already established drug use, including cigarette use, caffeine consumption, and use of alcohol. To varying extents, such behavior appears to contribute to disease. Similarly, stress may interfere with important health-maintenance activities: Exercise, diet, and other valuable behaviors may decrease or disappear during or after substantial stress. In addition, specific regimens designed to prevent or control already established disease may not be followed during stress-related episodes of negative affect or disruption of daily routine. Thus, maintenance of preventive behaviors or use of drugs to control diseases such as diabetes or hypertension may be more difficult during stress.

A third pathway is closely related to the second. Illness behavior, loosely defined as actions that characterize ill individuals or that affect treatment, also appears to be affected by stress. Use of insulin to control diabetes or adherence to antihypertensive medical regimens could also be considered here, but other aspects of illness behavior are affected as well. Seeking medical attention when symptoms warrant it, detection and interpretation of symptoms, adherence to various regimens, and several other aspects of effective health behaviors appear to be vulnerable to stress-derived interference.

The chapters in this book are concerned with these different pathways, focusing on direct effects of stress on the immune and endocrine systems, on behavioral factors in diseases such as cancer and diabetes, and with the general role of stress in illness processes. We believe that they push beyond the well-staked boundaries of traditional models of disease and that like the Academy of Behavioral Medicine Research meeting that the book is based on, the authors have a good deal to say that is new and important. Continued study of these and other stress-related processes will provide critical data for preventing and treating modern epidemics.

The Academy wishes to thank Cheryl Palacios and Sandra Racoobian for their help in producing this volume. As is so often the case, their contributions are essential but largely unrecognized.

Neil Schneiderman
Philip McCabe
Andrew Baum

LIST OF CONTRIBUTORS

ROBERT ADER Department of Psychiatry, University of Rochester School of Medicine and Dentistry, 300 Crittenden Boulevard, Box Psych., Rochester, NY 14642.

MICHAEL H. ANTONI Department of Psychology, University of Miami, P.O. Box 248185, Coral Gables, FL 33124.

ANDREW BAUM F. Edward Hébert School of Medicine, Uniformed Services University of the Health Sciences, 4301 Jones Bridge Road, Bethesda, MD 20814-4799.

FRANK BERKENBOSCH Department of Pharmacology, Free University, Van der Boechorststraat 7, 1081 BT Amsterdam, The Netherlands.

LILLY BOURGUIGNON Department of Medicine, University of Miami Medical School, Coral Gables, FL 33136.

NICHOLAS COHEN University of Rochester School of Medicine and Dentistry, Department of Microbiology and Immunology, 300 Crittenden Boulevard, Rochester, NY 14642.

BONITA FALKNER Department of Pediatrics, Medical College of Pennsylvania, 3300 Henry Avenue, Philadelphia, PA 19129.

MICHAEL D. FILI University of Miami School of Medicine, Coral Gables, FL 33101.

MARY ANN FLETCHER Department of Medicine (R-42), University of

Miami Medical School, 1600 N.W. 10th Avenue, Room 8166, Miami, FL 33136.

SONIA HULMAN   Department of Pediatrics, Hahnemann University, Philadelphia, PA 19102.

MICHAEL D. IRWIN   Veterans Administration Medical Center, Psychology 116A, 3350 La Jolla Village Drive, San Diego, CA 92161.

SUZANNE BENNETT JOHNSON   Department of Psychiatry, University of Florida Health Science Center, P.O. Box 10023-1, Gainesville, FL 32610-0234.

NANCY KLIMAS   Department of Medicine, R-42, University of Miami Medical School, P.O. Box 016960, Miami, FL 33101.

HARVEY KUSHNER   Department of Pediatrics, Hahnemann University, Philadelphia, PA 19102.

ANNETTE M. LA GRECA   Department of Psychology, University of Miami, P.O. Box 248185, Coral Gables, FL 33124.

ARTHUR LaPERRIERE   Department of Psychology, University of Miami, P.O. Box 248185, Coral Gables, FL 33124.

SANDRA M. LEVY   Pittsburgh Cancer Institute, University of Pittsburgh School of Medicine, 200 Meyran Avenue, Pittsburgh, PA 15213-2592.

JENNIFER B. MARKS   Behavioral Medicine Research Center, University of Miami Medical School, P.O. Box 016960, Miami, FL 33101.

PHILIP McCABE   Department of Psychology, University of Miami, P.O. Box 248185, Coral Gables, FL 33124.

CARRIE MILLON   Department of Medicine, University of Miami Medical School, P.O. Box 016960, Miami, FL 33101.

ROBERT MORGAN   Department of Medicine, University of Miami Medical School, P.O. Box 016960, Miami, FL 33101.

JAN A. MOYNIHAN   Department of Psychiatry, University of Rochester School of Medicine and Dentistry, 300 Crittenden Boulevard, Rochester, NY 14642.

DAWN C. ROBERTS Department of Psychology, The University of Iowa, Iowa City, IA 52242.

FERNANDO SALVATO Department of Medicine, University of Miami, P.O. Box 016960, Miami, FL 33101.

LAURA SCHNEIDERMAN Department of Medical Psychology, Uniformed Services University of the Health Sciences, 4301 Jones Bridge Road, Bethesda, MD 20814–4799.

NEIL SCHNEIDERMAN Department of Psychology, University of Miami, P.O. Box 248185, Coral Gables, FL 33124.

JAY S. SKYLER Behavioral Medicine Research Center, University of Miami Medical School, P.O. Box 016960 (D-110), Miami, FL 33101.

DANTE S. SPETTER Department of Psychology, University of Miami, P.O. Box 248185, Coral Gables, FL 33124.

ARTHUR A. STONE Departments of Psychiatry and Behavioral Science, State University of New York at Stony Brook, Putnam Hall, South Campus, Room 137, Stony Brook, NY 11794–8790.

EDWARD C. SUAREZ Department of Psychiatry, Duke University Medical Center, Box 3842, Durham, NC 27710.

RICHARD S. SURWIT Department of Psychiatry, Duke University Medical Center, Box 3842, Durham, NC 27710.

NOVELETTE E. THOMPSON Behavioral Medicine Research Center, University of Miami Medical School, P.O. Box 016960, Miami, FL 33101.

FLAVIA VAN RIEL Department of Medicine, University of Miami Medical School, P.O. Box 016960, Miami, FL 33101.

REDFORD B. WILLIAMS, JR. Department of Psychiatry, Duke University Medical Center, Box 3842, Durham, NC 27710.

1 Acute and Chronic Stress and the Immune System

Laura Schneiderman
Andrew Baum
Uniformed Services University of the Health Sciences

The relationship between stress and health has long been one block in the foundation of behavioral medicine research and intervention. The contribution of stress to a wide variety of physical illnesses and to mental health are widely believed to be important, and research has addressed stress as a factor in heart disease, hypertension, stroke, cancer, and many other illnesses. Hormonal changes, hemodynamic responses, and other bodily reactions during stress have been considered to be risk factors for illness. Of some interest is the relationship between stress and immunity and whether the changes that have been observed are meaningful. Yet, we still know relatively little about how stress affects immune function, why such effects occur, and whether these changes have any real clinical significance.

One problem has been the relative dearth of research on human subjects, at least until recently. Most work through the 1970s was concerned with animal populations and, although extremely important in revealing links between behavioral factors and immune response (Ader & Cohen, 1981), it provided an imperfect model of stress and immune function in humans. Related to this is the fact that most work with humans considered subjects who had been victimized or exposed to stressful conditions, be they bereaved, caregivers for seriously ill people, medical students facing examinations, or divorced and/or separated spouses. Relatively little research has addressed acute stress in humans and has examined the effects of experimentally applied stress on normal volunteers. The generalizability of the results of studies of intermediate or long-term stress on immunity to short-term events and the meaning of good or poor correspondence across stress durations remains undetermined. This chapter selectively reviews

1

research on animal and human immunological responses during acute and chronic stress to establish how well they correspond and whether one can consider acute and chronic stress as comparable in this instance.

Distinguishing between chronic and acute stress and gauging the severity and duration of stress effects is a complex task. Depending on an individual's experience when he or she is exposed to a stressor, the duration of the psychological and physiological responses may vary. This variation in response duration may depend on the ability of the organism to adjust to an event as much as on the duration or severity of the stressor (Baum, O'Keeffe, & Davidson, 1990). Acute stress may generate brief responses as the stressor passes or as adjustment to the event occurs. However, some acute events, such as traumatic events, may cause long-term responses that outlast the event itself. Similarly, chronic stressors may foster responses that last for a long time due to chronic exposure to an intractable situation or to failure to adjust, but may also lead to adaptation and cessation of stress responding while the stressor persists (Baum et al., 1990). Thus, acute stressors to which adjustment is difficult may generate long-term responses just as chronic stressors may cause chronic responses, and either may generate only brief responses. In addition, there are psychosocial mediators that affect adjustment to the stressful situation, by buffering the distress associated with the stressor (e.g., having perceived control over the stressor) or by augmenting distress associated with the stressor (e.g., by being lonely or depressed). Because it is likely that the duration of stress responding may affect the ways in which stress affects health, determination of these aspects of stress are important.

The complexity introduced by these concepts eliminates the elegance of simplicity, but increases their descriptive power. Although it may be more difficult to convince skeptics that basic stress–immune system relationships exist and are meaningful if we must qualify answers to these questions, the role of psychosocial mediation of this link provides clues as to preventive or ameliorative responses to stress-induced immunosuppression. Social support, efficacious coping, distress reduction, and other putative mediators of stress are potentially important in this effort.

We have divided the chapter into four sections, separately discussing animal and human studies of acute and chronic stress. It is difficult to classify some studies: Duration of stressor exposure varies greatly and distinctions between acute and chronic may become arbitrary at some level. Further, the duration of stress response does not necessarily match that of stressor exposure. These issues have led to extended analyses of chronic stress that are beyond the scope of this chapter (see Baum, 1990). Regardless, studies fall more or less into these categories and provide useful insights into the nature of stress and its health consequences.

ACUTE STRESSORS AND IMMUNITY

In psychophysiological studies of stress, acute laboratory exposure to stressful conditions is more common than are longer term or naturalistic studies of stress. This is particularly true of human studies where ethical and logistical concerns make the latter more difficult. In studies of stress and immune function, the reverse seems true; relatively few studies of acute stress and immune function in humans have been reported. To some extent this may be due to the time course of immune system changes: If these changes do not occur for several hours after exposure to a stressor, one must keep subjects in the laboratory and prevent potentially contaminating events for a long period of time. If they occur more rapidly, however, these studies can and should be pursued.

Animal Studies

In many animal studies simple physical events such as electric shock or immobilization have been used to generate stress and affect immune function (Gisler, 1974; Harmsen & Turney, 1985; Keller, Weiss, Schleifer, Miller, & Stein, 1983; Laudenslager, et al., 1988; Shavit, Lewis, Terman, Gale, & Liebeskind, 1984). For example, Harmsen and Turney (1985) exposed rats to 3 hours of intermittent shocks of one shock per minute. Neutrophil function was measured and results indicated that stressed rats demonstrated poor accumulation at a zymosan (yeast cell fragment) injection site compared to control rats. Acute physical stressors have also been found to decrease natural killer cell activity (Shavit et al., 1984) and lymphocyte proliferation to mitogen challenge (Keller et al., 1983). It is likely however, that physical stressors are emotionally arousing and that some of the consequences of these stressors are psychologically mediated (Mason, 1975). Being restrained or shocked is an aversive event that may involve psychological reactions as well as sensations associated with physiological changes.

The perception of a stressor as threatening may be necessary for stress responses to occur and therefore adjustment to a stressful event may only result if the stressor is no longer perceived as threatening (Mason, 1975). Kant and her colleagues (1984) have also suggested that response habituation results from behavioral experiences with a particular stressor, and not to biochemical adaptation or habituation of endocrine and neurotransmitter systems after repeated use. When rats were exposed to 15 minutes of restraint, footshock, or forced running for 10 consecutive days it was found that prolactin and pituitary cyclic AMP responses to each stressor gradually diminished and all but disappeared by the Day 10. However, those exposed to a novel stressor on Day 11 showed fully restored responses, whereas those exposed to the same stressor on Day 11 showed little response (Kant et al., 1984). Thus, exposure to a new stressor elicited an augmented hormonal and neurochemical response, whereas there was a diminished biochemical response to the same stressor experienced previously. This suggests that behavioral experiences with a particular stressor may lead to habituation but that this is not due to biochemical adaptation to stressors.

Acute psychosocial stressors have also been examined in animal populations and their relationship to changes in immunity measured. Fleshner, Laudenslager, Simons, and Maier (1988) studied immunological changes associated with brief bouts of territorial invasion. Rats living singly in plexiglass enclosures were divided into two groups: (a) animals who were directly exposed to aggressive rats living in a colony in pairs, and (b) animals who were separated from the colony groups by a barrier. Immediately before the first colony exposure, the intruders in both groups were immunized with keyhole limpet hemocyanin (KLH). The intruders were then exposed to five different colonies, each for 10 minutes. Intruders who directly interacted with aggressive colonies had lower levels of KLH serum IgG antibodies 1 and 2 weeks after immunization than the controls, suggesting that the animals exposed to a stressful situation (i.e., repeated confrontation with aggressive rats) were less able to launch an immune response against the KLH antigen. Apparently this was due to repeated exposure to dominant others, as those rats who reacted to the aggressive encounters by assuming more submissive postures had the lowest levels of antibody to KLH. Submissive posturing was associated with the frequency of being bitten but this variable was not correlated with KLH IgG levels. And, although the duration of the stressor exposure was acute (five, 10-minute exposures) differences in antibodies were still found 2 weeks later.

One way in which acute stressors may cause responses that outlast their physical presence is through conditioning, wherein neutral stimuli present during stressor exposure come to elicit responses independent of the stressor. Similar to the conditioned immunosuppression phenomenon (Ader & Cohen, 1981), the idea here is that the neutral stimuli could come to evoke immune responses or change responses when the stressor is no longer present. One study paired electric shock with an unrelated stimulus to determine if it would come to elicit similar immune changes when presented alone (Lysle, Cunnick, Fowler, & Rabin, 1988). Experimental animals were exposed to pairings of shock and either a clicking sound or flashing light. Ten presentations of the shock (5 seconds each) and conditioned stimulus (15 seconds each) were administered on consecutive days. Control animals were exposed to similar pairings of neutral and aversive stimuli but were not exposed to the conditioned stimulus (CS) during the test phase. After a

6-day recovery period the experimental group was given a test session of 10 presentations of the stimulus without shock.

Lymphocyte proliferation to mitogen challenge with concanavalin-A (Con A) and phytohemagglutinin (PHA) was suppressed following exposure to the CS. This suppression of proliferation was reduced during extinction when the conditioned stimulus was repeatedly presented in the absence of footshock. Additionally, pretreatment with repeated exposure to the conditioned stimulus before pairing with shock was found to lessen immune effects when the conditioned stimulus was later presented alone.

Psychosocial Mediators.   Psychosocial variables influence the impact of stressors and immunological sequelae of stress. Studies have examined psychological mediators that may buffer the effects of stressors; control or lack of control over stressors appears to be one such factor. Laudenslager (1983) observed lymphocyte proliferation to Con A and PHA following acute exposure to escapable or inescapable shock. Twelve rats were placed in a "wheel-turn" box and shock was given through tail electrodes on an average of one shock per minute for 80 minutes. The shock could be terminated by moving the wheel. Twelve more rats were each yoked with the escapable shock subjects and therefore received comparable amounts of inescapable shock. A home cage control group was also studied. Twenty-four hours later the rats in the two experimental groups were given five 5-second footshocks and blood was collected from all animals. Inescapable shock led to a suppression of lymphocyte proliferation to PHA in comparison to escapable shock and control procedures. The Con A-stimulated cultures revealed somewhat different results; inescapable shock depressed lymphocyte proliferation but escapable shock appeared to increase lymphocyte proliferation.

A similar study examined stressor (shock) controllability and its relationship to proliferation of lymphocytes to mitogen challenge (Mormede, Dantzer, Michaud, Kelly, & LeMoal, 1988). Splenic lymphocytes were examined instead of peripheral blood lymphocytes and in vivo antibody response to sheep red blood cells (SRBC) injected into the rats was measured as a function of stressor controllability. Animals in the controllable stressor group were able to postpone electric shocks by jumping over a barrier. Yoked animals were run at the same time and received the same amount of shock at the same intervals as the controllable stressor animals but were not able to regulate when the shocks would be administered. Control rats were placed in comparable settings but received no shock.

Lymphocyte response to PHA was significantly reduced in animals that had no control over the stressor relative to the controllable stressor or control groups, which were comparable. There were also significant differences in antibody titer levels to SRBC but these findings were seemingly inconsistent; animals in the controllable stressor group had lower antibody titers than did controls or animals in the uncontrollable stressor group. In observing decreases in antibody titer formation to SRBC in the controllable stressor group without changes in proliferation and depression of lympho-cyte proliferation to PHA it is important to note that consequences of controllability may vary depending on the type of immune response measured.

Uncontrollable shock may also affect immune-mediated health outcomes such as tumor development. Visintainer, Volpicelli, and Seligman (1982) examined tumor rejection in male rats exposed to inescapable or escapable shock, or not exposed to shock. Tumor cells were injected subcutaneously into the left lower anterior flank of each animal and 24 hours later each was exposed to shock or no-shock conditions. In the two shock conditions 60 random shock trials were delivered to the grid floor and sides of two identical chambers. Pressing a bar in the controllable shock chamber terminated the shock in both boxes, but depressing the bar in the inescap-able shock chamber had no effect. Only 37% of the rats exposed to escapable shock, compared to 46% of the rats given no shock and 73% of the inescapable shock animals developed tumors. Thus, rats exposed to inescapable shock were considerably less likely to reject the tumor as rats in the escapable shock condition. Visintainer et al. (1982) suggested that differences in immunocompetence was probably an important factor in fighting against the tumors.

Stressor predictability is related to control: Predictability may not increase instrumental control but appears to facilitate adaptation by permitting preparation and anticipating responses. It also appears to be related to immune system changes (Mormede et al., 1988). A predictable signaled shock condition featured a tone that was introduced 10 seconds before inescapable shock was delivered through a floor grid. In the unsignaled shock condition the tone was distributed randomly throughout the session. Lymphocyte response to Con A was 34% lower in the unsignaled shock than in the signaled shock condition. The same trend was found for lymphocyte responses to pokeweed mitogen (PWM) and PHA, although results were not significant. These results suggest that psycholog-ical interventions involving prediction or control may lessen the influence of a stressor on immune function.

The influence of predictability was significant only when cells were challenged with Con A, whereas controllability affected response to PHA. Mormede et al. (1988) suggested that these differences in response to the mitogens may reflect a variation in the sensitivity of the response to the mitogens depending on the conditions implemented during the sessions. This could indicate a differential involvement of immune cells including T lymphocyte subsets, such as helper T cells versus suppressor/cytotoxic T cells.

Conclusions. Animal models are useful in examining stress and immune activity as many of the variables involved in an experiment may be better controlled (e.g., life history, diet, and living conditions). However, use of animal models in studying the relationships between cognitive and emotional variables and immunity is limited by several factors. It is difficult to examine many psychological variables in relation to stress and immunity in animals because there are no ways to tap the phenomenological aspects of their experience. Depression, loneliness, and anxiety are just a few of the psychological variables that may require self-reports from humans in order to distinguish them and to fully understand their relationship to stress and immunity. Although, there have been some animal paradigms that have been used as models of depression and anxiety (e.g., Estes & Skinner, 1941; Maier, 1984) and these models are useful tools in gaining an understanding these phenomena, they may only model particular aspects of affect or dysfunction. It has been suggested for example, that learned helplessness is a good model for depression (e.g., Seligman, 1975). However, others have suggested that although learned helplessness may tap into some aspects of depression it does not duplicate the full clinical phenomena of depression. Learned helplessness results from exposure to uncontrollable situations and leads to debilitated escape learning during subsequent events that may reflect behavior common during depression. Also, changes produced in lever-pressing activities of rats in the Estes and Skinner (1941) experiments may be associated with some of the properties of anxiety, but again may not represent definitive characteristics of anxiety in all situations. It would be difficult to use these models to measure levels of anxiety or depression during stress because they were developed to examine the mechanisms involved in formation of emotional disturbances and not as quantitative indices of them during stress.

Physiological and psychological differences between animals and humans make comparisons between the two groups difficult. Human coping skills, adaptation, and emotionality appear to be different from those of most animal species, and immune systems may function differently across species. For example, Laudenslager (1983) and Mormede et al. (1988) found a decrease in proliferation of lymphocytes to PHA and/or Con A associated with uncontrollable shock in rats, whereas opposite results have been found in humans (Weisse et al., 1990). It is therefore critical that research be conducted with human subjects if the ultimate goal is application to them.

Human Studies

Research on acute human stress responses and immune function has not generally been as common as has work with animals. To some extent, this is due to the greater ease of obtaining measures of immune response and of controlling for genetic and behavioral history. Despite this, some studies have begun to appear and since the 1980s, our knowledge of how people respond during stress has expanded dramatically. There are still relatively few studies of controlled acute laboratory stressors and immune function in humans, however. Most of the recent work has been correlational, comparing stress and immune responses of selected groups of people.

One study of acute stress considered task performance and exercise and examined several indices of immunity (Landmann et al., 1984). Changes in numbers of lymphocyte subsets were measured in response to a cognitive conflict task (a modified version of the Stroop task; Stroop, 1935) and after bicycle ergometry performed to submaximal work capacity. Mean numbers of granulocytes were significantly higher after exercise stress than at baseline and all lymphocyte subtypes were increased. Following the cognitive conflict task, numbers of monocytes, B cells and, natural killer (NK) cells were significantly higher. Cell numbers increased during both the cognitive conflict task and the bicycle ergometry, although the types of cells differed. However, failure to adequately separate the two stressors, our lack of knowledge of the time course of changes in lymphocyte subpopulations, and the fact that no control group was included in the study design make interpretation of these findings difficult.

In an attempt to better understand how rapidly immune system changes occur in the face of stress and to examine controllability of a stressor as a mediator between stress and immunity, Weisse and colleagues (1990) exposed subjects either to a controllable noise/shock stressor or an uncontrollable noise/shock stressor. Subjects in the controllable stressor condition had to learn how many times they needed to press a button in order to terminate the stressor. Subjects in the uncontrollable stressor group were yoked to this group and were unable to control the noise/shock regardless of how many times they pressed the button. In order to control for time and blood drawing procedures subjects also participated in a baseline session in which they were not exposed to stressors.

Immune activity was not significantly altered by uncontrollable stress although mood and task performance on an anagram task were in predicted directions. However, subjects in the controllable stressor group exhibited a significant decrease in lymphocyte proliferation to Con A as well as in percentages of monocytes at the end of the session. Although clearly establishing an association between stress and immune system change in humans under controlled laboratory conditions, these results are not consistent with those reported by Laudenslager (1983) and suggest that important differences between animals and humans may be involved. It may be that mechanisms involved in controllability of a stressor and its effect on immune activity in rats may not be the same as in humans. Alternatively, the time frame involved in this study may explain these different findings. In the Laudenslager (1983) study blood was collected from the rats 24 hours after stress exposure, whereas Weisse (1989) collected blood samples within 2 hours of the stressor. The length of time in sampling in the Laudenslager (1983) study may have led to observations of different immune changes or responses. If so, the time course of these effects needs to be established. Biphasic effects of stress modulation of immunity would suggest a far more complex relationship than has generally been assumed.

A second controlled laboratory study of stress and lymphocyte proliferation also provided evidence of acute stress effects on blastogenic outcomes and suggests that these changes may occur very quickly (Zakowski, McAllister, Deal, & Baum, 1991). The stressor was a 7-minute combat surgery videotape and a memory test requiring subjects to report on details of the film. This procedure was administered twice, using the same film and memory task. The control group participated in similar procedures but viewed a film of landscape scenes with calming music. Self-report measures of stress were supplemented by plasma cortisol measures and heart rate and blood pressure assessments before and throughout the tasks.

Lymphocyte proliferation to Con A (5ug/ml) was significantly lower among subjects engaged in stressful procedures than among control subjects, and differences in proliferation to Con A (10ug/ml) was in the same direction although not significant. There were no differences in response to challenge with PHA. Individuals in the experimental group who were labeled as high reactors because they exhibited the largest changes in systolic and diastolic blood pressures during the film also showed significantly less lymphocyte proliferation to Con A than did lower reactors or controls. There were again no significant differences in response to PHA.

Failure to find effects with PHA after finding them with Con A are consistent with Weisse and colleagues (1990) and Mormede et al.'s (1988) findings. Cortisol levels were not significantly different between the two groups nor were they related to immune function. Consequently, this study suggests that stress exposure may affect immune function and that individuals with greater sympathetic reactivity to a stressor in particular show larger decreases in immune function compared to those who are not as reactive.

Conclusions.   To summarize, studies of animals have shown that there are changes in immune response following acute stressors such as shock, immobilization, territorial invasion, and exposure to a neutral stimulus previously paired with shock. Humans exposed to acute stressors also exhibit alterations in immune measures, although conditioned stress effects have not been demonstrated. These changes in immunity are presumably transient, although most studies have not followed responses for long enough periods to determine the actual duration of altered endocrine or immune responses. Psychological mediators such as the controllability or predictability of a stressor appear to buffer against the effect of stress on immunity in animals. However, controllability did not have similar effects in humans (Weisse et al., 1990). In addition, high reactors exhibiting larger changes in systolic and diastolic blood pressures during exposure to stressful procedures showed more stress-related deficits in lymphocyte proliferation than did lower reactors (Zakowski et al., 1991). This suggests that there may be physiological as well as psychological differences across individuals in response to stressful situations that may be related to changes in immunity, whereby some individuals react more dramatically to a stressor than others. The mechanisms involved should be investigated more fully.

CHRONIC STRESS AND IMMUNITY

As suggested earlier, chronic stress is a general category that covers a variety of types of events and reactions. Most studies of animals under chronic stress simply involve extending or increasing exposure to stressors used in studies of acute stress. In humans, however, such studies are exclusively naturalistic, considering independently applied stressors or persistent responses following shorter events. Consequently, the conditions under which these studies are done are not as controlled as are other studies, but potential applicability and significance for health may be greater.

Animal Studies

Research on chronic stress and immune function in animals must consider several potential barriers, including the effects of rapidly aging animals, habituation, and illness. Ghoneum, Gill, Assanah, and Stevens (1987) suggested that old rats subjected to stress have larger decreases in splenic and peripheral blood NK activity compared to young rats and this may be a factor in hesitancy of researchers to examine chronic stress in animals: Chronic stress studies may be impractical because animals of choice for these studies tend to age rapidly. However, if completed before the animal has reached "old age," studies lasting a period of months rather than a year or longer, depending on the species of animal may be feasible. If the studies are begun while the animal is still relatively young the effects of age may be avoided or controlled as well.

As we have suggested, acute stressors appear to suppress immune function. Some investigators, however, have argued that prolonged stressors (a month or longer) may increase functional indicators such as cell proliferation. Monjan and Collector (1977) examined the effects of a noise stressor over time and its relationship with immune function. In the experimental group, mice were subjected to 100 db of broad band sound for 5 seconds every minute for 3 hours a night. Animals varied in how many days they were exposed to the noise, up to 39 days. At the same time, control animals were subjected only to the normal activity of the animal room. In vitro lipopolysaccharide (LPS) was used to stimulate splenic B cell function and Con A was used to stimulate T cells. Also, T cell function was assessed by the lysis of P815 target cells in vitro. Exposure to the noise of 2 weeks or less was associated with lower lymphocyte proliferation to LPS and to Con A than was exposure to control conditions. Longer term exposure to noise (2–4 weeks) appeared to increase lymphocyte proliferation. Suppression of immune activity seemed to occur initially with shorter term noise stress, but gradually recovered and eventually exceeded original baseline levels with longer exposures, resulting in an apparent enhancement effect.

In an effort to explain the differential effect of the stressor on immunity over time, Monjon and Collector (1977) argued that animals exposed to noise stressors for more than 10 days are able to adapt and this adaptation is associated with reduced glucocorticoid levels, whereas acute stress increases levels of glucocorticoids, which presumably suppress immunologic responses. However, glucocorticoid levels were not associated with immunoenhancement following prolonged sound exposure. Riley (1981) also argued that these results were due to adaptation; animals were able to adjust to the stressor, gradually recovering function and briefly extending above baseline as normal responses were restored. Similarly, Borysenko and Borysenko (1982) suggested that the nature of the stressor, its duration, and the amount of time between the stress and immune measures may affect whether augmentation or suppression of immune activity is found. They noted that the findings in the Monjan and Collector study (1977) could have been due to rebound overshoot. Therefore, enhancement may not be due to prolonging the sound stressor but rather is a function of how long after exposure to a stressor immune measures are taken and whether adaptation is achieved.

Because there are so few animal studies examining chronic stress and immune activity it is difficult to assume that all forms of chronic stress would affect animals similarly. Because animal models are an important tool with which to examine immunity, the issue of whether different chronic stressors effect immune function similarly in animals must be addressed so that chronic stress and immunity can be better understood. Evidence that animals do not always adapt to chronic stressors or show apparent enhancement over time is provided by a study of 6-month stressor exposure, measuring immune function in rats undergoing escapable electric footshock (Odio, Goliszek, Brodish, & Ricardo, 1986). Four groups of 4-month-old male rats were used in the study. The stressor involved a variable interval schedule that shifted electrification from one half of the cage floor to the other. A tone was presented 1 second before each shift. Group I, the control group, received no shocks. Group II received 14 hours of shock exposure per week (2 hours of stress each day). Group III was exposed to 20 hours of stress per week with 4 hours of stress each day for 5 days each week. Group IV was exposed to 28 hours of stress per week with 4 hours of stress each day. These schedules were maintained for 6 months and animals received from 0 to 700 hours of shock exposure. One month after the last stress session the animals were sacrificed and their splenic lymphocytes examined.

All animals exposed to the stressor exhibited decreases in immune function. Exposure to long-term chronic stress resulted in a decrease in T lymphocyte proliferation to Con A and PHA even beyond the period of shock administration. Animals receiving only 14 hours of stress per week exhibited only moderate immunosuppression compared to other groups. Animals exposed to 20 or 28 hours of stress per week showed a 40% decrease in proliferative activities compared to controls.

These results suggest that immune system responses to stress are related to the amount of stressor exposure involved. That the suppression of immune function may extend beyond the time of the stressor application is also of interest. Monjan and Collector (1977) found that lymphocyte proliferation to Con A and LPS increased with long-term exposure to noise, but these measures were taken on the same day as the termination of the stressor, and it is difficult to reconcile the possible effects of a stressor on immune function at a later time with these results. The time course of immune system changes following a stressor still needs to be determined. Also, a dose response relationship may be important in the immune system's adaptation to a stressor. High stressor levels over time may continue to blunt immune activities and inhibit adaptation, whereas stressor levels in the Monjan and Collector study (1977) may not have been as resistant to adaptation and an overshoot in immune activity may have resulted.

Chronic stress in animals may also be associated with tumor growth. The ability of a tumor to develop is thought to be related to immune function by way of immune surveillance systems and therefore, effects of stress on immune function may be indirectly related to cancer progression. In a study by Riley (1975) stress-related tumor incidence in female mice infected with nodule-inducing virus was examined. Two groups of female rats (Groups A and B) who were infected with mammary tumor virus (MTV) were housed with males in standard stainless steel box cages. A third group (C) was infected with MTV and was housed without males, in plastic cages under protective conditions. A fourth group (D) was not infected with MTV and was randomly assigned housing with or without males in plastic cages under protective conditions. However, because all D subgroups had similar incidences of tumors, data on the subgroups were not given separately. Females in Groups A and B were exposed to handling, dust, odor, noise, and pheromones because they were housed in open racks. Females in Groups A, B, and C were handled weekly for tumor inspection and were frequently bled. In addition, females in Group A had one or more litters. Group C, however, was housed in plastic cages within ventilated shelves that protected them from environmental stress factors, although they were frequently weighed, inspected for tumors, and bled. Riley (1975) suggested that they experienced a moderate amount of stress compared to Groups A and B. Group D was thought to have experienced little or no stress as they also were housed in enclosed ventilated shelves and were rarely handled or bled.

Group A exhibited significantly earlier tumor appearance than did other groups with a median latent period of 276 days. Animals in Group B had a median latent period of 358 days, whereas animals in Group C had a median latent period of 566 days, significantly greater than Groups A and B. Animals in Group D still had no tumors at 400 days and their median latent period was greater than 800 days. Clearly, a dose response effect similar to that reported by Odio et al., (1986) indicated that increased stress was associated with greater tumor production or an inhibition of tumor rejection. Riley (1975) argued that although the milk-transmitted oncogenic Bittner mammary tumor virus is present in these mice from the time they are born, as long as immunologic surveillance systems are functioning properly the cells that are transformed and become malignant are recognized and destroyed. Under stressful conditions an increase in mammary tumor virus production may occur in the context of decreases in immunological control of malignant cells.

In another series of studies, Riley (1981) used rotation on a modified turntable as a stressor and examined lysis of lymphocytes, disintegration of the thymus and tumor growth in mice. The turntable was designed so that an entire cage of animals could be rotated without exposing animals to a novel environment or changing the availability of food and water. Following a rotation schedule of 10 minutes each hour at 45 rev/min over a 5-hour time period, substantial leukocytopenia was observed. Circulating lymphocyte damage occurred within 1 to 2 hours. Thymus involution followed, occurring within 24 hours. Riley (1981) suggested that because most of the circulating leukocytes lost were T cells and additional damage to the thymus could delay replacement, there was a significant effect on T cell-mediated immunity. In a subsequent study, half of a population of mice subcutaneously implanted with 6C3HED lymphosarcoma tumors were rotated at 45 rev/min for 10 minutes out of each hour for 3 days (Riley, 1981). Tumor growth was greater after 30 days among stressed mice compared to control animals. Decreased immunocompetency in the stressed mice may have resulted from the stress caused by the rotation, allowing increased tumor growth.

Conclusions.   Acute stressor exposure among animals has been associated with suppressed immune function, but responses to chronic stressors may be more complicated. In some cases, animal immune systems appeared to adapt to prolonged stressors over time, whereas in other situations their immune functions remained suppressed. There have been a variety of explanations for this discrepancy. The ability to adjust to stressors may depend on the nature of the stressor and/or its duration. In addition, immune system responses may be related to the amount of stressor exposure involved, where a dose response relationship may be important in adaptation or resistance to adaptation.

In some chronic stress studies it was observed that the administration of chronic stressors resulted in immune response changes that lasted longer than the presence of the stressor. However, not all studies measured immune responses beyond stressor administration and therefore conclusions cannot be made whether this phenomenon is always present. The time course of immune function changes needs to be further investigated.

In examining chronic stress and its affect on health, tumor growth was also found to correspond with chronic stressor administration. It has been suggested that tumor growth may be related to immunological control of malignant cells and therefore, the effects of stress on immunity may be related indirectly to cancer progression.

Human Studies

Many studies have investigated long-term stressors (either those of an intermediate duration or very long duration) in humans since the mid-1980s. Many have studied groups of students taking examinations (during semester midterms or finals) or a single major exam. We refer to these as *intermediate* because the period of threat or distress associated with an upcoming exam may last for a number of weeks, changing in stressfulness as exam time draws closer. However, these stressors may not have response durations as long as other stressors that last for months or years.

Intermediate Stress. A study conducted in Norway (Halvorsen & Vassend, 1987) considered undergraduates majoring in psychology who were required to take written exams for 2 days. Immune system activity was measured 6 weeks before the exams, 1 day before the exams, and 12–14 days after the examination. A group of students not taking exams served as controls. The State-Trait Anxiety Inventory (Spielberger, Gorsuch, & Lushene, 1970) was also administered on the days that immune measures were taken.

State anxiety increased significantly just before the exams, as did numbers of circulating monocytes compared to controls during the same time period and as compared to themselves 2 weeks later. However, the fraction of large helper/inducer T cells (larger cells indicate cell activation) was reduced just before the examination compared with 6 weeks before and 2 weeks after. The fraction of suppressor/cytotoxic T cells was also significantly reduced compared to 2 weeks after but was not significantly reduced when compared to rates obtained 6 weeks before. No differences in fractions were found in small (presumably inactive) cells.

It is possible that stress inhibited activation of these cells or, as Halvorsen and Vassend (1987) suggested, activated T cells are more strongly affected by stress than are inactive cells. That stress may inhibit activation is supported by the finding that the percentages of cells expressing IL-2 receptors was also reduced just before examinations. A delayed effect was also observed; a reduction in proliferation of T cells exposed to PHA, antigen (D. farinae), and pooled lymphocytes 2 weeks after the exams was found despite only a minimal nonsignificant reduction just before the examination period. This may have been due to an oral exam that students were scheduled to take shortly after the last blood draw but could have reflected long-term effects of the first set of exams. When these cells were cultured with IL-2 fortified medium, however, there was significantly less proliferation of T cells during the exam period compared to 6 weeks before.

In a study by Workman and La Via (1987), the effects of stress on T cell proliferation was examined in 15 medical students taking the National Board Medical Examinations. Blood drawing and questionnaire administration occurred the day before, and 1, 4, and 6 weeks after the exam. Fifteen age- and gender-matched controls also participated in the study. The Impact of Events Scale (IES; Horowitz, Wilner, & Alvarez, 1979) was used to measure overall stress as well as stress response styles in all of the subjects. The IES subscales include *avoidance,* made up of items assessing the extent in which a person attempts to avoid reminders of stressors (e.g., avoiding talking or thinking about the stressor) and *intrusion,* containing items that measure the extent to which a stressor intrudes into a persons thoughts, dreams, and so on. The Social Readjustment Rating Scale (SRRS) was also given to all subjects to measure life event stress during the previous 6 months.

Total scores for the IES were significantly higher for the experimental group than the control group the day before the examination but were not different after the exam. Students taking exams also exhibited significantly less T lymphocyte proliferation to PHA on the before the exams, and those with higher intrusion scores had the lowest T cell proliferation to PHA. A week later, students who had taken exams still showed significantly smaller proliferative responses to PHA mitogen compared to the control group. Partial recovery was observed after 4 weeks; T cell proliferative responses were significantly higher than they had been at 1 week after the examination but were still significantly lower than measures taken before the exam. At 6 weeks postexamination T cell responses were no longer different from preboard measurements, suggesting that it took about 6 weeks for immune function to return to normal after the stressor. The evidence for this recovery period is not definitive, however, as intervening conditions were not assessed following exams.

Kiecolt-Glaser, Glaser, and their colleagues have conducted several studies of medical students' immune function, and exam stress (Glaser, Kiecolt-Glaser, Stout, Tarr, Speicher, & Holliday, et al., 1985; Glaser, Rice, Speicher, Stout, & Kiecolt-Glaser, 1986; Glaser et al., 1987; Kiecolt-Glaser et al., 1984; Kiecolt-Glaser et al., 1986). Differences in NK activity have been observed during final examinations among medical students compared with measures taken 1 month before the exams (Kiecolt-Glaser, Garner, et al., 1984). Similarly, differences in numbers of NK cells, percentages of helper T cells, differences in lymphocyte proliferation to a mitogen challenge, and antibody titers to Epstein Barr virus (EBV) between examination and nonexamination periods have been reported (Glaser, Kiecolt-Glaser, Speicher, & Holliday, et al., 1985; Glaser et al., 1986; Kiecolt-Glaser et al., 1986). The EBV is used as a measure of cellular immune activity and cellular control over a latent virus (Glaser et al., 1987) and therefore, an inhibition of immune mechanisms that normally suppresses the virus may result in the increase of antibody titers to that virus.

Another study by this research team yielded some important evidence of immunological effects of psychological distress at the molecular level (Kiecolt-Glaser, Stephens, Lipetz, Speicher, & Glaser, 1985). The critical process of DNA repair in lymphocytes exposed to X-irradiation (in vitro) was examined in nonpsychotic psychiatric inpatients who had been divided into high- and low-distress subgroups according to measures on the Minnesota Multiphasic Personality Inventory (MMPI) Depression Scale 2. Significant differences were found in DNA repair between the high- and low-distress groups, with the high-distress group exhibiting significantly less DNA repair after 5 hours than the low-distress group. Kiecolt-Glaser and her colleagues (1985) suggested that this poor DNA repair may contribute to pathogenesis because faulty DNA repair may be related to increased occurrence of cancer. A concomitant decrease in NK cell activity with increased distress, as found in studies of examination stress in medical students, could result in markedly poorer destruction of transformed cells.

Psychosocial Mediators.   Studies examining the effects of stress on immune activity in humans have also reported data supporting the idea that psychological mediators may magnify or moderate responses to a stressor. For example in studies of medical students during and after exams, lonelier students had significantly higher antibody titers to EBV than did less lonely students. Loneliness also appeared to affect immune function in psychiatric inpatients; those scoring above the median on the UCLA Loneliness Scale

(Russell, Peplau, & Cutrona, 1980) had significantly lower NK activity and depressed T lymphocyte proliferation to PHA compared to those in the low loneliness group (Kiecolt-Glaser, 1984).

One important strength of the program of research by Kiecolt-Glaser, Glaser, and their colleagues is the demonstration that interventions to reduce distress block stress-related decreases in immune indicators or enhance them. Perhaps the clearest way to demonstrate that stress affects immunity is to reduce stress and measure simultaneous changes in immune function. One study examined the influence of relaxation techniques as a buffer from the stress of examinations in first-year medical students (Kiecolt-Glaser, Ricker, et al., 1986). Blood samples were collected 1 month before the examinations and again during the examination period. Half of the subjects received hypnotic/relaxation training during the interval between blood draws. Changes in distress levels were measured as were NK activity and lymphocyte subpopulations.

The two groups showed no significant differences before treatment on immunological measures or in self-reported distress. Further, there were no significant changes within the relaxation training group across the examination period. Subjects not learning relaxation, however, exhibited significant increases in anxiety and distress during the examination period. Although both groups showed a significant decrease in NK cell activity and percentages of helper/inducer cells during the examination period, the frequency of use of relaxation techniques was associated with percentages of helper/inducer cells during examinations.

A clearer instance of stress reduction and buffering of associated immune system changes was provided by a study of older people drawn from a geriatric population (Kiecolt-Glaser et al., 1985). The relaxation group in this study displayed a general increase in the T lymphocyte response to PHA, a significant increase in natural killer cell activity and a significant decrease in antibody titers to Herpes siplex virus compared to controls. Relaxation training was also associated with decreases in measures of distress.

Marital quality and separation/divorce can be considered more chronic than examination stress and have been studied as factors affecting immunity. Thirty-eight married women and 38 separated or divorced women who had been separated or divorced for 6 years or less participated in one study (Kiecolt-Glaser, Fisher, et al., 1987). The two groups were matched for age, socioeconomic status of the (ex)husband, education, number of children, and length of marriage. The results of the study indicated that poorer marital quality was related to higher levels of depression and lower T lymphocyte proliferation to Con A and PHA as well as an increase in antibody titers to EBV. More recent marital separation (1 year or less) and greater attachment to the (ex)husband lead to increased depressive symptoms and lower helper T lymphocytes and helper–suppressor ratios compared to the married controls. Also, the length of separation was significantly and positively related to lymphocyte response to PHA. Women who had been separated for 1 year or less also had significantly higher antibody titers to EBV and a significantly lower percentage of NH cells than did married women. Similar findings have been reported for divorced or separated men (Kiecolt-Glaser et al., 1988).

Chronic Stress.   Among the first prospective studies of immune function in relatively healthy people were studies of bereaved spouses. One, reported by Bartrop, Lazarus, Luckhurst, Kiloh, & Penny (1977), involved 26 surviving spouses, recruited for the study along with 26 control subjects who were matched for age, gender, and race. The first blood samples were taken within 3 weeks after the death of their loved one and the second were taken 6 weeks later. Control subjects had their blood drawn at the same times with assays performed on both groups simultaneously. Bereaved subjects exhibited significantly less lymphocyte transformation to PHA (at 10 and 20 ug/ml) and Con A (at 5 and 50 ug/ml) 6 weeks after the loss than did controls. Proliferation of cells to Con A challenge (at 5 and 50 ug/ml) was significantly lower 6 weeks after the loss than 3 weeks after among bereaved individuals, suggesting that lymphocyte proliferation to mitogens decreases over the first 6 weeks of bereavement rather than diminishing all at once and recovering slowly.

A prospective study of 15 husbands of women with advanced breast cancer also provided evidence of bereavement-induced immune system changes (Schleifer, Keller, Bond, Cohen, & Stein, et al., 1983). Prebreavement immune levels were compared to those after the death of a spouse. The number of T and B cells were not significantly different, but lymphocyte proliferation to Con A, PHA, and PWM were lower during the first 2 months of bereavement compared to before the death of their spouses. During the follow-up period of 4 and 14 months postbereavement lymphocyte stimulation responses were intermediate between before the spouses' death and during the first 2 months postbereavement. This study, however, did not include control subjects and therefore the pre- and postbereavement timepoints cannot be compared to individuals not experiencing the death of a loved one. Also, as the investigators note, a larger sample may be necessary to ascertain whether the responses observed during the follow-up periods exemplify subgroups, with some individuals exhibiting a recovery of lymphocyte responses and others having lower immune responses at later time points. Finally, depression and loneliness were not measured in the study, although these variables would be expected to be relevant during bereavement.

The role of depression in modulating immune function during bereavement appears to be important. In a study of bereaved women, Irwin, Daniels, Smith, Bloom, and Weiner (1987) measured NK cell activity and depressive symptoms at weekly intervals 1 to 2 months before the death of the husband and at least twice during the month following the spouses' deaths. Neither NK activity nor depression scores were significantly different from anticipatory to post-death bereavement periods. This may be due to the stress of anticipatory bereavement, which may also provide valuable time for coping and decrease the eventual impact of death. However, increases in depressive symptoms from before the death of the husband to after led to decreases in NK cell activity.

Recently, Stein (1989) has suggested that immune system changes may not be specific to depression but rather to subgroups of depressed individuals. It was proposed that altered immune measures may be present particularly in elderly, severely depressed individuals. Immune function in patients with major depressive disorder who were drug free, hospitalized, and ambulatory was examined (Schleifer et al., 1989). The patient sample consisted of a range of ages, gender, and illness severity. Depressed patients and age- and gender-matched controls showed no significant differences in the number of T and B lymphocytes, T4 or T8 cells, lymphocyte proliferation to PWM, Con A, and PHA, and NK cell activity. However, multiple regression analyses examining the contribution or age, severity of depression, gender, and hospitalization to immune status revealed that there were significant age-associated differences between depressed individuals and controls in number of T4 lymphocytes and in mitogen-induced lymphocyte activation. Similarly, severity of depression was significantly related to alterations in immune measures.

Very long-term stress and immunity have also been examined among family caregivers of Alzheimer's disease (AD) victims (Kiecolt-Glaser, Glaser, et al., 1987). The AD-afflicted individuals had been diagnosed for a mean of 2.83 years with some newly diagnosed and others diagnosed up to 11 years before, and stress associated with caring for these individuals may have continued for quite some time. Half of the subjects lived with the AD victim, 10 AD victims were in nursing homes, and 7 AD victims lived alone or with another relative. Control subjects were also studied; they were not caregivers of AD patients but were matched with the caregivers for age, years of education, and family income. Subjects' depressive symptoms were measured, as well as patterns of social contact, AD patient history, and current functioning information.

Caregivers exhibited significantly higher levels of depressive symptoms than did control subjects. Greater impairment of the AD patient was also associated with fewer social contacts by the caregiver. Significantly higher antibody titers to EBV and lower percentages of total T lymphocytes and helper T lymphocytes were found in caregivers compared to controls.

However, there were not significant differences in the percentages of suppressor T cells and NK cells. Caregivers who belonged to a social support group were also compared to those who did not and group members rated themselves as significantly less lonely and had a significantly larger percentage of NK cells than those who did not participate in a group.

In another study that measured very long chronic stress, people living near the Three Mile Island (TMI) nuclear power plant were compared to individuals living about 80 miles away (McKinnon, Weisse, Reynolds, Bowles, and Baum, 1989). The study was conducted more than 6 years after the accident at TMI and psychophysiological data collected over this 6-year period yielded evidence of continuing stress among residents of the TMI area (e.g., increased symptom reporting, elevated resting blood pressure, and catecholamine levels relative to controls). Individuals living near TMI also had significantly lower numbers of B lymphocytes, NK cells, and T-suppressor/cytotoxic lymphocytes compared to control subjects, and exhibited significantly greater antibody titers for herpes simplex virus and cytomeglavirus, both latent viruses, and no differences in titers for rubella virus, which is not latent. These data suggested that stress associated with the TMI accident and its aftermath may have suppressed key elements of the immune system, although possible radiation effects could not be evaluated.

Conclusions.   Animal studies have suggested that long-term stressors may decrease immune function or increase it above original baseline levels. If one allows for adaptation, other studies have found that animals exposed to long-term stressors exhibit decreases in immune function associated with the amount of stressor exposure. Over time, high stressor levels may continue to inhibit immune responses and lessen the ability to adapt, whereas lower stressor levels may be conducive to adaptation. Chronic stress has also been associated with tumor growth in mice (Riley, 1975, 1981), and is thought to be related to immune surveillance systems.

In humans, chronic stressors of an intermediate duration such as examination stress appear to affect immune function, including reducing numbers of large helper/inducer T cells, fractions of suppressor/cytotoxic T cells, proliferation of T cells to PHA, numbers of NK cells and their activity, and increasing antibody titers to EBV. Psychological mediators such as anxiety, loneliness, and intrusive thoughts may further affect immune function responses to stressors and interventions such as relaxation may buffer against stress and lessen the effects of stress on immune function.

Long-term chronic stressors such as separation/divorce or bereavement also appear to affect immunity. Differences between chronic stress and control groups in numbers of helper T lymphocytes, the fraction of helper/suppressor T cells, proliferation of lymphocytes to Con A, PWM, and PHA, numbers of antibody titers to EBV, and percentages and activity and of NK cells have been observed. Depression has been implicated as a psychological mediator that may play a role in further modulating immune function during stress.

STRESS AND IMMUNE FUNCTION

After reviewing studies of acute and chronic stress and immune function in animals and humans it is evident that both similarities and differences exist across stress durations as well as across species. There are a number of problems in making definitive statements about the comparability between these groups because there are large variations in types of stressors examined, as well as measures of immune function. In addition, physiological and psychological differences between animals and humans make comparisons between the two groups difficult.

Both animals and humans show changes in immune responses following acute stressors. These changes presumably last for short periods of time although responses have generally not been followed for long enough periods to determine the actual duration of immune response changes. There may be differences in the dynamics of stress-induced immune system changes, however. For example, the influences of controllability and predictability as buffers against the effects of acute stress on immunity appear to be clearer for animals than for humans. Those animal studies examining control and predictability have produced expected findings, whereas the few studies in humans have not. However, there is far too little work on these variables in humans to draw firm conclusions.

Both animal and human studies have shown that longer term stressors may have different effects on immune function depending on how long the exposure to the stressor is, the nature of the stressor, and the quantity of stress exposure. Higher stressor levels may inhibit the ability to adapt, whereas less severe stressors may lead to adaptation over time. The ability of human coping systems to adapt to long-term stressors has been observed; for example, alterations in immune response appear to lessen over time following divorce and/or separation (Kiecolt-Glaser, Fisher, et al., 1987). Other stressors may not be characterized by adaptation, such as the case of people living near Three Mile Island, where alterations in immunity were observed more than 6 years after the accident (McKinnon et al., 1989). Similarly, in animals a noise stressor may be more easily adapted to (Monjon & Collector, 1977) than electric shock (Odio et al., 1986) over long periods of time.

There are a number of reasons why acute and chronic stressors and associated immune system changes cannot be definitively compared. The nature of chronic stress is sufficiently complex to defy simple categorization. In this chapter, we have broken it down on a crude index of duration, comparing intermediate and long-term stressors and finding similar effects of both. However, we have not considered the many different sources of chronic stress. Are traumatic stress syndromes, wherein distress far outlasts the physical presence of an acute but powerful event, different from situations such as caregiving or occupational stress where stressors persist continuously for long periods of time? Studies of bereavement, divorce, caregiving, and the TMI situation suggest that they can have similar effects, but these different situations have not been studied systematically. If we are to arrive at a thorough and applicable understanding of stress and immune function, these and other questions must be addressed.

Similarly, the timing and selection of immune measures and neuroendocrine mediator indices must be considered more systematically. In studies of acute stress, such measures are typically collected during or shortly after challenge. Thus, these measures can be thought of as "reactivity" measures. Proliferation assessments in the Weisse and colleagues (1990) or Zakowski et al. (1990) studies involved measurement of cells challenged in vitro after they had been challenged in vivo. Studies of chronic stress are different in that they usually measure people at resting levels who have been challenged in the past. Thus, finding that people living near TMI exhibit elevated blood pressure and latent viral antibody titers 5 or 6 years after the accident cannot easily be compared with finding increased blood pressure or suppressed lymphocyte proliferation during or after acute laboratory stress. Whether these effects are comparable, whether different subsets of immune cells or factors are involved, and whether different mediators are involved are all questions that need to be answered.

Whether differences in acute or chronic stress-related changes in immune function are of clinical interest, provide insights into the basic mechanisms underlying appraisal or coping, or ultimately tell us about the stress response, they are useful objects of study. The lack of systematic consideration of these issues in favor of demonstration that such phenomena exist should no longer characterize research in this challenging area of research.

ACKNOWLEDGMENT

This chapter was supported in part by USUHS grants, CO7216 and R07265. The opinions and assertions contained herein are those of the authors and do not necessarily reflect those of the Department of Defense or the Uniformed Services University of the Health Sciences.

REFERENCES

Ader, R., & Cohen, N. (1981). Conditioned immunopharmacologic responses. In R. Ader (Ed.), *Psychoneuroimmunology.* New York: Academic Press.

Bartrop, R. W., Lazarus, L., Luckhurst, E., Kiloh, L. G., & Penny, R. (1977). Depressed lymphocyte function after bereavement. *Lancet, 1,* 834–836.

Baum, A. (1990). Stress, intrusive imagery, and chronic distress. *Health Psychology, 9*(6), 653–675.

Baum, A., O'Keeffe, M., & Davidson, L. M. (1990). Acute stressors and chronic response: The case of traumatic stress. *Journal of Applied Social Psychology, 20*(20), 1643–1654.

Borysenko, M., & Borysenko, J. (1982). Stress, behavior, and immunity: Animal models and mediating mechanisms. *General Hospital Psychiatry, 4,* 59–67.

Estes, W. K., & Skinner, B. F. (1941). *Journal of Experimental Psychology, 29,* 390.

Fleshner, M., Laudenslager, M. L., Simons, L., & Maier, S. F. (1985). Reduced serum antibodies associated with social defeat in rats. *Physiology and Behavior, 45,* 1183–1187.

Ghoneum, M., Gill, G., Assanah, P., & Stevens, W. (1987). Susceptibility of natural killer cell activity of old rats to stress. *Journal of Immunology, 60,* 461–465.

Gisler, R. G. (1974). Stress and the hormonal regulation of the immune response in mice. *Psychotherapy and Psychosomatics, 23,* 197 208.

Glaser, R., Kiecolt-Glaser, J. K., Speicher, C. H., & Holliday, J. E. (1985). Stress, loneliness, and changes in herpesvirus latency. *Journal of Behavioral Medicine, 8,* 249–260.

Glaser, R., Rice, J., Sheridan, J., Fertel, R., Stout, J., Speicher, C., Pinsky, D., Kotur, M., Post, A., Beck, M., & Kiecolt-Glaser, J. (1987). Stress-related immune suppression: Health implications. *Brain, Behavior, and Immunity, 1,* 7–20.

Glaser, R., Kiecolt-Glaser, J. K., Stout, J. C., Tarr, K. L., Speicher, C. E., & Holliday, J. E. (1985). Stress-related impairments of cellular immunity. *Psychiatry Research, 16,* 233–239.

Glaser, R., Rice, J. Speicher, C. E., Stout, J. C., & Kiecolt-Glaser, J. K. (1986). Stress depresses interferon production concomitant with a decrease in natural killer cell activity. *Behavioral Neuroscience, 100*(2) 675–678.

Halvorsen, R., & Vassend, O. (1987). Effects of examination stress on some cellular immunity functions. *Journal of Psychosomatic Research, 31*(6) 693–701.

Harmsen, H. G., & Turney, T. H. (1985). Inhibition of in vivo neutrophil accumulation by stress. Possible role of neutrophil adherence. *Inflammation, 9,* 9–20.

Horowitz, M., Wilner, N., & Alvarez, W. (1979). Impact of Events Scale: A measure of subjective stress. *Psychosomatic Medicine, 41,* 209–218.

Irwin, M., Daniels, M., Smith, T. L., Bloom, E., & Weiner, H. (1987). Impaired natural killer cell activity during bereavement. *Brain, Behavior, and Immunity, 1,* 98–104.

Kant, G. J., Eggleston, T., Landman-Roberts, L., Kenion, C. C., Driver, G. C., & Meyerhoff, J. L. (1984). Habituation to repeated stress is stressor specific. *Pharmacology, Biochemistry and Behavior, 22,* 631–634.

Keller, S. E., Weiss, J. M., Schleifer, S. J., Miller, N. E., Stein, M. (1983). Stress-induced suppression of immunity in adrenalectomized rats. *Science, 221,* 1301–1304.

Kiecolt-Glaser, J. K., Fisher, L. D., Ogrocki, P., Stout, J., Speicher, C. E., & Glaser, R. (1987). Marital quality, marital disruption, and immune function. *Psychosomatic Medicine, 49*(1) 13–34.

Kiecolt-Glaser, J. K., Garner, W., Speicher, C., Penn, G. M., Holiday, J. E., & Glaser, R. (1984). Psychosocial modifiers of immunocompetence in medical students. *Psychosomatic Medicine, 46,* 7–14.

Kiecolt-Glaser, J. K., Glaser, R., Shuttleworth, E. C., Dyer, C. S., Ogrocki, P., & Speicher,

C. E. (1987). Chronic stress and immunity in family caregivers of Alzheimer's Disease victims. *Psychosomatic Medicine, 49,* 523–35.

Kiecolt-Glaser, J. K., Glaser, R., Strain, E. C., Stout, J. C., Tarr, K. L., Holiday, J. E., & Speicher, C. E. (1986). Modulation of cellular immunity in medical students. *Journal of Behavioral Medicine, 9*(1) 5–21.

Kiecolt-Glaser, J. K., Kennedy, S., Malkoff, S., Fisher, L., Speicher, C. E., & Glaser, R. (1988). Marital discord and immunity in males. *Psychosomatic Medicine, 50,* 213–229.

Kiecolt-Glaser, J. K., Ricker, K., George, J., Messick, G., Speicher, C. E., Garner, W. & Glaser, R. (1984). Urininary cortisol levels, cellular immunocompetency, and loneliness in psychiatric inpatients. *Psychosomatic Medicine, 46*(1) 15–23.

Kiecolt-Glaser, J. K., Stephens, R. E., Lipetz, P. D., Speicher, C. E., & Glaser, R. (1985). Distress and DNA repair in human lymphocytes. *Journal of Behavioral Medicine, 8*(4) 311–320.

Landmann, R. M. A., Muller, R. B., Perini, C. H., Wesp, M., Erne, P., & Buhler, F. R. (1984). Changes of immunoregulatory cells induced by psychological and physical stress: Relationships to plasma catacholamines. *Clinical Experimental Immunology, 58,* 127–135.

Laudenslager, M. L. (1983). Coping and immunosuppression: Inescapable but not escapable shock suppresses lymphocyte proliferation. *Science, 221,* 568–570.

Laudenslager, M. L., Fleshner, M., Hofstadter, P., Held, P. E., Simons, L., & Maier, S. F. (1988). Stability under varying conditions. *Brain Behavior and Immunity, 2,* 92–101.

Lysle, D. T., Cunnick, J. E., Fowler, H., & Rabin, B. (1988). Pavlovian conditioning of shock-induced suppression of lymphocyte reactivity: Acquisition, extinction and preexposure effects. *Life Sciences, 42,* 2185–2194.

Maier, S. F. (1984). Learned helplessness and animal models of depression. *Progress in Neuro-Psychopharmacology and Biological Psychiatry, 8*(3), 435–446.

Mason, J. W. (1975). A historical view of the stress field. *Journal of Human Stress, 1,* 22–36.

McKinnon, W., Weisse, C. S., Reynolds, C. P., Bowles, C. A., & Baum, A. (1989). Chronic stress, leukocyte subpopulations, and humoral response to latent viruses. *Health Psychology, 8*(4) 389–402.

Monjan, A. A., & Collector, M. I. (1977). Stress-induced modulation of the immune response. *Science, 196,* 307–308.

Mormede, P., Dantzer, R., Michaud, B., Kelly, K. W., & LeMoal, M. (1988). Influence of stressor predictability and behavioral control on lymphocyte reactivity, antibody response and neuroendocrine activity in rats. *Physiology and Behavior, 43,* 577–583.

Odio, M., Goliszek, A., Brodish, A., & Ricardo, M. J., Jr. (1986). Impairment of immune function after cessation of long-term chronic stress. *Immunology Letters, 13,* 25–31.

O'Keefe, M., & Baum, A. (1990). Conceptual and methodological issues in the study of chronic stress. *Stress Medicine, 6,* 105–115.

Riley, V. (1975). Mouse mammary tumors: Alteration of incidence as apparent function of stress. *Science, 189,* 465–467.

Riley, V. (1981). Psychoneuroendocrine influences on immunocompetence and neoplasia. *Science, 212,* 1100–1109.

Russell, D., Peplau, L. A., & Cutrona, C. E. (1980). The revised UCLA Loneliness Scale: Concurrent and discriminant validity evidence. *Journal of Personality and Social Psychology, 39,* 472–480.

Schleifer, S. J., Keller, S. E., Bond, R. N., Cohen, J., & Stein, M. (1989). Major depressive disorder and immunity: Role of age, sex, severity, and hospitalization. *Archives of General Psychiatry, 46,* 81–87.

Schavit, Y., Lewis, J. W., Terman, G. W., Gale, P., & Liebeskind, J. C. (1984). Opioid peptides mediate the suppressive effects of stress on natural killer cell cytotoxicity. *Science, 223,* 188–190.

Seligman, M. E. P. (1975). *Helplessness: On depression, development, and death.* San Francisco: Freeman.

Speilberger, C. D., Gorsuch, R. L., & Lushene, R. E. (1970). In *STAI Manual for the State-Trait Anxiety Inventory.* Palo Alto: Consulting Psychologists Press.

Stein, M. (1989). Stress, depression, and the immune system. *Journal of Clinical Psychiatry, 50*(Suppl 5), 35-40.

Stroop, J. R. (1935). Studies of interference in serial verbal reactions. *Journal of Experimental Psychology, 18,* 643-662.

Visintainer, M. A., Volpicelli, J. R., & Seligman, M. E. P. (1982). Tumor rejection in rats after inescapable or escapable shock. *Science, 216,* 437-439.

Weisse, C. S., Pato, C. N., Littman, R., Brier, A., Paul, S. M., & Baum, A. (1990). Differential effects of controllable and uncontrollable acute stress on lymphocyte proliferation and leukocyte percentages in humans. *Brain, Behavior, and Immunity, 4*(4), 339-351.

Workman, E. A., & La Via, M. F. (1987). T-lymphocyte polyclonal proliferation: Effects of stress and stress response style on medical students taking national board examinations. *Clinical Immunology and Immunopathology, 43,* 308-313.

Zakowski, S. G., McAllister, C. G., Deal, M., & Baum, A. (1991). Stress, reactivity, and immune function. *Health Psychology.*

2 Stress and Immunity

Jan A. Moynihan
Nicholas Cohen
University of Rochester School of Medicine and Dentistry

Research conducted at three levels of biological complexity has revealed bidirectional communication between the central nervous system (CNS) and the immune system. Studies at the level of molecular and cellular events have pointed out that macrophages and lymphocytes express surface receptors for many neuropeptides and hormones (Bost, 1988), that macrophage-like glial cells of the CNS produce cytokines such as interleukin-1 (IL-1) and IL-6 (Beneviste, 1988), and that mitogen- or antigen-stimulated lymphocytes produce hormones including proopiomelanocortin-derived peptides, thyrotropin, prolactin, and growth hormone (Blalock, 1988). Numerous other studies have revealed that the interactions of hormones and neurotransmitters with their specific receptors on immunocytes signal alterations in immunologically relevant events such as lymphocyte proliferation, activity of natural killer (NK) cells, antibody production, the expression of cytokine receptors, and cytokine synthesis and release (Bernton, Bryant, & Holaday 1991; Goetzl, Turck, & Sreedharan, 1991; Heijnen, Kavelaars, & Ballieux, 1991; Kelley, 1991; Madden & Livnat, 1991; McCruden & Stimson, 1991; McGillis, Mitsuhashi, & Payan, 1991; Munck & Guyre, 1991; Ottaway, 1991). Experiments at the organ system level indicate that lymphoid tissues are richly innervated (Felten & Felten, 1991) and that abrogation of this sympathetic innervation alters immunity (Madden & Livnat, 1991). Thus, lines of communication between the nervous, endocrine, and immune systems are in place. Finally, experiments at the organismic level involving classical conditioning on the one hand, and "stress" on the other, point out that the immunomodulatory interactions between the CNS and the immune system are behaviorally driven and regulated (Ader & Cohen, 1984, 1991; Ader, Grota, Moynihan, & Cohen, 1991; Bohus & Koolhaas, 1991; Keller, Schleifer, & Demetrikopoulos, 1990; Shavit, 1991).

We have recently reviewed the immunological consequences of conditioning (Ader & Cohen, 1991); in this brief chapter, we highlight some of the extensive recent literature demonstrating that an organism's neuroendocrine responses to a perceived stressor can also be immunomodulatory. (Earlier studies of the effects of stress on immunity, infectious diseases, and cancer have been reviewed by Ader & Cohen, 1984). The studies described here involve different periods of exposure to either physical stimuli (e.g., electric shock, rotation, restraint, temperature, noise) or so-called psychosocial stressors (e.g., differential housing, maternal separation, handling, bereavement, divorce, and school examinations). In addition, different investigators, using different stress protocols, have measured either antibody and cell-mediated immunity in vivo or different leukocyte effector (e.g., cytotoxicity) and other physiological processes (e.g., proliferation) in vitro. To facilitate reading this chapter, it has been organized according to the particular kind of immune response that has been examined rather than according to the nature of the stressor, the species subjected to the stress protocol, or the putative neuroendocrine mediation of the stress effect.

STRESS-ASSOCIATED IN VIVO CHANGES IN CELL-MEDIATED IMMUNITY (CMI)

Thirty years ago, Wistar and Hildemann (1960) observed prolonged skin allograft survival, presumably resulting from depressed T cell activity, in an avoidance-learning paradigm with C57/BL or Swiss-Webster (SW) mice. More recently, Okimura, Ogawa, and Yamauchi (1986) reported that restraint was associated with suppression of the delayed-type hypersensitivity (DTH) response of BALB/c female mice following a challenge injection of sheep red blood cells (SRBC) given in the footpad 4 days after antigen priming. Suppression occurred regardless of whether animals were restrained (12 hours/day) for the 2 days immediately before or for the first 2 days after priming. Depressed DTH, again measured by footpad swelling, has also been observed in SW male mice that had been restrained for 2.5 hours either immediately prior to primary immunization or to test challenge with SRBC (Blecha, Barry, & Kelley, 1982; Blecha, Kelley, & Satterlee, 1982). It should be realized that during the restraint period, animals are unable to eat or drink. Moreover, restraint causes pathophysiological effects, for example, ulcers (Ader, 1971) or altered body core temperature (Selye, 1950), that could directly or indirectly affect the immune system.

Thermal changes have also been shown to modulate the DTH response.

For example, Blecha, Barry, and Kelley (1982) reported a depressed DTH when mice were exposed to the cold (5C) for 2 days prior to SRBC immunization. However, an increased rather than decreased footpad swelling was noted when the animals were kept at 5C throughout the entire experiment. Interestingly, an increased footpad DTH reaction was also recorded when the mice were exposed to an elevated temperature of 35C either for 2 days prior to immunization or throughout the period of primary immunization, secondary challenge, and subsequent evaluation of the DTH reaction. The use of cold or warm temperature as an "immunomodulatory stressor" in endothermic (warm-blooded) vertebrates is subject to a potential confound if significant deviations of ambient temperature might produce deviations of body core temperature that, in turn, directly affect the immune system (Hanson, Murphy, Silicano, & Shin, 1983; Lauwasser & Shands, 1979; Wang-Yang, Buttke, Miller, & Clem, in press). Low temperature-induced suppression and elevated temperature-induced enhancement of in vitro and in vivo immune reactivities of ectothermic vertebrates (e.g., fish, amphibians, and reptiles) are well documented (Clem, Miller, & Bly, in press).

Rabin and Salvin (1987) investigated the effects of housing on resistance of mice to an intravenous (iv) injection of Candida albicans. Immediately after the mice were received from the supplier, they were housed either one or five per cage; they were injected with the yeast either 5, 10, 14, 16, or 20 days later. C3H/HeJ male mice housed in a group for 10 days displayed lower resistance than did mice of the same strain and sex that had been housed individually for the same period of time. No significant differences between individually and group-housed animals were apparent after the other periods of housing, and no differences attributable to housing for any time period were noted with either C3H/HeJ females or with male C57BL/6 animals. It should be noted that in these and in other experiments addressing the effects of differential housing on immunity, it is difficult, if not impossible, to determine which housing situation serves as the control or the experimental group (i.e., does isolation and/or social interaction provide the potentially immunomodulatory stimuli?).

In vivo CMI in humans undergoing stressful experiences has been studied, albeit indirectly. Glaser, Kiecolt-Glaser, Speicher, and Holliday (1985) and Kiecolt-Glaser et al. (1986) reported an increase in serum antibody to the Epstein-Barr virus (EBV) capsid antigen (VCA) and Type 1 herpes simplex virus (HSV-1) antigens in medical students subjected to examination stress. Similar increases in anti-VCA antibody have been observed in subjects whose marriages were psychometrically characterized as poor, and in women who had been separated or divorced 1 year or less, compared with a group of sociodemographically matched married women (Kiecolt-Glaser et al., 1987). The stress-associated increase in antibody to antigenic epitopes associated with these latent viruses has been interpreted as a reflection of a stress-induced suppression of CMI leading to increased viral activation and a concomitant increase in anti-viral antibodies (Glaser & Gottleib-Stematsky, 1982).

STRESS-ASSOCIATED CHANGES IN HUMORAL IMMUNITY

Psychological Stressors

In an early study, Yamada, Jensen, and Rasmussen (1964) investigated the effects of avoidance-learning stress in a shuttlebox apparatus on the antibody response to vesicular stomatitis virus (VSV). Female SW mice were subjected to the stressor for 6 hours a day beginning either 2 or 15 days prior to inoculation with VSV and continuing until the day of sacrifice. No difference in the titer of antibody from stressed and control mice was observed. However, muscles from the stressed mice contained significantly more virus than control muscle. Although it is unknown whether this reflected a suppressed CMI to virus-infected cells, when this same avoidance-learning protocol was followed several years earlier by Wistar and Hildemann (1960), it was, in fact, associated with prolonged skin allograft survival in SW mice.

Beden and Brain (1982, 1984) have used an attack/aggression model to investigate the effects of social stress on humoral immunity. They housed male "TO" strain mice individually and then paired each of them with a trained "attacker mouse" in the attacker's home cage. This was done one, three, or five times in a single day. Each encounter was ended when the intruder mouse was defeated. The defeated mice were then injected with SRBC and their sera were collected for antibody titration 4 days later. Mice that had either three or five defeats had a significantly reduced primary anti-SRBC antibody response. Differences between the secondary response of these and control animals, however, were not observed.

Ito, Mine, Ago, Nakagawa, Fujiwara, and Ueki (1983) exposed male Wistar rats for 1 hour to a trained aggressive animal on each of 3 consecutive days before they were injected with the hapten, dinitrophenyl (DNP) coupled to *Ascaris* to elicit either a primary or secondary IgE antibody response. Stress prior to priming was without apparent effect. When antigen-primed animals were stressed prior to a secondary immunization, however, a significant decrease in the antibody response was noted. Interpretation of this and other studies using an aggression protocol are potentially complicated by the possibility that wounding of the experimental animals might itself be associated with immune changes.

Fleshner, Laudenslager, Simons, and Maier (1989) explored the effect of defeat associated with territorial defense on the serum antibody response of male rats to the thymus-dependent protein antigen, keyhole limpet hemocyanin (KLH). Pairs of rats formed "colonies" that remained undisturbed for 3 to 6 months. These colonies were then repeatedly exposed to intruders until the dominant male consistently attacked 9 of 10 intruders. Animals that were to serve as experimental intruders were maintained undisturbed for 2 to 3 weeks in individual cages. They were then randomly divided into two groups. One group, which served as a control, consisted of animals that were exposed to, but physically separated from, the colony by an air-permeable plexiglass barrier. Animals in the experimental group were physically exposed to the established colony (i.e., the barrier was removed). Immediately before the first colony exposure, all intruders were immunized subcutaneously (sc) at the base of the tail with 50 ug KLH. Experimental intruders were then given five successive 10-minute exposures to different aggressive colonies. After animals were removed from the last colony, they were picked up and visually inspected for wounds; any animals that evidenced signs of having been wounded were eliminated from the study. The entire procedure was repeated 1 week later with exposure to different colonies but without KLH immunization. Blood samples were drawn from the tail vein 1, 2, and 3 weeks postimmunization. The introduction of intruder rats into aggressive colonies for 50 minutes immediately following immunization and for 50 minutes 1 week later was associated with a significantly reduced level of IgG anti-KLH antibodies at each postimmunization interval tested. Interestingly, the best predictor of the level of serum antibody was the total time the intruders spent in submissive (i.e., defeat) postures at the time of the first series, but not the second series, of exposures to the aggressive colonies that immediately followed immunization. That is, serum antibody titers of intruder animals who fell below the group median of the amount of time spent in a submissive posture of defeat in their encounter shortly after immunization, did not differ from control antibody titers.

Coe, Rosenberg, Fisher, and Levine (1987) evaluated humoral immune responses in 6-month-old squirrel monkeys that had been separated from their mothers for 7 days prior to being immunized with a bacteriophage. Experimental groups included infant monkeys that were separated and housed alone in a familiar setting; housed alone in an unfamiliar setting; and housed with familiar infants in their home setting. A significant decrease in antibody response to the phage was observed only in separated monkeys that were maintained alone in an unfamiliar environment.

The effects of early maternal deprivation on humoral immunity have also been studied in outbred SW mice (Michaut et al., 1981). In the experimental group of randomized and mixed sex litters, mothers were removed for 4 hours a day during the offsprings' first week of life and for 8 hours a day during their second. These litters were also weaned precociously at Day 15. When they were 8 weeks old, experimental and age-matched control mice (weaned at 21 rather than 15 days of age), were injected with SRBC. Serum antibody titers and numbers of splenic cells producing specific antibody in vitro (i.e., plaque-forming cells or PFCs), measured 4 days after immunization, were reduced in the experimental animals.

The effects of housing different numbers of animals in a cage on antibody responsiveness have been studied in several laboratories. Vessey (1964) individually housed weanling C3H male mice. Experimental animals were switched to a group-housing situation (six per cage) for 4 hours daily throughout the experiment; controls were unmanipulated. On the fifth day, all animals were immunized with bovine serum. Antibody titers, determined at various times postimmunization, were attenuated in intermittently group-housed mice relative to the individually housed and unmanipulated controls.

Rabin, Lyte, Epstein, and Caggiula (1987) and Rabin and Salvin (1987) investigated the effects of group versus individual housing on the in vitro PFC response of SRBC-immunized mice. Male and female C3H or male C57BL/6J mice were housed individually or five per cage immediately after they were received from the supplier. Mice were immunized after 5, 8, 12, 14, 25, or 32 days, and their spleens were harvested for PFC assays 4 days later. Male C3H mice, group housed for 8 days prior to immunization, had fewer PFCs relative to individually housed controls. After 25 days of group housing, however, PFCs in experimentals and controls did not differ. This housing effect showed the same strain and sex dependency that was previously described for resistance to *Candida* in that PFCs in group and individually housed female C3H mice or male C57BL/6J mice did not differ.

In a related study, Edwards, Rahe, Stephens, and Henry (1980) investigated changes in housing on the primary and secondary antibody responses to bovine serum albumin (BSA) in CBA/USC male mice. These animals were housed individually from weaning to 16 weeks of age. At this time, all mice were immunized and some of them were placed into population cages with "socialized" females. After 7 days, a second injection of antigen was given and half of the group-housed males in the population cages were returned to isolation. Serum antibodies were titrated 1 week later. Mice that were exposed to the group-housing environment and then returned to individual housing had a significantly depressed anti-BSA antibody titer compared to all other males.

We have studied the effects of handling on serum antibody response to KLH in C3H/HeJ male mice (Moynihan, Koota, Brenner, Cohen, & Ader, 1989) and BALB/c female mice (Moynihan, Brenner et al., 1990). Simply picking up individually housed C3H/HeJ mice as if to inject them every day for 2 weeks prior to actually immunizing them intraperitoneally (ip) was associated with a depressed IgM and IgG anti-KLH antibody response relative to home-caged unmanipulated controls. We also determined, in C3H/HeJ mice, that actual ip injections of saline, given as infrequently as every fourth day for 2 weeks prior to immunization, similarly attenuated the anti-KLH primary antibody response. Using BALB/c females housed six to a cage, we demonstrated that holding mice gently in the palm of the hand for 2 minutes a day for 2 weeks prior to immunization with KLH, reproducibly depressed the primary IgG (but not IgM) anti-KLH response. The secondary anti-KLH IgG response was measured in one experiment and was also found to be depressed.

Early experiences have been demonstrated to affect antibody responses. For example, Solomon, Levine, and Kraft (1968) placed individual group-housed Fisher rat pups in boxes for 3 minutes a day from birth until weaning. All animals received a primary and secondary immunization with flagellin at 9 and 13 weeks of age, respectively. Both the primary and secondary serum antibody titers to flagellin were higher in "handled" rats than in unmanipulated controls.

Raymond, Reyes, Tokuda, and Jones (1986) also examined the effects of early handling by placing individual BALB/c and C57BL/10J mouse pups in a bare metal cage for 3 minutes a day from birth to weaning. A suppression of the 5-day splenic PFC response of handled C57BL/10J mice relative to unhandled controls was reported; however, no differences between handled and control BALB/c mice were observed.

Endothermic vertebrates are not the only animals whose immune system can be compromised by "stress." Aquaculture of fish often requires that the animals be handled and transported, procedures that have been correlated with an increase in morbidity and mortality associated with bacterially and virally mediated diseases. It has been postulated for fish, as well as for endotherms, that increased susceptibility to infectious agents may result from stress-mediated immunosuppression (Wedemeyer, 1970). Recently, Elssaesser and Clem (1986) developed a laboratory model of handling/transport to determine whether stress affects various parameters of immunity in teleosts. Laboratory-acclimated individually housed 1.5 kg channel catfish were bled to provide baseline hematological and immunological measurements and were then individually placed in 150 liter tanks that were aerated. These tanks were then wheeled up and down a hallway on a cart for 15 minutes after which time the fish were returned to their home tanks. At 18–24 hours later, and again at 4 weeks, the fish were again bled and various hematological and immunological assays performed. These included in vitro production of antibody and accessory cell function (as well as differential blood counts and mitogen responses described later). "Transport stress" was associated with a dramatic reduction in the primary in vitro plaque forming cell responses of PBLs to the trinitrophenyl hapten (TNP) coupled to the thymus dependent (TD) carrier, KLH, or to the thymus independent (TI) carrier, lipopolysaccharide (LPS). By 4 weeks, primary PFC responses had returned to baseline levels.

Unpublished observations on catfish by Ellsaesser and Clem (personal communication, April 4, 1990) reveal that an iv injection of a physiological concentration of cortisol (defined according to Ellsaesser & Clem, 1987, as "the amount necessary to achieve at 30 minutes after injection the serum levels of cortisol observed 30 minutes after transport stress") eliminated the generation of in vitro primary antibody responses of peripheral blood leukocytes to TNP coupled to either TD or TI carriers. When the same concentration of cortisol was added directly to primary antibody forming cell cultures of lymphocytes from the peripheral blood of nonstressed animals, no inhibition of antibody was seen. Interestingly, when cortisol was added to cultures of lymphocytes from the pronephros (a major lymphopoietic organ in teleosts), in vitro primary antibody responses to TNP-LPS but not to TNP-KLH were suppressed. Tripp, Maule, Schreck, and Kaattari (1987) have also reported that addition of physiological levels of cortisol suppressed the in vitro primary anti-TNP-LPS responses of pronephric lymphocytes in trout (neither peripheral blood responses nor responses to TNP coupled to a TD carrier were examined).

Other than the clinical studies revealing stress-associated increases in antibodies to latent viruses described earlier (Kiecolt-Glaser & Glaser, in press), we are unaware of any experiments with humans dealing with the effects of stress on humoral immunity to exogenously administered antigens. However, salivary IgA, which is important in the prevention of respiratory tract infections, was found to be decreased in a population of dental students during their academic examinations (Jemmott et al., 1983). Although this finding was not corroborated by another study involving medical students (Kiecolt-Glaser et al., 1984), this latter population actually had increased concentrations of IgA in their serum during examinations.

Physical Stressors

The effect of thermal stress on antibody responses has been examined in calves that were housed during the first week after their birth in environmental chambers set at either 21C or 1C (Olson & Bull, 1986). They were then immunized with DNP-KLH and maintained in groups at 15C. No differences in antibody titers were seen. Kelley, Osbourne, Evermann, Parish, and Gaskins (1982) measured immunoglobulin levels (as opposed to specific antibody) in calves that had been reared at 35C or − 5C for 2 weeks. Plasma levels of IgG, but not IgM, were depressed in the calves exposed to elevated temperatures but were unaffected by the cold.

Solomon (1969) explored the influence of three different stressors on the primary and secondary antibody responses to polymeric flagellin in male Fisher rats. Signaled footshock, administered for five 15-second pulses per hour for 8–10 hours, was initiated 1 week prior to immunization and was continued throughout the course of immune measurements performed approximately 6 weeks later. The amperage was increased over time to decrease habituation. At the concentrations of antigen used, no differences in either primary or secondary antibody titers were noted. In contrast, rats subjected to a change in housing from two per cage to five or six per cage for 1 week prior to immunization, did display a significantly depressed primary and secondary anti-flagellin response. Finally, rats placed on either a large or small platform in an pan of water for 2 days before and 2 days after primary and secondary immunization with flagellin, had a depressed primary but an unaffected secondary response. Thus, this study clearly demonstrates that different stressors can affect the same parameters of immunity quite differently.

Okimura and Nigo (1986) reported that restraint stress (12 hours a day for 2 consecutive days) depressed the PFC response of BALB/c mice to SRBC, but did not affect their antibody response to ficoll, a Type 2 TI antigen. Thus, whether a given restraint protocol affects humoral immunity may depend on the nature of the antigen being used to evoke antibody production. The effect of restraint on the anti-SRBC antibody response was noted when the animals were restrained before, but not after, immunization. It should be recalled, however, that 2 consecutive days of stress for 12 hours a day administered either for the first 2 days before or for the 2 days immediately following priming with SRBC, was effective in depressing the DTH response to a subsequent challenge with SRBC (Okimura et al., 1986b).

Okimura, Satomi-Sasaki, and Ohkuma (1986a) used the same 12-hour restraint protocol and immunized mice with KLH following two stress sessions. Two days later, spleen cells were harvested and cultured for 4 days with either TNP coupled to the TD carrier KLH, or with DNP or TNP coupled to the TI carriers, ficoll or LPS, respectively. The anti-TNP-KLH response was diminished in stressed animals; the response to DNP-ficoll was unaffected; and there was a significant enhancement of the response to TNP coupled to LPS, a Type 1 TI carrier. Whether stress effects on thymus independent responses are more easily revealed with Type 1 TI antigens that activate relatively more immature B cells remains to be determined.

Esterling and Rabin (1987) used a rotation (100 rpm) stress model with either three (beginning 24 hours after immunization with SRBC) or four (beginning on the same day as immunization) rotation sessions. Each rotation session involved five 60-minute cycles. Each cycle consisted of 10 minutes of rotation followed by 50 minutes of rest over a 5-hour period.

The serum antibody and PFC responses in the stressed SW mice were measured 4 days after immunization with SRBC. There was no effect of stress when it was administered beginning at the time of immunization; however, the PFC and serum antibody titers were significantly depressed in mice for whom rotational stress began 24 hours after immunization. Thus, there appear to be critical periods relative to immunization when the physiological responses to a stressor can culminate in a demonstrable effect on antibody formation.

Zalcman, Minkiewicz-Janda, Richter, and Anisman (1988) have also provided evidence of a critical period when footshock of male CD-1 mice affects humoral immunity. Mice were subjected to 360 shocks, each of 2 seconds duration (0.15 or 0.3 mA), at either 0, 24, 48, 72, or 96 hours after immunization with SRBC. The anti-SRBC PFC response was assayed 96 hours after immunization. A significant reduction of serum antibody titers and the number of PFCs was noted, but only when the one session of footshock was administered 72 hours after immunization. The suppression of the splenic PFC response occurred regardless of whether the footshock session at 72 hours was escapable or inescapable. It was not indicated whether "control" over the stress situation had any effect on serum antibody responses. Indeed, whether the ability to control shock has any influence on the immune parameter being measured is still an open issue (Maier & Laudenslager, 1988; Mormede, Dantzer, Mischaud, Kelley, & Le Moal, 1988).

Subsequently, Zalcman, Richter, and Anisman (1990) showed that the footshock-induced suppression of anti-SRBC serum antibody and PFC responses could be conditioned. That is, a suppressed antibody response was observed in previously shocked mice after they were immunized with SRBC and exposed to the conditioned stimuli of stress-related cues. Conditioned footshock-induced suppression of the anti-SRBC response has also been observed in male Lewis rats by Lysle, Cunnick, Fowler, and Rabin (1988). It is unknown whether the immunosuppressive effects of the physical stressor and the conditioned stimuli are mediated through the same CNS pathways and neuropeptides.

Laudenslager et al. (1988) exposed male Sprague-Dawley rats to inescapable tailshock (100 shocks of 5 seconds each with shock intensity increasing from 0.8 to 1.6 mA every 25 shocks). Experimental animals received either one or three shock sessions a week for 2 consecutive weeks. Prior to the first shock session of Weeks 1 and 2, the rats were injected sc with 1 mg KLH to elicit a primary antibody response. Eight weeks after the initial KLH injection, the rats were given a third injection of 1 mg KLH ostensibly (see later) to elicit a secondary response. Serum anti-KLH antibody titers were determined following the second and third injections. A significantly depressed IgG anti-KLH antibody response was observed after the second and third injections of KLH regardless of whether the rats received one or three shock sessions on 2 consecutive weeks. It is unclear whether this protocol effected suppression of true secondary as well as primary antibody responses because the primary antibody response in shocked and control animals had not yet fully waned by the time the animals received the third injection of KLH.

In another footshock paradigm, Moynihan, Ader, Grota, Schachtman, and Cohen (1990) have demonstrated an antigen concentration-dependent suppressive effect on the secondary antibody response following primary immunization with a very small amount of KLH. Specifically, mice were primed with 1 ug KLH (or less), a dose that by itself did not elicit a primary response detectable by an enzyme-linked immunoassay (ELISA). This low priming dose contrasts with a primary immunization protocol involving 100–1000 ug KLH that is commonly followed in other investigations. Signaled footshock was administered as 60 ten-second pulses of 0.6 mA at random intervals during a 90-minute period. Initially, a suppressive effect on the secondary IgM and IgG response to 1 ug KLH (injected 23 days after priming) was demonstrated when shock was delivered on each of 7 consecutive days before and 7 days after antigen priming. It was subsequently determined in four of four experiments, that a single shock session delivered 24 hours after low dose antigen priming also resulted in a significant depression of the secondary anti-KLH antibody response. The effect of 14 footshock sessions on the secondary response was dependent on the amount of antigen used to evoke the secondary response. That is, a depressed secondary anti-KLH antibody response was demonstrable when the primed and stressed mice were challenged with 1 ug KLH but not with 5 ug KLH. This suggests that some immunomodulatory effects of a stressor may be subtle and could be masked when an investigator selects a concentration of antigen to inject based on what elicits an "optimal response" in the laboratory rather than what might be more equivalent to physiological concentrations of antigens encountered in the real world.

STRESS-ASSOCIATED CHANGES IN MITOGEN-STIMULATED LYMPHOCYTE PROLIFERATION IN VITRO

One of the most commonly chosen outcome measurements of the effects of stress on the immune system is the proliferative response of lymphocytes cultured with T cell mitogens such as phytohemagglutinin (PHA) and concanavalin A (Con A) and B cell mitogens such as LPS and dextran sulfate (DxS). Although stress-associated alterations in mitogen-driven lymphoproliferation are often considered to be synonymous with altered immune function, it should be understood that mitogen-stimulated lymphocyte division (as opposed to antigen-specific proliferation) does not reflect specific immune function per se. For example, whereas less than 1% of the B cells from an immunized animal might be stimulated by the immunizing antigen (in conjunction with accessory cells and antigen-specific T cells), LPS can drive proliferation of 20% of the B cells from a nonimmune animal, and the combination of LPS plus DxS can trigger proliferation of 80% of the B cells, even in the absence of T cells and macrophages (Feldbush, Stunz, & LaFrenz, 1986). Thus, in principal, one could observe a 25% change in tritiated thymidine incorporation in Con A stimulated splenocytes or peripheral blood lymphocytes (PBLs) from a stressed animal that is quite capable of responding to a thymus-dependent antigen by producing specific antibody with the same kinetics and the same titer as an unstressed control. On the other hand, stress-altered mitogenesis may well provide some indication of significant changes in either the numbers of leukocytes in a particular lymphoid compartment, a limited availability of different leukocyte-derived cytokines needed for proliferation, and/or an altered physiological state of the responding lymphocyte itself (e.g., altered expression of relevant cytokine and/or antigen receptors). The following studies should be reviewed with these caveats in mind.

Keller, Weiss, Schleifer, Miller, and Stein (1981) have investigated the effects of low (0.8–1.2 mA current) versus high (1.6–3.0 mA) tailshock (plus mild restraint) on immune parameters in W/Fu rats. In their paradigm, shock was administered over a 20-hour period, and the intensity was increased over time. Rats were sacrificed at the end of the shock period and the mitogen responses of their PBLs was examined. In one set of experiments, whole blood was incubated with two different concentrations of PHA. The two shock groups differed significantly from each other and the responses in both were significantly lower than the home-caged controls. Specifically, the high shock intensity resulted in the lowest proliferative responses. In a second set of procedures, PBLs were purified and cultured at fixed cell concentrations. Under these circumstances, proliferative responses of lymphocytes from both the high and low intensity shock groups still differed from the home-caged animals; however, they no longer differed from each other. The authors suggested that the lack of a difference between the responses of PBLs from animals in the two shock groups might have been the result of the addition of fetal bovine serum (FBS) to the cultures because FBS did have some stimulatory effects by itself. It also seems plausible that differences between whole blood responses of the two shock groups resulted from a differential reduction of the numbers of mitogen-reactive cells actually being placed in culture, a difference that no longer existed when the numbers of purified PBLs put into culture were equivalent. Because differences between the mitogen responsiveness of purified PBLs lymphocytes from the shocked and home caged groups were not eliminated when equal numbers of PBLs from animals in these groups were cultured, the suppressed responses may reflect qualitative rather than quantitative changes in the mitogen-reactive cell populations themselves. Subsequent studies by Keller, Weiss, Schleifer, Miller, and Stein (1983) with adrenalectomized rats indicated that this stress-induced suppression of the PHA response of peripheral blood was not mediated by adrenally derived "stress hormones" (e.g., catecholamines, glucocorticoids).

Lysle, Lyte, Fowler, and Rabin (1987) investigated the effects of different numbers of signaled footshocks (4, 8, or 16 shocks of 1.6 mA, each of 5 seconds duration) and different numbers of footshock sessions (1, 3, or 5 daily sessions) on the Con A-induced proliferative responses of whole blood and splenic leukocytes from Lewis strain male rats. Mitogenesis was measured immediately following the last shock exposure. Con A responses in whole blood were significantly suppressed by 1, 3, or 5 daily sessions when 8 or 16 shocks per session were administered, but there was no difference between controls and animals that received only four shocks per session. Splenic mitogen responses were similarly unaffected by four shocks per session regardless of the number of sessions. Interestingly, however, the suppression of the splenic Con A response to 8 or 16 shocks per session decreased as a function of the number of sessions such that the response had recovered to control levels following five sessions. These important observations suggest that alterations in the mitogen-induced in vitro proliferative response can be different in different lymphoid compartments and that these differences may reflect different underlying mechanisms. These investigators have also demonstrated that shock-induced depression of the T cell mitogen response can be conditioned (Lysle et al., 1988; Rabin, Cohen, Ganguli, Lysle, & Cunnick, 1989).

Studies of Monjan and Collector (1977) and Lysle et al. (1987) suggest that there may be habituation to stressful responses as determined by mitogen responses of splenocytes. Monjan and Collector (1977) also demonstrated that stress can be associated with enhanced as well as depressed in vitro mitogenesis. In these early studies, AKR or C57BL/6 mice were subjected to auditory stimulation for 5 seconds every minute during a 1- to 3-hour period for various periods of time before being sacrificed. Spleen cells were cultured with Con A or LPS. Short-term exposure to noise produced a striking suppression of mitogen responses. After approximately 20 days, the mitogen responses returned to control levels. Between 20 and 40 days, however, there was actually an enhanced response to both the T cell and B cell mitogens. Thus, there appeared to be an interaction between the number of exposures to the auditory stressor and the direction of the modulated mitogen response.

Kelley et al. (1982) measured PHA- and Con A-induced mitogenesis in calves exposed to thermal stress (see earlier for effects of this stressor on bovine humoral immunity). Neither heat nor cold stress altered the proliferative responses of purified PBLs. However, when plasma from heat-exposed calves was added to cultures of cells from normally maintained calves, consistently enhanced proliferative responses were seen relative to the effects of plasma from cold-stressed or thermoneutrally maintained calves.

Using the previously described protocol in which mice were handled daily for 2 minutes for 2 weeks, Moynihan, Brenner et al. (1990) harvested splenocytes 24 hours after the last handling session and demonstrated a significant decrease in the Con A response of spleen cells from handled mice. No group differences were noted in the responses to B cell mitogens (LPS plus DxS). Lown and Dutka (1987) used a different "handling" protocol in which individual mice were placed into different cages for 10 minutes a day either every day from weaning until Day 60 in studies with adult mice, or every day from birth to weaning in studies with neonates. These investigators reported no effect of "handling" on the Con A and LPS responses of spleen cells from adult C3H/St male and female group-housed mice. However, handling of neonates significantly enhanced mitogen responses when the animals reached 60 days of age.

Hardy, Quay, Livnat, and Ader (1990) have studied effects of social conflict (dominance/submission) on Con A and PHA responses. After 14 daily 10-minute encounters between two male C3H/HeJ mice, the submissive member of the pair had lower splenic mitogen responses.

The effect of social conflict on in vitro mitogenesis has also been examined in the teleost fish, *Tilapia* (Faisal, Chiapelli, Ahmed, Cooper, & Weiner, 1989). Pairs of temperature- and aquarium-acclimated fish were separated by a partition for 1 week. The partition was then removed for 5–10 hours and the fish were characterized as being either dominant or submissive. The mean PHA-, Con A-, or LPS-induced proliferative responses of lymphocytes harvested from the pronephros were similar for cells from the dominant and control fish; however, the responses of lymphocytes from submissive animal to all three mitogens were significantly reduced. In a second experiment, sera were harvested from control, dominant, and submissive fish and added, together with mitogens, to cultures of pronephric leukocytes from fish in each of the three groups. Serum from submissive fish suppressed the proliferative responses of cells from control and dominant fish to the T cell mitogens but not to LPS. This suppressive effect of serum was lost when the fish were injected with naltrexone prior to the onset of social conflict.

A dramatic reduction (relative to "pre-stress baseline values") of LPS- and Con A-induced mitogenesis of peripheral blood lymphocytes harvested from "transported" channel catfish was noted 18 hours after they were returned to their home tanks (Ellsaesser & Clem, 1986). Indeed, a significant reduction was often seen as early as 3 hours after the animals were returned. By 3 or 4 weeks, mitogen responses showed a variable degree of recovery. Depending on the fish, they either significantly exceeded responses noted 18 hours after the end of the stress, or they had returned to baseline, or, in fact they actually exceeded baseline measurements by twofold. It is important to note that successive bleedings without the intermediate handling and transport manipulations did not affect mitogen responsivity. It is also noteworthy from a mechanistic perspective that depressed mitogen reactivities could not be attributed to a stress-associated increase in a putative suppressor population. That is, the addition of "stressed cells" to populations of mitogen-stimulated peripheral blood lymphocytes from unmanipulated controls did not effect a reduction of mitogen responses. In addition, the loss of Con-A reactivity did not appear to result from a stress-associated change in the function of accessory cells (i.e., adherent macrophages) that are requisite for catfish lymphocytes to respond to mitogens. Thus, macrophages from stressed fish permitted macrophage-depleted peripheral blood lymphocytes to display normal Con A responses, and macrophages from unstressed fish did not cause an increase in the Con A responses of macrophage-depleted lymphocytes harvested from stressed animals. These findings imply that the putative neuroendocrine factors associated with transport stress were acting directly on catfish T and B cells rather than on catfish macrophages. Just what neuroendocrine factors are involved in mediating the constellation of stress-associated immunological effects in catfish are is not clear. It is known, however, that unmanipulated fish that received an iv injection of a dose of cortisol equivalent to that found in a transport-stressed fish, displayed the same degree of mitogen suppression noted with transport stress (as well as lymphopenia and neutrophila). However, the addition of the same physiological concentration of cortisol directly to mitogen-treated cultures of lymphocytes from unmanipulated catfish was without effect (Ellsaesser & Clem, 1987). The authors interpret these observations as an indication of indirect immunomodulatory effects of endogenous glucocorticoids.

A number of studies have addressed the effects of stress on several in vitro properties of human PBLs including numbers of T cells, NK cell number and activity, and mitogen responses to Con A, PHA, and the human B cell mitogen pokeweed mitogen (PWM) (Kiecolt-Glaser & Glaser, in press). In an early publication, Bartrop, Luckhurst, Lazarus, Kiloh, and Penney (1977) reported that bereaved spouses had lower mitogen responses than nonbereaved comparison subjects. In a prospective study, Schleifer, Keller, Camerino, Thornton, and Stein (1983) examined the mitogen responsivity of ficoll hypaque-purified PBLs from 15 males before and after their spouses died from breast cancer. Using a full dose range of each of the mitogens, these investigators observed significant decreases, relative to prebereavement measurements, in proliferation of cells obtained within the first 2 months following their loss. Follow-up measurements were made between 4 and 14 months after their spouses died, and the mitogen-induced proliferative responses were intermediate between, but not significantly different from, pre- and early postbereavement responses. Interpretation of these data is complicated by the fact that the mitogen response data from a group of normal males with healthy spouses were not included as a comparison control (although the relevant data were collected as a control for interassay variability). Thus, it is not known whether the mitogen responses of males prebereavement were also suppressed compared to the control population, and whether the degree of suppression might be a function of the length of their spouses' illness.

Glaser, Kiecolt-Glaser, Stout et al. (1985) compared the Con A and PHA responses of PBLs from 40 medical students 6 weeks before and during final exams. Using three concentrations of each of the mitogens, these investigators demonstrated reduced responses during exams relative to pre-examination measurements. Corroborative data on examination stress has been provided by Workman and LaVia (1987) who measured the PHA-induced proliferative response of whole blood lymphocytes from 15 medical students 1 day before and 1, 4, and 6 weeks after they took National Board Medical Examinations. A significant suppression of the PHA response persisted for about 4 weeks after they took the Boards; by 6 weeks, the responses were comparable to those observed 1 day prior to the taking the exams.

Finally, reduced mitogen responses have been noted in primary caregivers of Alzheimer's patients (Kiecolt-Glaser & Glaser, in press) and in women who had been divorced or separated for 1 year or less (Kiecolt-Glaser et al., 1987).

STRESS-ASSOCIATED CHANGES IN NUMBERS AND SUBSET DISTRIBUTION OF T AND B LYMPHOCYTES

Several investigators have addressed the issue of whether stress-associated changes in mitogen reactivity might result from a change in either the actual number of lymphocytes available in the lymphoid compartment being examined, a change the percent of T cells relative to B cells, and/or an alteration of the number or relative percents of various T cell subsets. The following studies have involved physical and psychological stimuli in experimental animals and man.

After 11–12 days of restraint for 3 hours each day, female Lewis rats had fewer CD4[+] and CD8[+] peripheral blood T cells, but the percentage of T cells remained unchanged (Steplewski & Vogel, 1986; Steplewski, Vogel, Ehya, Poropatich, & Smith, 1985). Following a 12-day recovery period, the total number and percentage of total T cells and T helper cells in the blood was significantly increased. Whether these changes also occurred in other lymphoid compartments is unknown.

Esterling and Rabin (1987) used the rotation stress model described previously and observed that male SW mice had a decreased number of splenic T helper cells following either three or four rotation sessions. Numbers of cytotoxic/suppressor splenic T cells were decreased only in animals that received a total of four rotation sessions.

Keller et al. (1981) and Keller, Schleifer, and Stein (1984), who investigated the effects of low versus high intensity tailshock on several immune parameters (see earlier), found no differences in the number of T cells in blood from shocked and control rats. However, there was a marked lymphocytopenia in both low and high intensity shock groups. Although this suggests that the number of B cells must have been differentially effected, no data on numbers of B cells were presented.

Moynihan, Brenner et al. (1990) did not observe differences in total spleen cell number of numbers of CD4[+] and CD8[+] T cells and surface IgM[+] B cells in the spleens of BALB/c mice following 2 weeks of daily handling. Again, no other lymphoid compartments were examined.

In the fish model of social conflict previously discussed within the context of mitogen responses, it was noted that submissive *Tilapia* exhibited a reduction in the number of pronephric mononuclear cells and a concomitant increase in polymorphonuclear leukocytes (Ghoneum, Faisal, Peters, Ahmed, & Cooper, 1988; Peters & Schwarzer, 1985). Peripheral blood from channel catfish subjected to transport stress was also characterized by a marked (50%) reduction in the number of peripheral blood leukocytes and a concomitant increase in the number of neutrophils that was independent of the bleedings at immediately before and shortly after transport (Bly, Miller, & Clem, in press; Ellsaesser & Clem, 1986). These investigators further demonstrated that the leukopenia preferentially resulted from lymphocytopenia (approximately a 65% reduction) and that both T and B cell numbers were depressed. All hematological values returned to normal by 4 weeks after stress.

Stress-associated hematological changes have also been noted in clinical studies. For example, the percentages of total T cells and of CD4[+] helper and CD8[+] cytotoxic/suppressor peripheral blood T cells were lower in medical students during an examination period relative to samples obtained during a relatively nonstressful pre-exam period (Glaser, Kiecolt-Glaser, Speicher et al. 1985; Glaser, Kiecolt-Glaser, Stout et al., 1985). In their aforementioned study of marital quality and divorce, Kiecolt-Glaser et al.

(1987) found that women who had been separated 1 year or less had, in addition to poorer mitogen responses and apparently decreased cell-mediated responses to EBV VCA, a significantly lower numbers of helper T cells than the control matched married group. There were no differences between the two groups in the percentage of cytotoxic/suppressor CD8$^+$ T cells or in the helper–suppressor ratio. In contrast, in their prospective study of men whose spouses died of breast cancer, Schleifer et al. (1983) found no changes in either percentages or absolute numbers of peripheral blood T and B lymphocytes prior to or after the time their subjects became widowed.

STRESS-ASSOCIATED CHANGES IN NATURAL KILLER (NK) CELL CYTOTOXICITY

An animal's ability to nonspecifically kill tumor cells or virally infected cells in a nonspecific fashion is considered to be a phylogenetically early defense mechanism (Evans & McKinney, in press). NK cells are large granular lymphocytes that appear to serve this cytotoxic function, at least in vitro as assayed by the release of radioactive isotope from ^{51}Cr-labelled target tumor cells (e.g., YAC-1 mouse lymphoma cells). By and large, physical stressors are associated with diminished NK cytotoxicity. For example, Aarstad, Gaudernack, and Seljelid (1983) demonstrated reduced NK activity of splenocytes from C57BL/10 male mice that had been immersed in cold water twice daily for 5 minutes for 1 to 8 days. Shavit et al. (1986) observed suppressed NK activity in Fisher 344 female rats that had been footshocked (2.0mA) for 1 to 5 seconds for 10 minutes a day for either 4, 14, or 30 days. Suppressed NK cytotoxicity has also been demonstrated in BALB/c female mice by Okimura, Ogawa, and Yamauchi et al. (1986b) and in female Lewis rats by Steplewski and Vogel (1986) using the restraint protocols described earlier. Pollock, Babcock, Romsdahl, and Nishioka (1984) and Pollock, Lotzova, Stanford, and Romsdahl (1987) observed suppression of NK cell activity in (C57BL/6 × DBA/2)F$_1$ hybrid female mice during the first 12 days following surgery.

In experimental animals, psychological stressors such as handling and differential housing have not always resulted in NK suppression. Ghoneum, Gill, Assanah, and Stevens (1987) studied the effects of differential housing in young and aged (12-month-old) Sprague-Dawley male rats. The animals were first group-housed for 1 week and then housed in groups or individually for an additional week. NK cell activity was depressed in the aged and individually housed rats compared to group-housed aged rats. However, there were no housing-related differences in NK cell function in spleen cells from young animals. In the previously described handling protocol of

Moynihan, Brenner et al. (1990), which resulted in reduced serum antibody titers and altered mitogen responses, NK cell activity was not affected (unpublished observations).

Social stress in *Tilapia* was also associated with a marked reduction in the NK-like killing of YAC target cells by nonimmune pronephric leukocytes from both the dominant and the submissive fish. However, suppression appeared greatest in the submissive animals. Injection of the fish with naltrexone 1 hour prior to the onset of social conflict maintained the cytotoxic responses of the dominant fish at control levels and somewhat blocked the suppression seen in the submissive animals. As seen with mitogens, the sera from submissive fish appeared capable of suppressing NK-like killing by pronephric cells from control fish; this inhibitory effect was also blocked by when the fish were pretreated with naltrexone (Faisal et al., 1989).

Several of the previously described clinical populations such as medical students undergoing examinations and subjects with poor marriages, have also been characterized by a depressed number of Leu-11b[+] NK cells and depressed NK mediated cytotoxicity (Glaser, Kiecolt-Glaser, Speicher et al., 1985; Glaser, Kiecolt-Glaser, Stout et al., 1985; Glaser, Rice, Speicher, Stout, & Kiecolt-Glaser, 1986). Levy, Herberman, Lippman, and D'Angelo (1987) have reported, in breast cancer patents, a correlation of "stress factors" with depressed NK cell cytotoxicity and poor prognosis. Whether these latter observations reflect a reduced percentage of these cells in the peripheral blood and/or an actual decrease in killing ability is not clear. Obviously, it is also not known whether stress-associated changes in NK activity in clinical populations would also be noted in lymphoid compartments other than the peripheral blood.

CNS-MEDIATION OF STRESS-ASSOCIATED CHANGES IN IMMUNITY

This review does not attempt to provide a detailed summary or synthesis of the rapidly expanding body of information about the CNS mediation of the behavioral regulation of immunity (for reviews see Dantzer & Kelley, 1989; Khansari, Murgo, & Faith, 1990; Rabin et al., 1989; Sklar & Anisman, 1981). We do, however, highlight some of the major lines of research that are currently being pursued, and some of the complexity and confusion that has already resulted from this research.

The hypothalamo-pituitary-adrenal (HPA) axis is clearly involved in stress and immunomodulation. Because of the involvement of the HPA axis in stress-induced analgesia, the role of endogenous opioids in stress-associated immunomodulation has been examined in a variety of species from fish to man. Cunnick, Lysle, Armfield, and Rabin (1988) and Shavit,

Yirmiya, and Beilin (1990) have recently reviewed the effects of opioids on NK cell cytotoxicity and tumor growth. Lewis, Shavit, Terman, Gale, and Liebeskind (1983); Shavit et al. (1986); Ghoneum et al. (1987); and Faisal et al. (1989) have all reported that the stress-induced depression of NK cytotoxicity they observe in various physical and psychological stress paradigms can be blocked by naloxone or naltrexone and mimicked by exogenous opioids such as endorphins and morphine. However, Ben-Eliyahu, Yirmiya, Shavit, and Liebeskind (1990) have recently reported a stress-induced suppression of NK cell cytotoxicity that does not appear to be opioid mediated.

Although there is evidence for adrenal corticosteroid mediation of some immunomodulatory stress effects (Blecha, Kelley, & Satterlee, 1982), several studies with adrenalectomized animals indicate that the relationship between stress, adrenal hormones, and immune changes is still an open issue (Esterling & Rabin, 1987; Keller et al., 1983). Indeed, Moynihan et al. (1989) have recently shown that mice handled for 2 weeks, and therefore exhibiting a depressed anti-KLH antibody response, actually had an attenuated glucocorticoid response compared with previously unhandled mice immediately prior to primary immunization.

The role of catecholamines and other neurotransmitters in the stress response is well-known. A number of studies have investigated the role of neurotransmitters such as norepinephrine on immune function (for a review see Madden & Livnat, 1991). Far fewer studies, however, have attempted to correlate stress-induced changes in plasma catecholamines with altered immune function (Landmann et al., 1984).

Finally, there is conflicting evidence that neurotransmitters such as gamma-amino-butyric acid (GABA) may play a role in stress effects on immune function. Okimura and Nigo (1986) reported that the anti-anxiolytic drug, diazepam, which binds to the benzodiazepine receptor, could prevent restraint-induced suppression of the anti-SRBC antibody response. In contrast, Cunnick et al. (1988) reported that diazepam could not prevent footshock-induced suppression of the mitogen response of splenocytes.

CONCLUDING REMARKS

In this review, we have selectively highlighted some immunological conse-quences of "stress" in a variety of species including humans, subhuman primates, rats, mice, and fish. Despite the phylogenetic constancy of the fact that "stress" can have an effect on the immune system, and that in many studies, this effect translates into a reduction in the response parameter being investigated, it is difficult, if not misleading, to speak categorically about the nature and "direction" of these stress effects (Ader & Cohen, 1984). Indeed, the wealth of published studies indicate that a given stressor can be associated with an enhancement as well as a depression of an immune response (Okimura & Nigo, 1986) and that different stressors can have different qualitative, and perhaps even quantitative effects on a single immune parameter (Solomon, 1969). Indeed, the magnitude and direction of a behaviorally driven deviation of immune function from "normalcy" appears to be related to the factors such as: the duration of exposure to the stressor (Monjan & Collector, 1977; Moynihan, Ader et al., 1990); the timing of stress administration relative to the time of antigenic exposure (Esterling & Rabin, 1987; Okimura & Nigo, 1986; Zalcman et al., 1988); the time of immunological assay after exposure to the stressor (Schleifer et al., 1983); the immune status of the animal being stressed (Edwards et al., 1980; Laudenslager et al., 1988; Moynihan, Ader, Grota, Schachtman, & Cohen, 1990; Solomon, 1969); the concentration of antigen used to elicit an antibody response in a stressed animal (Moynihan et al., 1990); and perhaps the coping behavior of the organism (Maier & Laudenslager, 1988; Mormede et al., 1988).

By choice, we have not attempted to review the large body of literature indicating the constellation of effects that diverse stress hormones (e.g., catecholamines, steroids, proopiomelanocortin-derived peptides, prolactin, growth hormone, etc.) can have on immunity (reviewed in Ader, Felten, & Cohen, 1990; see also citations in the introduction). Neither have we attempted to review in any detail the somewhat conflicting literature dealing with correlations between stress-associated changes in an immune parameter and changes in endogenous neuropeptides (e.g., endogenous opioids) or hormones (e.g., glucocorticoids). At this time, we believe that there are still too many gaps in our knowledge to allow us to present anything resembling a clear picture of cause and effect. We do anticipate, however, that with the expanding interest in the basic and clinical ramifications of psychoneuroimmunology that the next decade of stress-immune response research will clearly reveal what neuroendocrine changes are evoked by which stressor, how these changes modify components of the immune system, and how these changes in the immune response are causally related to increased morbidity and mortality.

ACKNOWLEDGMENTS

Research cited from the authors' laboratory has been supported by grant MH–45681 from the National Institutes of Mental Health.

REFERENCES

Aarstad, H. J., Gaudernack, G., & Seljelid, R. (1983). Stress causes reduced natural killer cell activity in mice. *Scandanavian Journal of Immunology, 18,* 461–464.

Ader, R. (1971). Experimentally-induced gastric lesions: Results and implications of studies in animals. *Advances in Psychosomatic Medicine, 6,* 1–39.

Ader, R., & Cohen, N. (1984). Behavior and the immune system. In W. D. Gentry (Ed.), *Handbook of behavioral medicine* (pp. 117–173). New York: Guilford Press.

Ader, R., & Cohen, N. (1991). The influence of conditioning on immune responses. In R. Ader, N. Cohen, & D. L. Felten (Eds.), *Psychoneuroimmunology* (2nd ed., pp. 611–646). New York: Academic Press.

Ader, R., Felten, D. L., & Cohen, N. (1990). Interactions between the brain and the immune system. *Annual Review Pharmacology and Toxicology, 30,* 561–602.

Ader, R., Grota, L. J., Moynihan, J. A., & Cohen, N. (1991). Behavioral adaptations in autoimmune disease-susceptible mice. In R. Ader, N. Cohen, & D. L. Felten (Eds.), Psychoneuroimmunology (2nd ed., pp. 685–708). New York: Academic Press.

Bartrop, R., Luckhurst, E., Lazarus, L., Kiloh, L., & Penney, R. (1977). Depressed lymphocyte function after bereavement. *Lancet, 1,* 834–836.

Beden, S. N., & Brain, P. F. (1982). Studies on the effect of social stress on measures of disease resistance in laboratory mice. *Aggressive Behavior, 8,* 126–129.

Beden, S. N., & Brain, P. F. (1984). Effects of attack-related stress on the primary immune response to sheep red blood cells in castrated mice. *IRCS Medical Science, 12,* 675.

Ben-Eliyahu, S., Yirmiya, R., Shavit, Y., & Liebeskind, J. C. (1990). Stress-induced suppression of natural killer cell cytotoxicity in the rat: a naltrexone-insensitive paradigm. *Behavioral Neuroscience, 104,* 235–238.

Beneviste, E. M. (1988). Lymphokines and monokines in the neuroendocrine system. In J. E. Blalock & K. L. Bost (Eds.), *Neuroimmunoendocrinology progress in allergy* (Vol. 43, pp. 84–120). New York: Karger.

Bernton, E. W., Bryant, H. Y., & Holaday, J. W. (1991). Prolactin and immune function. In R. Ader, N. Cohen, & D. L. Felten (Eds.), *Psychoneuroimmunology* (2nd ed., pp. 403–428). New York: Academic Press.

Blalock, J. E. (1988). Production of neuroendocrine peptide hormones by the immune system. In J. E. Blalock & K. L. Bost (Eds.), *Neuroimmunoendocrinology progress in allergy* (Vol. 43, pp. 1–13). New York: Karger.

Blecha, F., Barry, R. A., & Kelley, K. W. (1982). Stress-induced alterations in delayed-type hypersensitivity to SRBC and contact sensitivity to DNFB in mice. *Proceedings of the Society of Experimental Biology and Medicine, 169,* 239–246.

Blecha, F., Kelley, K. W., & Satterlee, D. G. (1982). Adrenal involvement in the expression of delayed-type hypersensitivity to SRBC and contact sensitivity to DNFB in stressed mice. *Proceedings of the Society of Experimental Biology and Medicine, 169,* 247–252.

Bly, J. E., Miller, N. W., & Clem, L. W. (in press). A monoclonal antibody specific for neutrophils in normal and stressed channel catfish. *Developmental and Comparative Immunology, 14.*

Bohus, B., & Koolhaas, J. (1991). Psychoimmunology of social factors in rodents and other subprimate vertebrates. In R. Ader, N. Cohen, & D. L. Felten (Eds.), *Psychoneuroimmunology* (2nd ed., pp. 807–830). New York: Academic Press.

Bost, K. L. (1988). Hormone and neuropeptide receptors on mononuclear leukocytes. In J. E. Blalock & K. L. Bost (Eds.), *Neuroimmunoendocrinology progress in allergy* (Vol. 43, pp. 68–83). New York: Karger.

Clem, L. W., Miller, N. W., & Bly, J. E. (in press). Evolution of lymphocyte subpopulations, their interactions, and temperature sensitivities. In G. W. Warr & N. Cohen (Eds.), *Phylogenesis of immune functions.* Boca Raton, FL: CRC Press.

Coe, C. L., Rosenberg, L. T., Fisher, M., & Levine, S. (1987). Psychological factors capable of preventing the inhibition of antibody responses in separated infant monkeys. *Child Development, 58,* 1420–1430.

Cunnick, J. E., Lysle, D. T., Armfield, A., & Rabin, B. S. (1988). Shock-induced modulation of lymphocyte responsiveness and natural killer activity: differential mechanisms of induction. *Brain, Behavior, and Immunity, 2,* 102–113.

Dantzer, R., & Kelley, K. W. (1989). Stress and immunity: an integrated view of relationships between the brain and the immune system. *Life Sciences, 44,* 1995–2008.

Edwards, E. A., Rahe, R. H., Stephens, P. M., & Henry, J. P. (1980). Antibody response to bovine serum albumin in mice: The effects of psychosocial environmental change. *Proceedings of the Society of Experimental Biology and Medicine, 164,* 478–481.

Ellsaesser, C. F., & Clem, L. W. (1986). Haematological and immunological changes in channel catfish stressed by handling and transport. *Journal of Fish Biology, 28,* 511–521.

Ellsaesser, C. F., & Clem, L. W. (1987). Cortisol-induced hematologic and immunologic changes in channel catfish *(Ictalurus punctatus). Comparative Biochemical Physiology, 87A,* 405–408.

Esterling, B., & Rabin, B. S. (1987). Stress-induced alteration of T-lymphocyte subsets and humoral immunity in mice. *Behavioral Neuroscience, 101,* 115–119.

Evans, D. L., & McKinney, E. C. (in press). Phylogeny of cytotoxic cells. In G. W. Warr & N. Cohen (Eds.), *Phylogenesis of immune functions.* Boca Raton, FL: CRC Press.

Faisal, M., Chiapelli, F., Ahmed, I. I., Cooper, E. L., & Weiner, H. (1989). Social confrontation "stress" in aggressive fish is associated with an endogenous opioid-mediated suppression of proliferative responses to mitogens and nonspecific cytotoxicity. *Brain, Behavior, and Immunity, 3,* 223–233.

Feldbush, T. L., Stunz, L. L., & LaFrenz, D. E. (1986). Memory B-cell activation, differentiation, and isotype switching. In J. C. Cambier (Ed.), *B-lymphocyte differentiation* (pp. 135–162). Boca Raton, FL: CRC Press.

Felten, S. Y., & Felten, D. L. (1991). The innervation of lymphoid tissue. In R. Ader, N. Cohen, & D. L. Felten (Eds.), *Psychoneuroimmunology* (2nd ed., pp. 27–70). New York: Academic Press.

Fleshner, M., Laudenslager, M. L., Simons, L., & Maier, S. F. (1989). Reduced serum antibodies associated with social defeat in rats. *Physiology and Behavior, 45,* 1183–1187.

Ghoneum, M., Faisal, M., Peters, G., Ahmed, I. I., & Cooper, E. L. (1988). Suppression of natural cytotoxic cell activity by social aggressiveness in *Tilapia. Developmental and Comparative Immunology, 12,* 595–602.

Ghoneum, M., Gill, G., Assanah, P., & Stevens, W. (1987). Susceptibility of natural killer cell activity of old rats to stress. *Immunology, 60,* 461–465.

Glaser, R., & Gottlieb-Stematsky, R. (1982). *Human herpesvirus infections: Clinical aspects.* New York: Marcel-Dekker.

Glaser, R., Kiecolt-Glaser, J. K., Speicher, C. E., & Holliday, J. E. (1985). Stress, loneliness, and changes in herpesvirus latency. *Journal of Behavioral Medicine, 8,* 249–260.

Glaser, R., Kiecolt-Glaser, J. K., Stout, J. C., Tarr, K. L., Speicher, C. E., & Holliday, J. E., (1985). Stress-related impairments in cellular immunity. *Psychological Research, 16,* 233–239.

Glaser, R., Rice, J., Sheridan, J., Fertel, R., Stout, J., Speicher, C., Pinsky, D., Kotur, M., Post, A., Beck, M., & Kiecolt-Glaser, J. (1987). Stress-related immune suppression: Health implications. *Brain, Behavior, and Immunology, 1,* 7–20.

Glaser, R., Rice, J., Speicher, C. E., Stout, J., & Kiecolt-Glaser, J. K. (1986). Stress depresses interferon production by leukocytes concomitant with a decrease in natural killer cell activity. *Behavioral Neuroscience, 100,* 675–678.

Goetzl, E. J., Turck, C. W., & Sreedharen, S. P. (1991). Production and recognition of neuropeptides by cells of the immune system. In R. Ader, N. Cohen, & D. L. Felten (Eds.), *Psychoneuroimmunology* (2nd ed., pp. 263–282). New York: Academic Press.

Hanson, D. F., Murphy, P. A., Silicano, R., & Shin, H. S. (1983). The effects of temperature on the activation of thymocytes by interleukins I and II. *Journal of Immunology, 130,* 216–221.

Hardy, C., Quay, J., Livnat, S., & Ader, R. (in press). Altered T lymphocyte response following aggressive encounters in mice. *Physiology and Behavior,* 1245–1251.

Heijen, D. J., Kavelaars, A., & Ballieux, R. E. (1991). CRH and POMC-derived peptides in the modulation of immune function. In R. Ader, N. Cohen, & D. L. Felten (Eds.), *Psychoneuroimmunology* (2nd ed., pp. 429–446). New York: Academic Press.

Ito, Y., Mine, K., Ago, Y., Nakagawa, T., Fujiwara, M., & Ueki, S. (1983). Attack stress and IgE antibody response in rats. *Pharmacology, Biochemistry, and Behavior, 19,* 883–886.

Jemmott, J. B., Borysenko, J. Z., Borysenko, M., McClelland, D. C., Chapman, R., Meyer, D. J., & Benson, H. (1983). Academic stress, power motivation, and decrease in secretion rate of salivary secretory immunoglobulin A. *Lancet 1,* 1400–1402.

Keller, S. E., Schleifer, S. J., & Demetrikopoulos, M. K. (1991). Stress-induced changes in immune function in animals: hypothalamic-pituitary-adrenal influences. In R. Ader, N. Cohen, & D. L. Felten (Eds.), *Psychoneuroimmunology* (2nd ed., pp. 771–788). New York: Academic Press.

Keller, S. E., Schleifer, S. J., & Stein, M. (1984). Stress-induced suppression of lymphocyte function in rats. In E. L. Cooper (Ed.), *Stress, immunity, and aging* (pp. 109–121). New York: Marcel Dekker.

Keller, S. E., Weiss, J. M., Schleifer, S. J., Miller, N. E., & Stein, M. (1981). Suppression of immunity by stress: effects of a graded series of stressors on lymphocyte stimulation in the rat. *Science, 213,* 1397–1400.

Keller, S. E., Weiss, J. M., Schleifer, S. J., Miller, N. E., & Stein, M. (1983). Stress-induced suppression of immunity in adrenaectomized rats. *Science, 221,* 1301–1304.

Kelley, K. W. (1991). Growth hormone in immunobiology. In R. Ader, N. Cohen, & D. L. Felten (Eds.), *Psychoneuroimmunology* (2nd ed., pp. 377–402). New York: Academic Press.

Kelley, K. W., Osbourne, C. A., Evermann, J. F., Parish, S. M., & Gaskins, C. T. (1982). Effects of chronic heat and cold stressors on plasma immunoglobulin and mitogen-induced blastogenesis in calves. *Journal of Dairy Science, 65,* 1514–1528.

Khansari, D. N., Murgo, A. J., & Faith, R. E. (1990). Effects of stress on the immune system. *Immunology Today, 11,* 170–175.

Kiecolt-Glaser, J. K., Fisher, L. D., Ogrocki, P., Stout, J. C., Speicher, C. E., & Glaser, R. (1987). Marital quality, marital disruption, and immune function. *Psychosomatic Medicine, 49,* 13–34.

Kiecolt-Glaser, J. K., Garner, W., Speicher, C., Penn, G. M., Holliday, J., & Glaser, R. (1984). Psychosocial modifiers of immunocompetence in medical students. *Psychosomatic Medicine, 46,* 7–14.

Kiecolt-Glaser, J. K., & Glaser, R. (in press). Stress and immune function. In R. Ader, N. Cohen, & D. L. Felten (Eds.), *Psychoneuroimmunology* (2nd ed.). New York: Academic Press.

Kiecolt-Glaser, J. K., Glaser, R., Strain, E., Stout, J., Tarr, K., Holliday, J., & Speicher, C. (1986). Modulation of cellular immunity in medical students. *Journal of Behavioral Medicine, 9,* 5–21.

Landmann, R. M. A., Muller, F. B., Perini, C., Wesp, M., Erne, P., & Buhler, F. R. (1984). Changes of immunoregulatory cells induced by psychological and physical stress: Relationship to plasma catecholamines. *Clinical and Experimental Immunology, 58,* 127–135.

Laudenslager, M., Fleshner, M., Hofstadter, P., Held, P. E., Simons, L., & Maiers. (1988). Suppression of specific antibody production by inescapable shock: stability under varying conditions. *Brain, Behavior, and Immunity, 2,* 92–101.

Lauwasser, M., & Shands, J. W., Jr. (1979). Depressed mitogen responsiveness of lymphocytes at skin temperature. *Infectious Disease, 24,* 454–458.

Levy, S., Herberman, R., Lippman, M., & D'Angelo, T. (1987). Correlation of stress factors with sustained depression of natural killer cell activity and predicted prognosis in patients with breast cancer. *Journal of Clinical Oncology, 5,* 348–353.

Lewis, J. W., Shavit, Y., Terman, G. W., Gale, R. P., & Liebeskind, J. C. (1983). Stress and morphine affect survival of rats challenged with a mammary ascites tumor (MAT 13762B). *Natural Immunity and Cellular Growth Regulation, 3,* 43–50.

Lown, B. A., & Dutka, M. E. (1987). Early handling enhances mitogen responses of splenic cells in adult C3H mice. *Brain, Behavior, and Immunity, 1,* 356–360.

Lysle, D. T., Lyte, M., Fowler, H., & Rabin, B. S. (1987). Shock-induced modulation of lymphocyte reactivity: suppression, habituation, and recovery. *Life Sciences, 41,* 1805–1814.

Lysle, D. T. Cunnick, J. E., Fowler, H., & Rabin, B. S. (1988). Pavlovian conditioning of shock-induced suppression of lymphocyte reactivity. Acquisition, extinction, and preexposure effects. *Life Sciences, 42,* 2185–2194.

Madden, K. S., & Livnat, S. (1991). Catecholamine action and immunologic activity. In R. Ader, N. Cohen, & D. L. Felten (Eds.), *Psychoneuroimmunology* (2nd ed., pp. 283–310). New York: Academic Press.

Maier, S. F., & Laudenslager, M. L. (1988). Inescapable shock, shock controllability, and mitogen-stimulated lymphocyte proliferation. *Brain, Behavior and Immunity, 2,* 87–91.

McCruden, A. B., & Stimson, W. H. (1991). Sex hormones and immune function. In R. Ader, N. Cohen, & D. L. Felten (Eds.), *Psychoneuroimmunology.* (2nd ed., pp. 475–494). New York: Academic Press.

McGillis, J. P., Mitsuhashi, M., & Payan, D. G. (1991). Immunologic properties of substance P. In R. Ader, N. Cohen, & D. L. Felten (Eds.), *Pychoneuroimmunology* (2nd ed., pp. 209–224). New York: Academic Press.

Michaut, R., Dechambre, R., Doumerc, S., Lesourd, B., Devillechabrolle, A., & Moulias, R. (1981) Influence of early maternal deprivation on adult humoral immune response in mice. *Physiology and Behavior, 26,* 189–191.

Monjan, A. A., & Collector, M. I. (1977). Stress-induced modulation of the immune response. *Science, 196,* 307–308.

Mormede, P., Dantzer, R., Mischaud, B., Kelley, K., & Le Moal, M. (1988). Influence of stressor predictability and behavioral control on lymphocyte reactivity, antibody responses, and neuroendocrine activation in rats. *Physiology and Behavior, 43,* 577–583.

Moynihan, J., Brenner, G., Koota, D., Breneman, S., Cohen, N., & Ader, R. (1990). The effects of handling on antibody production, mitogen responses, spleen cell number, and lymphocyte subpopulations. *Life Sciences, 46,* 1937–1944.

Moynihan, J., Koota, D., Brenner, G., Cohen, N., & Ader, R. (1989). Repeated intraperitoneal injections of saline attenuate the antibody response to a subsequent intraperitoneal injection of antigen. *Brain, Behavior, and Immunity, 3,* 90–96.

Moynihan, J. A., Ader, R., Grota, L. J., Schachtman, T. R., & Cohen, N. (1990). The effects of stress on the development of immunological memory following low-dose antigen priming in mice. *Brain, Behavior, and Immunity, 4,* 1–12.

Munck, A., & Guyre, P. M. (1991). Glucocorticoids and immune function. In R. Ader, N. Cohen, & D. L. Felten (Eds.), *Psychoneuroimmunology* (2nd ed., pp. 447–474). New York: Academic Press.

Okimura, T., & Nigo, Y. (1986). Stress and immune responses. I. Suppression of T cell functions in restraint-stressed mice. *Japanese Journal of Pharmacology, 40,* 505–511.

Okimura, T., Ogawa, M., & Yamauchi, T. (1986). Stress and immune responses III. Effect of restraint stress on delayed type hypersensitivity (DTH) response, natural killer (NK) activity, and phagocytosis in mice. *Japanese Journal of Pharmacology, 41,* 229–235.

Okimura, T., Satomi-Sasaki, & Ohkuma, S. (1986). Stress and immune responses II. Identification of stress-sensitive cells in murine spleen cells. *Japanese Journal of Pharmacology, 40,* 513–525.

Olson, D. P., & Bull, R. C. (1986). Antibody response in protein-energy restricted beef cows and their cold-stressed progeny. *Canadian Journal of Veterinary Research, 50,* 410–417.

Ottaway, C. (1991). Vasoactive intestinal peptide and immune function. In R. Ader, N. Cohen, & D. L. Felten (Eds.), *Psychoneuroimmunology* (2nd ed., pp. 225–262). New York: Academic Press.

Peters, G., & Schwarzer, R. (1985). Changes in hematopoetic tissue of rainbow trout under influence of stress. *Diseases of Acquatic Origin, 1,* 1–10.

Pollock, R. E., Babcock, G. F., Romsdahl, M. M., & Nishioka, K. (1984). Surgical stress-mediated suppression of murine natural killer cell cytotoxicity. *Cancer Research, 44,* 3888–3891.

Pollock, R. E., Lotzova, E., Stanford, S. D., & Romsdahl, M. M. (1987). Effect of surgical stress on murine natural killer cell activity. *Journal of Immunology, 138,* 171–178.

Rabin, B. S., Cohen, S., Ganguli, R., Lysle, D. T., & Cunnick, J. E. (1989). Bidirectional interaction between the central nervous system and the immune system. *Critical Reviews in Immunology, 9,* 279–312.

Rabin, B. S., Lyte, M., Epstein, L. H., & Caggiula, A. R. (1987). Alteration of immune competency by number of mice housed per cage. *Annals New York Academy of Science, 496,* 492–500.

Rabin, B. S., & Salvin, S. B. (1987). Effect of differential housing and time on immune reactivity to sheep erythrocytes and *Candida. Brain, Behavior, and Immunity, 1,* 267–275.

Raymond, L. N., Reyes, E., Tokuda, S., & Jones, B. C. (1986). Differential immune response in two handled inbred strains of mice. *Physiology and Behavior, 37,* 295–297.

Schleifer, S. J., Keller, S. E., Camerino, M., Thornton, J. C., & Stein, M. (1983). Suppression of lymphocyte stimulation following bereavement. *Journal of the American Medical Association, 250,* 374–377.

Selye, H. (1950). *Stress.* Montreal, Canada: ACTA.

Shavit, Y. (in press). Stress-induced immune modulation in animals: Opiates and endogenous opioid peptides. In R. Ader, N. Cohen, & D. L. Felten (Eds.), *Psychoneuroimmunology* (2nd ed.). New York: Academic Press.

Shavit, Y., Terman, G. W., Lewis, J. W., Zane, C. J., Gale, R. P., & Liebeskind, J. C. (1986). Effects of footshock stress and morphine on natural killer lymphocytes in rats: studies of tolerance and cross-tolerance. *Brain Research, 372,* 382–385.

Shavit, Y., Yirmiya, R., & Beilin, B. (1990). Stress neuropeptides, immunity, and neoplasia. In S. Frier (Ed.), *The neuroendocrine-immune network,* (pp. 163–175). Boca Raton, FL: CRC Press.

Sklar, L. S., & Anisman, H. (1981). Stress and cancer. *Psychological Bulletin, 89,* 369–406.

Solomon, G. F. (1969). Stress and antibody response in rats. *International Archives of Allergy, 35,* 97–104.

Solomon, G. F., Levine, S., & Kraft, J. K. (1968). Early experience and immunity. *Nature,*

220, 821–822.

Steplewski, Z., & Vogel, W. H. (1986). Total leukocytes, T cell subpopulation, and natural killer (NK) cell activity in rats exposed to restraint stress. *Life Sciences, 38,* 2419–2427.

Steplewski, Z., Vogel, W. H., Ehya, H., Poropatich, C., & Smith, J. M. (1985). Effects of restraint stress on inoculated tumor growth and immune response in rats. *Cancer Research, 45,* 5126–5133.

Tripp, R. A., Maule, A. G., Schreck, C. B., & Kaattari, S. L. (1987). Cortisol mediated suppression of salmonid lymphocyte responses *in vitro. Developmental and Comparative Immunology, 11,* 565–576.

Vessey, S. H. (1964). Effects of grouping on levels of circulating antibodies in mice. *Proceedings of the Society of Experimental Biology and Medicine, 115,* 252–255.

Wedemeyer, G. (1970). The role of stress in the disease resistance of fishes. In S. F. Snieszko (Ed.), *A symposium on diseases of fish and shellfishes* (Special Pub. 5, pp. 35–35). Washington, DC: American Fisheries Society.

Wistar, Jr., R., & Hildemann, W. H. (1960). Effects of stress on skin transplantation immunity in mice. *Science, 131,* 159–160.

Workman, E. A., & LaVia, M. F. (1987). T lymphocyte polyclonal proliferation: effects of stress response style on medical students taking national board examinations. *Clinical Immunology and Immunopathology, 43,* 308–313.

Yamada, A., Jensen, M. M., & Rasmussen, A. F., Jr. (1964). Stress and susceptibility to herpes simplex in mice subjected to avoidance-learning stress or restraint. *Proceedings of the Society of Experimental Biology and Medicine, 96,* 183–189.

Zalcman, S., Minkiewicz-Janda, A., Richter, M., & Anisman, H. (1988). Critical periods associated with stressor effects on antibody titers and on the plaque-forming cell response to sheep red blood cells. *Brain, Behavior, and Immunity, 2,* 254–266.

Zalcman, S., Richter, M., & Anisman, H. (1990). Alterations of immune functioning following exposure to stressor related cues. *Brain, Behavior, and Immunity, 3,* 99–110.

3 Selected Methodological Concepts: Mediation and Moderation, Individual Differences, Aggregation Strategies, and Variability of Replicates

Arthur A. Stone
State University of New York at Stony Brook

There is little doubt that the field of psychoncuroimmunology (PNI) has made tremendous strides since the 1980s. Reports of PNI research have been frequent in topnotch journals, funding for PNI research has increased greatly, and there is a new journal devoted exclusively to the topic. Despite these achievements, many reasonable criticisms have been leveled at research conducted in this area. The identified problems include, but are not limited to, absence of the measurement of disease outcomes in studies, the meaning of immune measures and their relationship to disease processes, issues concerning the generalizability of laboratory studies, and the potential confounding of stress–immune system relationships by health-related behaviors, sleep, and so forth. My goal in this chapter is not to examine these potential problems, as that has been done in published reviews of the literature and in articles and chapters (including some in this volume) specifically addressing issues facing PNI researchers. Rather, the aim of this chapter is to describe methods of possibly improving PNI research by employing concepts from the psychological literature that may have thus far been overlooked by the field. I present this information not to criticize the field, but in the spirit of making the most of what psychology can offer PNI.

I suggest that there is much psychology has to offer to the PNI field. Already, PNI has incorporated psychological concepts such as stress, moderators of the stress response (such as social supports or loneliness), and ways of measuring mental health, but these are only a few of the potential contributions that psychology can make to the field. In this chapter I focus on four concepts from psychology that may be revelant for the PNI field: mediation and moderation of immune effects, individual differences in response to stress, aggregation strategies for improving reliability of immune measures, and variability in replicate assays. To illustrate the potential impact of the concepts, data are presented from several of my own studies exploring stress-immune reactions both in field and in controlled laboratory settings. The data presented are not intended to confirm or refute previous findings in the area; rather, they are meant to serve as a vehicle for explicating the concepts.

MEDIATION AND MODERATION

The first concept concerns how we conceptualize the relationships among the variables studied in PNI experiments. In the causal chain that leads to disease onset, there are usually several variables that are hypothesized to affect disease onset. For example, we may hypothesize that negative life events produce a change in immune function and that, in turn, leads to an increased susceptibility to disease. This linear model is a simplistic description of the process. However, for both practical reasons such as funding levels and for technical reasons such as the inability to measure what we would like, it may be as complex a model as we are likely to investigate. For explanatory purposes, an additional factor, gender, is also included in the model and we hypothesize that life events have a different impact on illness susceptibility for males than for females.

The task of understanding the influence of gender, life events, and immune function on disease susceptibility boils down to assessing statistical moderation and mediation. There has been considerable confusion about this issue in the field of psychology where the terms have often been interchanged and, perhaps more serious than simple linguistic confusion, often moderation and mediation have not been properly assessed. Several articles have brought this to the attention of psychologists recently, such as one by Baron and Kenny (1986) in the *Journal of Personality and Social Psychology.*

Despite the discussion of these concepts in recent literature, PNI investigations have not been attentive to the appropriate methods of analyzing mediation and moderation. A basic theoretical question for PNI is that of mediation. Generically, mediation occurs when the effect of a predictor on an outcome measure is the result of the predictor variable influencing a third variable that, in turn, affects the outcome. In other words, the effect of a predictor on outcome is not direct, but is mediated by the third variable. A typical question for PNI is: Does stress (predictor) affect the immune system (third variable) and do these changes then impact on health (outcome)? More often than not, PNI studies evaluate the relationships among stress, immune function, and disease with univariate correlations or with analysis of variance schemes and show, for example, that a group experiencing an experimental stressor has a change in immune function and a change in susceptibility to disease. In contrast, a nonstressed control group shows a stable pattern of results: Immune function remains at baseline levels as does susceptibility to disease. This is usually the extent of the analyses seen in the PNI literature, and authors of these studies conclude that immune function is mediating the link between stress and susceptibility to disease.

But has immunological mediation of the stress–disease link been demonstrated by these analyses? Closer inspection suggests it has not. Although immune change has *covaried* with stressor status in the expected direction, the notion that the immunological change is epiphenomological cannot be ruled out. Immune function may have been influenced by another variable that has gone unmeasured or the impact of stress on illness may be independent of the effect of stress on the immune system.

Statistical techniques involving regression modeling are available for evaluating the mediator status of immune function in this instance (see Fig. 3.1). Briefly, regression equations are estimated with stress predicting immune function (Model A), stress predicting disease (Model B), and, finally, stress and immune function predicting disease (Model C). To receive the designation of mediator, the following conditions must be met: Stress must be significantly related to immune function; stress must be significantly related to disease; and there must be a reduction in the magnitude of the regression coefficient of the stress variable in the last equation (Model C) relative to the value of the coefficient in the first equation.

A complete reduction of the magnitude of the stress regression coefficient

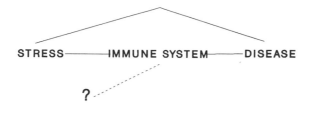

STRESS————IMMUNE SYSTEM————DISEASE

?

Regressions	Mediator Status
(A) Stress--› Immune	1. (A) significant
(B) Stress--› Disease	2. (B) significant
(C) Stress + Immune--› Disease	3. Decrease in Stress regression coefficient in (C) relative to (A)

FIG. 3.1. Summary of method for testing mediational effects among three variables.

indicates a unitary mediator: wonderful, but highly unlikely in these undoubtedly multiple cause systems. A substantial reduction of the stress regression coefficient indicates that disease is partially mediated by immune function, an outcome that we may reasonably hope to achieve. Finally, no change in the coefficient indicates a third variable explanation of the relationship of stress and health. This last outcome is important because it suggests that we search for that more potent, "unknown" variable (indicated by a "?" in the figure). I think that we must use these or other stringent tests in evaluating our mediational hypotheses. Clearly, bivariate correlational analyses do not allow for the evaluation of three or more variables, a condition that is required to properly evaluate mediation.

What are the implications of not thoroughly assessing mediation with appropriate statistical models? The ANOVA models mentioned earlier do indicate that an association exists between immune function and health, yet do not indicate that immune function is a causal link, as hypothesized, in the stress–immune–health nexus. Thus, inaccurate conclusions may be drawn about the role of immune function when the regression modeling described here is not used.

Moderation is conceptually distinct from mediation. When a variable influences the relationship between two other variables, moderation is occurring. In the PNI example described earlier, if gender influences the relationship between stress and health, it would then be considered a moderator variable. Moderators are in many ways easier to assess than mediators: They are often, but not always, stable characteristics of subjects such as the demographic attributes, income, or living conditions, or they may be personality characteristics such as locus of control or Type A behavior. Statistically, moderator effects are assessed in regression or ANOVA models by the interaction effect of the potential moderator (gender) and the predictor variable (stress) on the outcome (health). A significant interaction effect indicates moderation.

Perhaps it is in some sense flashier to focus solely on mediators, because they address more central hypothesized linkages. This might be true, if it were not for the fact that there is conceptual interplay between moderators and mediators. Moderators can inform us of the potential existence of mediator variables. In the case of gender, why might the relationship between stress and health be different for males and females? We know that the genders differ in many important ways including levels of circulating hormones (e.g., Collins & Frankenhauser, 1978; Frankenhauser, 1975). Perhaps these hormonal differences are mediating the stress–health relationship. A logical step in the research program would be to design a study exploring the effects of an experimental stressor and covarying levels of, for instance, testosterone using both a between- and a within-group design. The relative ease with which moderators may be assessed suggests that a search for variables acting in this capacity is a reasonable, cost-effective approach in a search for potent mediators (Baron & Kenny, 1986).

INDIVIDUAL DIFFERENCES

The second methodological issue explores a particular kind of mediational variable, individual differences, and may suggest alternate ways of testing PNI hypotheses. We know that all people do not respond in exactly the same manner to stressful stimuli: Some people report more subjective distress than others, some people become more cardiovascularly aroused than others, and some secrete more epinephrine than others (e.g., Glass, Lake, Contrada, Kehoe, & Erlanger, 1983). These individual differences in response to a stressor may be a major aid in understanding PNI processes. Although nomothethic views of the effects of stressors may provide a first glimpse of the underlying psychological state of affairs, they are unlikely to provide a very deep understanding of these processes. Conversely, individual differences may allow us to test hypotheses in a correlational fashion utilizing specific groups of individuals who naturally vary in characteristics related to the hypotheses.

Analyses reported in the PNI literature are usually at the nomothetic level in both study design and analytic methods. Typically, subjects are exposed to some experimental stressor or subjects' reactions to a stressful situation are monitored, and conclusions are advanced that an immune process either was or was not affected by the stressor. It is rare in PNI research to predict variability in the immunological outcomes, using either subjective responses to the stressor, physiological responses to the stressor, or other psychosocial or physiological qualities of the individual. Exploration of individual differences is, however, more common in studies of naturally occurring stressors (see Jemmott & Locke, 1984).

Are individual differences approaches relevant for PNI researchers? Given their importance for psychological research in general, it is likely that they are of considerable importance in PNI research. An example with data from my own lab demonstrates how this kind of approach can influence our interpretation of a fairly typical PNI finding. We recently conducted a study with 36 undergraduates at State University of New York at Stony Brook (Valdimarsdottir, Stone, Neale, & Cox, in preparation). All subjects were seen several times during a 3-week period prior to the day stressors were administered. A blood sample was drawn 2 days before the stress session to assess baseline immunological levels.

The stress session proceeded as follows: Subjects came to the lab individually and were allowed to relax for 15 minutes. During this time blood pressure and heart rate were measured, and these measures continued to be taken at intervals throughout the subsequent 2 hours. Subjective reports of tension and distress were also obtained. Electrodes were placed on subjects arms, and subjects were told that a painful shock would accompany poor performance in the upcoming tasks. The Stroop color word task was then administered for 15 minutes (a word that describes a color is projected on a screen, yet the word printed in another color, while the subject hears yet another color spoken over headphones; the task is to name the actual color of the word), then 15 minutes of mental arithmetic (counting backward by 13s), and, finally, another 15 minutes of the Stroop task. At preselected times the experimenter provided feedback that the subject was performing poorly and was in jeopardy of being shocked. Blood was drawn immediately after, 30 minutes after, and 60 minutes after the stress exposure concluded.

Reactions to the stressor include heightened tension, heart rate, and blood pressure as shown in Fig. 3.2. The two immune measures explored in this study, lymphocyte proliferation to the mitogen, Concanvalin A (Con A), and functional IL-2 produced to the Con A stimulation are shown in Fig. 3.3. A rebound effect for lymphocyte stimulation is quite clear; a similar result has recently been reported by another research team using a similar experimental task (Weisse, Pato, McAllister, & Paul, 1989). However, the point is not the actual pattern of the result or its relationship to previous findings. Rather, the point is that it is tempting to conclude that subjective and cardiovascular responses to the stressor, which are clearly associated with the stressor, are responsible for the immune changes. However, this finding is only implied by the pattern of results and has not specifically been tested.

One method of testing the association of the psychophysiological mea-

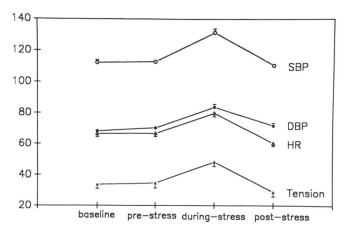

FIG. 3.2.   Reactions to psychological stress: subjective tension (Tension), blood pressure (systolic [SPB] and diastolic [DBP]), and heart rate (HR) at baseline, prestress, during-stress, and poststress.

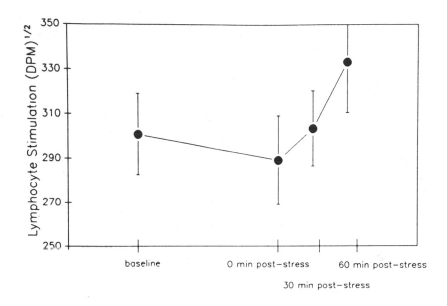

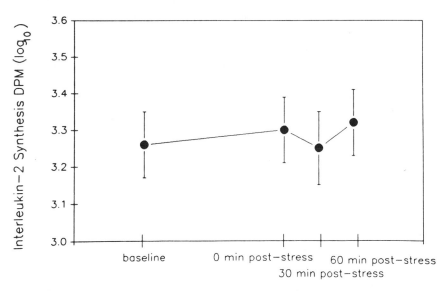

FIG. 3.3.   Reactions to psychological stress: Immune functioning at baseline and at three periods poststress (0, 30, and 60 minutes).

sures change and immune change is by making use of the variability of psychophysiological reactivity to the stressors. As indicated by the standard deviations in the figure, subjects responded with considerable diversity to the stressors. If these individual differences are affecting immune responsivity, we would expect little immune change for those subjects who were relatively nonreactive (say, cardiovascularily), and relatively larger changes for those who are more reactive.

Analyses presented in Fig. 3.4 explored this hypothesis. Subjects were divided into reactive and nonreactive groups based on subjective tension and systolic blood pressure changes in response to the stressor, and the resulting immune patterns were plotted. Expectations were not borne out: There is little difference in the pattern of immune response of the groups created by scores on the individual differences analyses. These analyses suggest that blood pressure and subjective tension are not responsible for the observed immune changes. (An alternative, and probably preferable, method of exploring these questions is with the regression strategy described in the previous section for assessing mediation. For the sake of explication, subgroups of the data were compared, instead.)

When we are forced into a situation in which we can only run a single group and no control group (and there are many examples of this in the PNI literature), I suggest that we attempt to disect our findings by subdividing on variables that we presume have been important in the causal chain leading to the observed immune response or by including these variables in the appropriate regression models (as described in the previous section of the chapter). For example, in a natural observation study that followed the course of a traumatic event that produced, on average, a large increase in negative affect followed by an immune decrement, exploring individual differences in mood reactivity could buttress a conclusion that negative mood was related to the immune change. On the other hand, we may be surprised by findings that presumed individual differences in factors expected to relate to the outcome are not related, leading us to reconsider some of our theories about the processes studied.

AGGREGATION

The third methodological issue I discuss is part of a field that has been of considerable interest to psychologists for many years — psychometrics. Psychometrics concerns the study of the measurement properties of the concepts we quantify in our studies, ranging from formal, standardized questionnaires such as the MMPI to the measurement of global behavior such as children's on-task behavior. There is little question that various psychometric concepts pertaining to reliability and validity are very important in the conduct and interpretation of psychological research and to biomedical research in general.

There is a relative absence of psychometric procedures in the PNI field, but they could be extremely useful. I refer here not so much to the

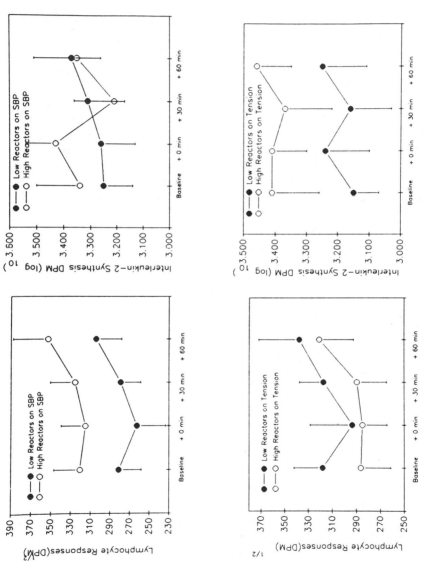

FIG. 3.4. Immune response (Lymphocyte Proliferation and Interleukin-2) for low and high reactivity groups as defined by systolic blood pressure (Panels A & B) and by subjective tension (Panels C & D).

63

psychological variables (e.g., stress, affect, personality, etc.), which often have published validity and reliability statistics available in the literature, but to the immunological measures themselves. Several reviews of PNI have discussed the unreliability of immunological measures (Hall, 1985); perhaps this is because the original assays were not designed for quantitative research, but rather for clinical purposes where minor fluctuations in the assay are acceptable.

Very little information is available on the reliability of many of the immune assays. For example, we know little about temporal stability. Some PNI studies are essentially one group designs and assume high temporal stability in the immune measures studied. Often such technically flawed designs are unavoidable for practical reasons, yet no evidence is presented for the critical, unstated assumption that the immune measures studied would not have changed in magnitude had no intervention occurred. For this reason, it is useful to have information about the various levels of reliability of immune measures. Unfortunately, much of this information simply is not currently available, and, perhaps somewhat pessimistically, it is likely that most immune measures are less reliable than we think. Apart from improving the technical aspects of the assay, which may be contributing error to the measure, what can be done to improve reliability?

There is one approach to the problem that emerged out of a controversy that raged in the psychological journals a decade ago. The controversy concerned the ability of traits, or relatively stable personality structures, to predict behavior, broadly defined as cognition, physiological states, and observable actions. Personality could predict behavior, but not very well: Correlations between traits and behaviors rarely exceeded .3 or 9% of the outcome's variance.

In the late 1970s, Seymour Epstein (1979) wrote a series of papers that attempted to support the validity of traits by advancing an argument concerning the reliability of the behaviors that were serving as outcome measures. To summarize his position: Epstein stated that single-point measurement of behavior is relatively unreliable and this unreliability is the limiting factor for traits predicting behavior. Concerning behavior observed in a laboratory in particular, Epstein stated: "Given the esteem in which laboratory experimental procedures have been held, who would have dared to think that they often fail to meet one of the most fundamental scientific tests of all, temporal reliability?" (p. 1121). As mentioned earlier, there has been relatively little work concerning the reliability of immunological assays, and I suspect that Epstein's comments apply to PNI measures.

The solution to the unreliability issues was extraordinarily simple and founded on basic statistical concepts: To increase reliability, increase the number of observations used to compute dependent variable scores. Whereas a single measurement has a certain component of error inherent in the score, the mean of two measurements will have relatively less error because the error in each measurement will, on average, cancel out. As the number of observations increase, error contributes proportionately less to the variance of the mean.

A summary of a portion of Epstein's results is presented in Fig. 3.5 to demonstrate what may be achieved with this method. The data are the observations subjects made on 30 or so consecutive days. The ordinate presents the number of observations making up the dependent measure, for example, 3 indicates that three daily observations were averaged (say, Days 1, 3, and 5) and correlated with another average of 3 different days (say Days 2, 4, 6), which is an odd–even test–retest reliability. Increasing the number of observations dramatically increases the reliability of the measure. Note that the reliability of a single observation varies by the content of the variable: Emotions are the most reliable, whereas situations are least reliable. Also note that the curves are asymptotic: After 9 or 10 observations are averaged, little additional increment in reliability is gained. Epstein found that trait–behavior validity correlations all increased, and some dramatically, with the aggregation procedure. That is, personality measures now predicted behavior beyond the .30 threshold.

Aggregation techniques can readily be applied to PNI research in several ways. In research examining how various demographic factors such as age, gender, or marital status relate to immune function, obtaining several immune measures on different occasions and averaging them into a single measure should yield higher correlations because reliability has been improved. In process-oriented research, increased reliability may be obtained in the same manner. For example, a researcher could obtain and average several immune assays obtained during a single day for several days, creating a more reliable daily variable. Obviously, the drawback to

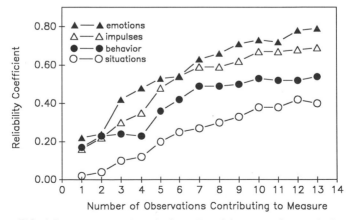

FIG. 3.5.   Summary of results from Epstein's aggregation method.

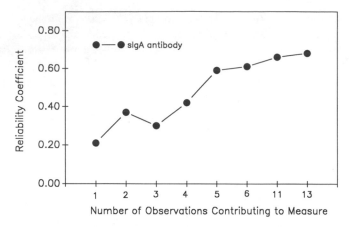

FIG. 3.6.   Aggregation of sIgA antibody over several days.

this method is effort and expense: Multiple assays can be quite expensive and difficult to obtain even if resources allow for them.

I demonstrate this procedure with longitudinal data from a sample of dental students obtained several years ago. Thirty students had saliva drawn from their parotid gland three times weekly for 8 ⅓ weeks (see Stone, Cox, Valdimarsdottir, Jardorf, & Neale, 1987). Subjects ingested rabbit albumin daily during this period, which enabled us to explore secretory IgA antibody response to the albumin with ELISA and RID assays. Figure 3.6 is organized in the same manner as the previous figure. Reliability for antibody on a single occasion was dismal: .2. However, a reliability coefficient of above .6 was achieved by averaging five observations — certainly a substantial gain. With 13 observations, a maximal reliability of .7 was achieved. The decision to obtain additional observations to maximize reliability is aided by the figure: At some point it is simply too expensive to obtain additional data for the increment in reliability.

Thus, I suggest that, when possible, we assess the reliability of the immune measures we employ and, if needed, perhaps improve reliability by this aggregation procedure.

REPLICATE ANALYSES OF ASSAY RESULTS

The last issue to be discussed in this chapter concerns another technique for improving reliability of immunological measures that has recently been explored by my research group at Stony Brook (Stone, Schwartz, Valdimarsdottir, Napoli, Neale, & Cox, 1990). Generally, immune assays such as lymphocyte proliferation, NK, and so forth, are performed in duplicate, triplicate, or quadruplicate in order to help reduce the error inherent in running assays. By averaging the replicate assays from a single sample, error is reduced much in the same manner as averaging across occasions to obtain improved reliability as in Epstein's work. A review of the PNI literature where lymphocyte proliferation with mitogens was used as a dependent measure indicated that all of the studies averaged or took the median of the duplicate or triplicate assays that were performed. Somewhat surprisingly, in no study were any samples discarded or rerun on the basis of the replicate information.

At first glance, the averaging of replicates appears perfectly consistent with the aggregation approach just described, and in some ways it is. However, with extreme outliers, as may be found in abberant assay replicates, and with Ns of three or four replicates, the averaging procedure may be problematic, because the possibility that a replicate is an outlier is not evaluated. Moreover, there is information available with the replicate sets for improving assay reliability that might, for instance, suggest rejecting the sample or discarding a replicate assay. For example, there are patterns of results that would make it difficult to believe that an average properly represented the central tendency of the sample. Take the case where four replicates have been run and two values are relatively high, whereas the remaining two values are relatively low. Which is correct and is the mean a reasonable estimate of the sample value? This is probably a case where rerunning the assay is appropriate.

Another example of a pattern of replicates that might be considered questionable is the case where they are spread quite far apart, that is, they have a large standard deviation. Although the average of the three replicates may represent central tendency, just how much variability in the assays are we willing to accept? At some point rejection of the set of replicates may be wise. Alternatives include rerunning the assays or simply entering a missing code into our analysis. Another characteristic of replicates is that duplicate samples carry relatively little information about outliers because their within-sample variability is based on only two measurements. They can indicate a problematic situation, however, when the absolute distance between the two points is very large. In such cases, the researcher should consider rerunning the assays.

The points just mentioned suggest that some sort of rules for taking a closer look at replicate data are in order to make the most of the information contained in the replicates and for standardizing treatment of replicates. Rather than simply "eyeballing" the data and using arbitrary and probably inconsistent decision rules for excluding data points, I discuss a very simple rule that we created and illustrate the effect that application of the rule has on a sample of data. The rule is this: For each sample, compute the median from whatever number of replicates you have, and then create a "window of acceptance" around that median, much as you would create a confidence interval around a mean. The size of the window is based on generally agreed upon standards for defining outliers (Tukey, 1977), although the exact size should be influenced by the degree of reliability you feel is achievable with the assay or perhaps by some absolute standard that is felt to define the minimally acceptable variability. Next, reject any samples that fall outside of this window and take the average of the remaining samples. The value resulting from this process serves as the dependent variable.

The rule is illustrated in Fig. 3.7. Outliers (circled in the figure) are eliminated and only "good" or within-the-window values contribute to the average. It is possible that none of the replicate values will be retained, that is, that they all fall outside the window and the sample is rejected as too variable. The case of four replicates of which two are high and two are low probably will also be rejected as being too variable. Thus, the rule handles many of the issues just mentioned.

A more sophisticated rule may also be employed that acknowledges that the variability around a given point is likely to increase as the magnitude of the point increases and, hence, the window of acceptance should perhaps be narrower below the median than above the median so as not to reject too many large magnitude values. Complex rules taking this into account by predicting the expected variability can also be created, and we have explored these as well as the simple rule (Stone et al., 1991). The results from the simple and complex rules were comparable and are not presented here.

The study that I use to exemplify the replicate exclusionary rule employed the medical student exam paradigm: A group of 15 students gave blood samples several weeks prior to an examination period and then again during the examinations. Lymphocyte proliferation to Con A was the dependent

Replicate Analyses

Single Sample in Quadruplicate	"Ideal" Result
Case I: 130 140 160 170	Take Average
Case II: 50 140 160 250	Reject extremes
Case III: 50 140 150 170	Reject outlier
Case IV: 50 60 200 210	Reject entire sample

Compute the Median of the Replicates
Create a "window" of X% around that average
Reject replicates beyond outside of the window
Compute the average of remaining replicates

FIG. 3.7.   Summary of replicates exclusionary rule.

measure used in the study, and the assays were run at one point in time in quadruplicate. Figure 3.8 presents the data for both prestress and stress periods. The first row of the table is the mean of the replicates and we see that lymphocyte stimulation declined during the exams. A measure of central tendency that is less sensitive to outlying values is the median and the mean of the replicate medians is similar to the mean of the replicate means at both time points.

Stimulated and unstimulated assays were run yielding two sets of four replicates for each sample. An exclusionary rule specifying a window of 50% of the mean was applied. This is rather liberal rule that we expected would not affect a large proportion of the data. It yielded the following results: 27% of the 30 samples at Time 1 had at least one of the four replicates rejected. At Time 2, 47% had at least one replicate rejected, but more significantly, one entire sample was eliminated by the procedure. On examination, the mean of one sample was quite low relative to the other samples, yet the exclusionary rule did not use this information about level; rather, it used the within-sample variability as described earlier.

The last row of the figure presents the results of the 14 subjects who remained in the analysis after the application of the rule. We see that there is no longer a substantial decline in the measure of lymphocyte stimulation, a surprising finding indeed. We had expected that the reliability of the samples would be influenced by the procedure such that within-sample standard deviations would decrease, which they indeed did. We did not expect that the magnitudes of immune response would be affected by the exclusionary rule.

The analyses presented were solely for the purpose of exposition and no statistical analyses were computed on the effects. My point here is not to

Mean, Median, and Mean of Replicates
After the Exclusionary Rule at Both Time Points

	Time 1	Time 2
Mean of the Replicate Means	69,826	63,101
Mean of Replicate Medians	71,231	64,158
Mean of All Replicates After Rule is Applied *	70,955	68,565

N=15. * N=14, 1 sample eliminated

FIG. 3.8.   Data from lymphocyte proliferation study with and without the use of replicates rule.

support or refute the effect of exam stress on lymphocyte stimulation. Rather, I wish to emphasize the potential usefulness of the information contained in replicate assays. Certainly the application of the exclusionary rule described here, or of other similar rules, has the potential not only to increase reliability of the immune measures, but also to impact on the levels of immune responsiveness.

CONCLUSION

The concepts presented here are quite familiar to scientists working in psychology and they have proved to be useful for testing hypotheses in those fields. Psychoneuroimmunology is both a new and interdisciplinary field that combines conceptual and methodological concepts from the many of the disciplines contributing to the area. The purpose of this chapter was to highlight four concepts, mediation versus moderation, individual differences, aggregation, and replicates, that have been important to psychology and to suggest that they may have a place in PNI research.

ACKNOWLEDGMENTS

The author thanks Heiddis Valdimarsdottir, Eileen Kennedy-Moore, Anthony Napoli, and Joseph Schwartz for their helpful comments on an earlier draft.

This research was supported, in part, by grant MH39234 from the National Institutes for Mental Health.

REFERENCES

Baron, R. M., & Kenny, D. A. (1986). The moderator–mediator variable distinction is social psychological research: Conceptual, strategic, and statistical considerations. *Journal of Personality and Social Psychology, 51,* 1173–1182.

Collins, A., & Frankenhauser, M. (1978). Stress response in male and female engineering students. *Journal of Human Stress, 4,* 43–48.

Epstein, S. (1979). The stability of behavior: I. On predicting most of the people much of the time. *Journal of Personality and Social Psychology, 7,* 1097–1126.

Frankenhauser, M. (1975). Experimental approaches to the study of catecholamine and emotions. In L. Levi (Ed.), *Emotions: Their parameters and measurement* (pp. 209–234) New York: Raven Press.

Glass, D. C., Lake, C. R., Contrada, R. J., Kehoe, K., & Erlanger, L. R. (1983). Stability of individual differences in psychological responses to stress. *Health Psychology, 2,* 317–341.

Hall, J. G. (1985). Emotions and immunity. *Lancet, 2,* 326–327.

Jemmott, J. B., III., & Locke, S. F. (1984). Psychological Factors, Immunologic Mediation, and Human Susceptibility to Infectious Diseases: How much do we know. *Psychological Bulletin, 1,* 78–108.

Stone, A. A., Cox, D., Valdimarsdottir, H., Jandorf, L., & Neale, J. M. (1987). Evidence that secretory IgA is associated with daily mood. *Journal of Personality and Social Psychology, 5,* 988–993.

Stone, A. A., Schwartz, J. E., Valdimarsdottir, H. B., Napoli, A., Neale, J. M., & Cox, D. S. (1991). Treatment of replicate sample data in psychoimmunology studies. *Journal of Immunological Methods, 136*(1) 111–117.

Tukey, J. W. (1977) *Exploratory data analysis.* Reading, MA: Addison-Wesley.

Valdimarsdottir, H. B., Stone, A. A., Neale, J. M., & Cox, D. S. (in preparation). *The effects of experimental stressors on the immune system.* New York: SUNY at Stonybrook.

Weisse, C., Pato, C. N., McAllister, C., & Paul, S. M. (1989, August). *Differential effects of controllable and uncontrollable acute stress on immune function in humans.* Symposium at the annual meeting of the American Psychological Association, New Orleans, LA.

Corticotropin-Releasing Factor and Catecholamines: A Study on Their Role In Stress-Induced Immunomodulation

4

Frank Berkenbosch
Free University, Amsterdam, Holland

Recently, there has been a growing body of interest in the interaction between stress, psychosocial factors, behavior, and the immune system. A major premise underlying this relationship is that stressors may increase vulnerability to certain diseases intimately connected with immunologic mechanisms such as infection, malignancy, and autoimmune disorders. However, as yet, no conclusive studies have been undertaken to prove the existence of this relationship. In fact, although many observations have been published demonstrating the immunosuppressive effect of chronic laboratory stressors in mammals (e.g., Keller, Weiss, Schleifer, Miller, & Stein, 1981, 1983), no detailed findings have been delineated to examine the relationship between immune parameters and the intensity, quality, and duration of stress. Moreover, although many in vitro studies have shown immunoregulatory potencies of stress-labile substances from neural and endocrine origin (e.g., Chang, 1984; Coffy & Hadden, 1985; Johnson, Smith, Torres, & Blalock, 1982), little evidence has been presented demonstrating the role of such substances in stress-induced changes in immunity in vivo. In this chapter, we review our studies on effects of acute stress on secretion of propiomelanocortin (POMC)-derived peptides from the pituitary gland and of catecholamines from the sympatho-adrenomedullary system. Moreover, we show that acute emotional stressors can enhance cellular and humoral immune responses and that neuroendocrine mechanisms are involved in these responses. In fact, our data favor the view that peptides derived from POMC, the production and release of which is controlled by hypothalamic corticotropin-releasing factor (CRF), may mediate enhanced immune response in acutely stressed animals.

PRO-OPIOMELANOCORTIN-DERIVED PEPTIDES

The pituitary gland of most species contains two cell types designated as corticotrophs of the anterior lobe and melanotrophs of the intermediate lobe (intermediate zone in man) that both synthesize a precursor protein called pro-opiomelanocortin (POMC). In both cell types, POMC precursor is processed by enzymes resulting in glycosylation and/or phosphorylation, cleavage, formation of aminated and acetylated peptides (Eipper & Mains, 1980; Hope & Lowry, 1981). Although both melanotrophs and corticotrophs synthesize POMC, the major POMC-derived peptides produced by these cells are different. Thus, cell-specific differences in the enzymatic machinery appear to be involved in processing of POMC. The final products of POMC processing are indicated in Fig. 4.1.

Although the highest concentrations of POMC-derived peptides exist in the pituitary gland, considerable amounts are also found in the brain, gastrointestinal tract, testis, female reproductive tract, thyroid, placenta (see for review O'Donohue & Dorsa, 1982) and in lymphoid tissue (Blalock & Smith, 1985; Kavelaars, Berkenbosch, Croiset, Ballieux, & Heijnen, 1990; Smith, Morrill, Meyer, & Blalock, 1986). Details about the processing of POMC precursor in most of these tissue has been reviewed elsewhere (O'Donohue & Dorsa, 1982).

The diversity of distribution of POMC-derived peptides may be indica-

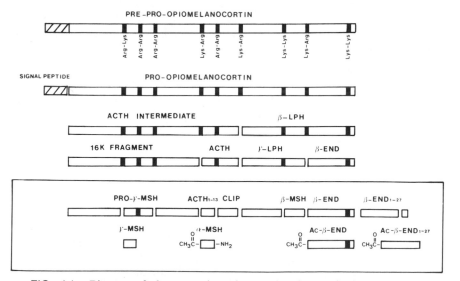

FIG. 4.1. Diagram of the processing of pro-opiomelanocortin in the pituitary gland. Pairs of basic aminoacids are indicated by black blocks. In the rectangle bottom: cleavages and modifications that occur in the melanotrophs of the intermediate lobe but not in the corticotrophs of the anterior lobe. Ac = acetate; NH2 = amide.

tive for a broad range of different biological activities. However, besides the clear biological function of ACTH being its capacity to regulate the synthesis and release of adrenal glucocorticoids, no undisputed biological functions of the other POMC-derived peptides have been described (for review see O'Donohue & Dorsa, 1982). For instance, the melanocyte-stimulating properties of MSH are important in reptiles and amphibians, but are obscure in higher vertebrates. Beta-endorphin exhibits clearly potent opiate activity when injected into the brain, but such function cannot be described for the circulating beta-endorphin forms. Therefore, the question arises: "Do the different POMC-derived peptides have a clear biological function at every site where they are produced or should the wide tissue distribution be considered as part of evolutionary abundance"?

CATECHOLAMINES

Circulating catecholamines originate from the sympatho-adrenomedullary system. The sympathetic part of this system is composed primarily of norepinephrine containing neurons with cell bodies located in sympathetic ganglia and paravertebral ganglia and projections to various peripheral organs. Evidence is presented that sympathetic control of innervated tissues is to a large extend mediated by nonsynaptic neurotransmission (Schipper & Tilders, 1982). Therefore, norepinephrine released from sympathetic nerves may enter a large extracellular compartment from which it easily penetrates the general circulation. Thus, by this nonsynaptic pathway, neuronal norepinephrine may exert control over organs that are not or only poorly innervated.

The chromaffin cells of the adrenal medulla is considered to be the endocrine part of the sympatho-adrenomedullary system. Immunocytochemical evidence have indicated that the adrenal medulla contains two cells that produce norepinephrine or epinephrine respectively (Verhofstad et al., 1983). No studies are available indicating that the release of catecholamines from these cells is under differential control.

SECRETION OF POMC-DERIVED HORMONES AND CATECHOLAMINES DURING ACUTE STRESS

Experimental procedures such as handling, transport, or injections cannot easily be avoided when rats are exposed to conventional laboratory stressors such as restraint, electric footshocks, psychosocial interactions, and others. These manipulations by themselves can activate the neuroendocrine systems, thereby complicating the interpretation of the neuroendocrine response to the actual stressor. It appears that the novelty or unpredictability of the experimental manipulation forms the major clue for this response because repeated exposure can lead to full extinction of the endocrine reaction. For instance, rats subjected for 3 consecutive days, twice daily to procedures that consist of opening the cage, handling, and intraperitoneal injection show full habituation as indicated by low corticosterone and ACTH plasma levels (Berkenbosch, Tilders, & Vermes, 1983; Berkenbosch, Vermes, & Tilders, 1984).

It is generally accepted that the classical neuroendocrine response to a stimulus associated with a real expected damage or life-threatening situation consists of a rapid release of ACTH from the corticotrophs of the anterior pituitary gland. However, over the years, our studies have demonstrated that a variety of stressors additionally induces instantaneous secretion of POMC-derived peptides from the melanotrophs of the intermediate lobe (Berkenbosch et al., 1983; Berkenbosch et al., 1984). Such stimuli, resulting in a threefold to tenfold increase in circulating ACTH as well as MSH end endorphin concentrations are for instance mild electric footshocks or physical restraint during 2–5 minutes. By inference, stimuli such as laparotomy or formalin injection under pentobarbital anesthesia hardly stimulate POMC-peptide secretion from the intermediate lobe. As a consequence, the source of endorphin and related peptides in the circulation during stress is dependent on the nature of the stressor. These findings are in line with an old and classical division of stress stimuli into emotional or neurogenic stressors (restraint, electric footshocks) and somatic or systemic stimuli (laparotomy, formalin injection; Fortier, 1966). The data strongly indicate that a intrinsic relationship exists between emotional stimuli and secretion of POMC-derived peptides from the intermediate lobe. The intermediary role of the sympathetic nervous system in this response is discussed later.

That emotions elicit secretion of epinephrine from the adrenal medulla was recognized as early as 1911 (Cannon & De La Paz, 1911). Over the years, evidence has accumulated that a variety of exogenous stimuli and/or learned emotional reactions lead to a rapid and concerted activation of the sympathetic nervous system and chromaffin cells of the adrenal medulla. Consequently, circulating levels of norepinephrine and epinephrine rapidly increase following exposure of an organism to a stressor (Kvetnansky et al., 1978). Although the sympathetic nerves and adrenal medulla are simultaneously activated during stress, the contribution to circulating catecholamines responses may vary and appear to be dependent on the nature and duration of the stressor (McCarthy & Kopin, 1979). Moreover, the ratio of circulating norepinephrine/epinephrine appear to correlate with coping behavior. For instance, Henry (1980) presented evidence that high norepinephrine levels are associated with aggressive behavior or challenge to control, whereas loss of control is associated with relatively high epinephrine levels.

FACTORS CONTROLLING SECRETION OF POMC-DERIVED PEPTIDES DURING ACUTE STRESS

Various lines of evidence indicate that a 41-aminoacid peptide designated corticotropin-releasing factor is a prominent regulator of POMC secretion from the pituitary gland (for reviews see Makara, Antoni, Stark, & Karteszi, 1984; Tilders, Berkenbosch, & Smelik, 1985;). After the isolation and characterization of CRF by Vale, Spiess, Rivier, and Rivier (1981), synthetic peptides became available and antibodies have been raised to visualize and quantitate CRF. At least four systems have been described in the rat brain as reviewed elsewhere (Tilders, Berkenbosch, Vermes, Linton, & Smelek, 1986). The system controlling POMC secretion from the pituitary gland, called the paraventricular-infundibular system consists of approximately 2,000 cells located in the parvocellular part of the hypothalamic paraventricular nucleus projecting predominantly to the external zone of the median eminence. On their route, most fibers pass the retrochiasmatic area, which has been shown earlier to be essential for stress-induced secretion of POMC-derived peptides (Makara et al., 1984; Tilders et al., 1986). The paraventricular-infundibular system is clearly involved in controlling secretion of POMC-derived peptides because adrenalectomy, hypophysectomy, and glucocorticoid treatments have clear effects on the activity of this system (Berkenbosch & Tilders, 1988; Schipper et al., 1984). In vitro data have provided evidence that CRF may control POMC secretion of the corticotrophs and of the melanotrophs (Tilders, Tatemoto, & Berkenbosch, 1984; Vale et al., 1983). However, approximately 100–1,000 times higher concentrations of CRF are necessary to cause release POMC-derived peptides from the melanotrophs. At date, the best procedures to show that CRF plays a physiological role in stress-induced secretion of pituitary hormones are based on the use of specific polyclonal or monoclonal antibodies to CRF. These studies have shown that CRF is indispensable for ACTH release during restraint stress (see also Fig. 4.4), formalin stress, ether stress, and infusion of epinephrine and after administration of the cytokine interleukin-1 (Linton et al., 1985; Oers, Tilders, & Berkenbosch, 1989; Berkenbosch, Van Oers, Del Rey, Tilders, Besedovsky, 1907; Tilders et al., 1985). In addition, CRF appears to drive the high resting ACTH levels found in adrenalectomized rats (Berkenbosch & Tilders, 1988; Rivier, Rivier, & Vale, 1982). In contrast, antisera to CRF do not neutralize peak MSH levels in response to restraint stress (e.g., Fig.

4.4). These observations led us to conclude that CRF does not play a physiological role in the acute response of the intermediate lobe to stress.

CRF administration into the brain has been shown to activate the sympatho-adrenomedullary system and to elicit a number of behavioral reactions that also occur during stress (for review see Vale et al., 1983). The observation that alpha-helical CRF9-41, a CRF analog with CRF antagonistic properties, when administered in the brain, can suppress stress-induced behavioral and physiological responses (Brown, Fisher, Webb, Vale, & Rivier, 1985) has led to the hypothesis that brain CRF systems play a central role in the coordination of the response to stress.

As pointed out earlier, a special relationship exists between emotional stress and reflex activation of the melanotrophs of the intermediate lobe. Emotional stressors such as restraint stress activate the sympatho-adrenomedullary system and lead to a rapid increase in circulating catecholamines (Kvetnansky et al., 1978; see also Fig. 4.4). By infusion experiments of epinephrine, we have demonstrated that these circulating concentrations are sufficient to stimulate POMC-peptide secretion from the corticotrophs and melanotrophs (Berkenbosch, Vermes, Binnekade, & Tilders, 1981; Tilders, Berkenbosch, & Smelik, 1982). The action of catecholamines on POMC-secretion from the melanotrophs involves beta-adrenoceptors (Berkenbosch et al., 1981) that have been localized on the intermediate lobe and the activation of which leads to an increased peptide secretion (Cote et al., 1982). Studies with the beta-blockers propranolol and timolol led us to conclude that stress-induced secretion of POMC-derived peptides from the intermediate lobe is mediated by catecholamines (Berkenbosch et al., 1983; Berkenbosch et al., 1984). In order to study involvement of the adrenal medulla, we studied the stress-induced MSH response in rats with adrenal enucleation. The results demonstrated that the epinephrine released from the adrenal medulla directly affects POMC-hormone secretion from the melanotrophs (Kvetnansky et al., 1987). This mechanism, which we named *adrenomedullary-pituitary-axis* is schematically presented in Fig. 4.2. Some authors have suggested that the adrenomedullary axis may also be involved in stress-induced POMC secretion from the corticotrophs (Axelrod & Reisine, 1984). However, detailed observations of our group have shown that epinephrine only plays a minor role in stress-induced ACTH release (Berkenbosch et al., 1984; Kvetnansky et al., 1987).

IMMUNOMODULATORY EFFECTS OF ACUTE STRESS

In man as well as in animals, most researchers have focused their research on studying the effects of long-term stress on immune function. No systematic studies are available to delineate effects of acute and relatively

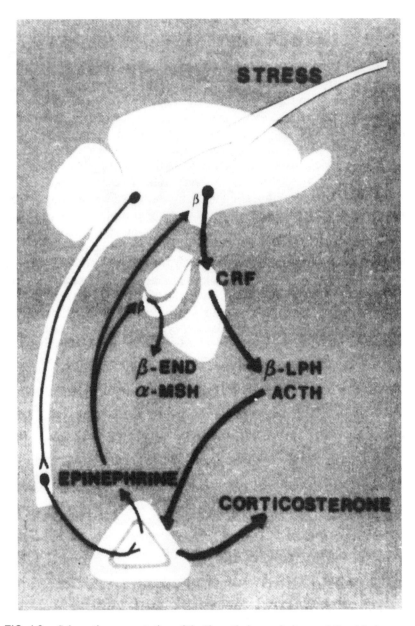

FIG. 4.2. Schematic representation of the "hypothalamo-pituitary-axis" and "adreno-medullary-pituitary axis" in stress-induced secretion of POMC-derived peptides from the pituitary gland.

mild forms of emotional stress on immune measures, although it can be anticipated that such situations reflect stress stimuli encountered in daily life. To determine whether mild acute emotional stressors can affect a cellular immune response, we studied spleen cells from stressed and unstressed Wistar rats for their capacity to proliferate in vitro in response to the specific T cell mitogen concanavalin-A (Con A). Because our rats are handled for reasons described earlier, we first studied the effects of daily handling on immune responses. However, a 4-day handling period did not significantly affect a variety of immune responses as described previously (Berkenbosch, Heijnen, Croiset, Revers, Ballieux et al., 1986). However, to our surprise, we systematically observed that handled rats subjected to restraint stress of short duration (2–5 minutes) showed enhancement of splenic T cell proliferation (e.g., Fig. 4.3). Similar results could be obtained by using electric footshock (0.5 mA, 5 second one per minute, 5 minute duration), a stressor that shows a similar pattern of hormonal activation to that of restraint stress (Berkenbosch et al., 1984). As yet, we do not know whether these changes are caused by changes in the cellular composition due to stress-induced redistribution of lymphocytes or whether they are caused by changes at the level of lymphocyte function. Preliminary experiments indicate that both phenomena may play a role in immunomodulation in response to acute stress (Miller & Berkenbosch, unpublished observations). Because mitogen-stimulation of splenic cells is primarily an in vitro T cell response, we examined in the next series of experiments, whether a 5 minute restraint stress might also affect a functional immune parameter being the number of plaque forming cells (PFC) secreting antibodies to sheep red blood cells (SRBC), primarily being a B cell response.

As with T cell proliferation, restraint stress was found to augment the number of splenic cells secreting specific antibodies to SRBC as measured at the maximum of the humoral response (Fig. 4.3, lower panel). This effect varies from a twofold to sixfold enhancement over the PFC response found in nonstressed animals and is independent of the concentration of SRBC cells administered (5×10^8 cells/ml; 5×10^9 cells/ml). Moreover, restraint stress does not alter the time course of the humoral response to SRBC (Berkenbosch, Wolvers, Derijk, 1991). Also, other immune responses are modulated by restraint stress. In preliminary experiments, we found enhanced activity of natural killer cells (NK cells) isolated from peripheral blood from rats subjected to restraint stress compared to nonstressed controls. In summary, these data show that acute stress (restraint, electric footshocks) is capable of augmenting the immune response in vitro as well as in vivo. These data can be looked upon as being on a continuum with the immunosuppressive effects of long-term and repeated stress. Recently, we studied immune responses in rats after single and repeated social confrontation. In these experiments, intruder male rats are placed in territorial cages of dominant rats, which leads to an immediate aggressive confrontation. The confrontation usually continues until defeat of the intruder. Repeated loser experience can be obtained by placing the intruder (e.g., once daily for 30 minutes) in cages of different territorial dominant males. Although the behavior of the intruder rat is changing during repeated confrontation (from active defense to passive defense), the intensity of the confrontation seems largely dependent on the aggressiveness of the territorial male. It is worth noting in this respect, that the intruder does not show endocrine habituation during repeated confrontations, indicating the inability of the intruder to actively or passively cope with this stress situation. The results of these experiments show that primary humoral responses are enhanced after a single loser experience, but are dramatically reduced after repeated loser experience. Our preliminary data indicate that mitogen-induced proliferation of T cells obtained from the spleen is similarly affected by single or repeated confrontation respectively. Moreover, the stress-induced effects on the humoral response seems the dependent on the time interval between the confrontation and the immunization. No immunoenhancing or immunosuppressive effects are found when the interval between confrontation and immunization exceeds a time period longer than 1 day. Therefore, these data suggest that (a) the direction of immunomodulatory effects of stress is determined by duration of the stressor, and (b) the ability of the stressor to influence the immune response is largely dependent on the time interval between stress and antigenic stimulation.

INVOLVEMENT OF BETA-ADRENOCEPTORS

The consecutive changes in endocrine and immunological parameters in response to acute stress suggest that both events may be casually related. Since sympathetic-adrenomedullary activation as well as release of POMC-derived peptides from the pituitary gland are critical responses to acute stress as described earlier, we were interested in investigating their role in the immuno-enhancing effects of restraint stress. In support of this notion of a sympathetic–immune interaction, immunocytochemical data have shown the presence of sympathetic nerve fibers innervating the parenchymal fields of lymphocytes in several lymphoid organs, including the spleen (Felten, Felten, Carlson, Olschowka, & Livnat, 1985). However, evidence regarding the role of the sympathetic-adrenomedullary system with respect to the immune response is still confusing (Livnat, Felten, Carlson, Bellinger, & Felten, 1985), partly due to the use of highly toxic drugs to cause sympathectomy. These drugs (e.g., 6-OHDA, guanethidine) only partially cause depletion of adrenergic stores in nerve terminals, and result in a compensatory increased catecholamine synthesis by the adrenal

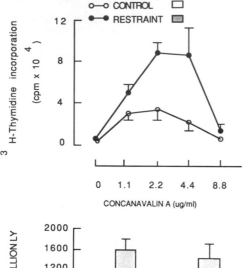

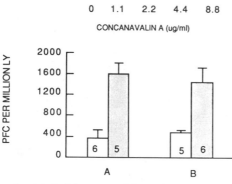

FIG. 4.3. Effect of restraint stress on the concanavalin-A (Con A) induced proliferation of splenic T cells (upper panel) and the plaque-forming response of spleen cells to immunization with sheep red blood cells (SRBC). Male Wistar rats (160 to 180 g) were housed and adapted to experimental conditions as described (Berkenbosch et al., 1984). Briefly, the animals were kept, two per cage, in a quiet room under a 12-h light, 12-h dark regimen in which the light period was from 7 a.m. to 7 p.m. Food and water were available ad libitum. To adapt the rats to handling procedures, they were injected intraperitoneally with 1 ml of sterile saline on at least 3 to 4 consecutive days before the experiments. To expose rats to restraint stress, they were placed in front of a translucent perspex restraint box (inner size: 14.5 × 6.4 × 5.4 cm). After spontaneous entry, the boxes were closed for 5 minutes unless otherwise stated. After removal from the boxes, the rats were either immediately sacrificed by decapitation or immunized with antigen. Rats decapitated within 10 seconds after transfer from an adjacent room served as control. For Con A stimulation, spleens were removed directly after sacrifice and minced through a mesh wire into ice cold RPMI-medium supplemented with penicillin/streptomycin. Spleen cells were stimulated with Con A (Difco) as described (Croiset, Heijnen, Veldhuis, De Wied, & Ballieux, 1987). SRBC (Bloedtransfusiedienst, Amsterdam) were used as antigen to immunize rats. The red blood cells were washed three times with saline and, thereafter, 1 ml of a cell suspension containing 5×10^8 (A) or 5×10^9 (B) cells were injected intraperitoneally into control rats or into rats immediately after exposure to restraint stress. Plaque-forming cells (PFC) were determined as described (Croiset et al., 1987) using splenic cells taken 5 days after injection of SRBC. The number of plaques were expressed as $PFC/10^6$ splenic cells. *Upper panel:* Each point represents the mean and SEM of six animals. Data were evaluated with analysis of variance with repeated measures ($F = :8.4; p < .01$). *Lower panel:* Each point represents the mean of five to six animals. Nonresponders were excluded from the statistical evaluation. Analysis of all experiments performed showed that nonresponders were equally distributed over the stressed and nonstressed rats. Data was evaluated by two-way analysis of variance with Duncan range test for multiple comparison. Significance between restraint groups versus control groups were defined at the 0.05 level (*).

medulla (Mueller, Thoenen, & Axelrod, 1969) and/or increased sensitivity of beta-adrenoceptors for catecholamines (Levitzki, 1978), making meaningful interpretation of data difficult. Various studies have demonstrated that lymphocytes possess large numbers of beta-adrenoceptors that are linked to adenylate cyclase (Coffy & Hadden, 1985). Because beta-adrenoceptors are targets for CA released from the sympathetic-adrenomedullary system, we set out to conduct a series of experiments on the effect of beta-adrenoceptor blockade on basal immune responses as well as stress-induced changes in these responses. As discussed earlier, our previous studies have shown that administration of beta-adrenoceptor blockers, like timolol or propranolol, to handled rats do not elicit changes in blood concentrations of POMC hormones, catecholamines or prolactin. As illustrated in Table 4.1, the peripheral acting beta-adrenoceptor blocker, timolol, clearly reduces the number of splenic cells secreting specific antibodies to SRBC in nonstressed rats. Nevertheless, in timolol-treated rats we still could see enhanced humoral responses to restraint stress. In fact, the stress-induced increments in timolol- versus saline-treated rats are not significantly different (Table 4.1). Similar results can be obtained by using the beta-adrenoceptor blocker propranolol. The doses of timolol or propranolol were chosen based on the capacity to fully block tachycardia in response to a maximally effective dose of the beta-adrenoceptor agonist

TABLE 4.1

Effect of Beta-Adrenoceptor Blockade on the Plaque-Forming Cell Response of Spleen Cells to Immunization with Sheep Red Blood Cells in Restraint Stressed and Nonstressed Animals.

Treatment	Controls	Restraint	Increment
Saline	312 + 15	1120 + 96	808 + 97
Timolol	100 + 26 #	640 + 62 #	540 + 68 NS
Saline	308 + 15	1312 + 92	984 + 92
Propranolol	140 + 36 #	878 + 123	733 + 110 NS

Male Wistar rats were housed and adapted to experimental conditions as described in the legend to Fig. 4.3. On the day of the experiments, groups of rat ($n = 6$) were injected intraperitoneally with saline or saline containing the beta-adrenoceptor blocker timolol (1 mg mg/kg) or propranolol (2.5 mg/kg). After 40 minutes, two groups of rats were subjected to restraint stress of 5 minutes duration. After termination of the stressor, they were injected intraperitoneally with 1 ml of a cell suspension containing 5×10^9 SRBC/ml. The nonstressed groups were only injected with 5×10^9 SRBC/ml and are indicated as control. Plaque-forming cells (PFC) were determined using splenic cells taken 5 days after immunization as indicated in the legend of Fig. 4.3. The number of plaque-forming cells are expressed as PFC/10^6 splenic cells. Data represent the mean and S.E.M. of five to six animals are evaluated by two-way analysis variance with Duncan range tests for multiple comparison. Significance was defined at the 0.05 level and is indicated by asterisks. Increments were obtained by subtracting the means of the saline or adrenergic blocker treated non-stressed controls from their matched stressed groups and differences were evaluated by Student t statistics. (NS: non significant).

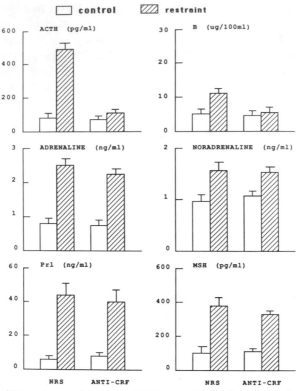

FIG. 4.4. Effect of normal rat serum (NRS) or antiserum for CRF levels on plasma adrenaline, noradrenaline, ACTH, corticosterone (B), Prolactin (PrL), and melanocyte-stimulating hormone (MSH) concentrations in peripheral blood in nonstress rats and rats subjected to restraint stress. See for rats and their environmental conditions and handling procedures legend of Fig. 4.3. To obtain a homologous antiserum to CRF, female Wistar rats (180–240 g) were actively immunized by repeated intraperitoneal administration (4-week intervals) of 25 ug rat CRF (Peninsula Labs) conjugated to bovine thyroglobulin by using glutaraldehyde. The first dose was emulsified in complete Freund's adjuvant (1:1 v/v), four subsequent boosters were given in incomplete Freund's adjuvant. After the third booster, rats were screened for their plasma corticosterone responses to ether stress. In addition, plasma samples obtained were screened for rCRF-binding capacity using radiolabeled rCRF. Blood plasma was obtained by tail vena sampling. All animals developed antibodies binding to rCRF and showed reduced plasma corticosterone concentrations after stress exposure. The rat with the highest antibody titer as well as the lowest plasma corticosterone response to ether stress, was decapitated 10 days after the fourth booster and serum was stored at −20C. Rats immunized with Freund's complete and incomplete according to the same schedule were used as a source of control serum (NRS). To verify the potency and selectivity of the antiserum (titer based on binding to radiolabeled CRF: 1:1600), 0.2 ml of antiserum or control serum respectively, was injected intravenously to groups of male Wistar rats (160–180 gram, n = 4) prior to stress exposure. Five minutes after restraint stress, the animals were decapitated for collection of trunk blood and head blood. Plasma was stored at −70 C until assayed for hormones. Control animals injected with antiserum were decapitated within 10 seconds after transfer from the adjacent room. Plasma obtained from the head was used for determination of the

84

isoproterenol (Tilders et al., 1982). Therefore, these data do not support the notion that the restraint stress-induced augmentation of splenic antibody formation is due to stimulation of immunocyte beta-adrenoceptors by catecholamines released from the sympathetic-adrenomedullary system. Nevertheless, catecholamines do appear to have a role in a beta-adrenoceptor-mediated tonic influence on the humoral response. As discussed earlier, it is worth noting that beta-adrenoceptor blockade also attenuates the increase in alpha-MSH and endorphin secretion by the rat intermediate lobe in response to restraint stress. Such blockade has no effect on the basal secretion of these intermediate lobe hormones. It has been suggested that alpha-MSH functions as an endogenous inhibitor of certain immunomodulatory and inflammatory activities of interleukin-1 in vivo and in vitro (Cannon, Tatro, Reichlin, & Dinarello, 1986; Daynes, Robertson, Cho, Burnham, & Newton, 1987). However, the inability of beta-adrenergic blockers to abrogate stress-induced increases of the humoral response to SRBC, as shown in this chapter, challenges the view that intermediate lobe hormones have a primary role in acute stress-induced alterations of the humoral response.

INVOLVEMENT OF CORTICOTROPIN-RELEASING FACTOR

In attempting to study the role of anterior pituitary corticotrophs in stress-induced changes in humoral responses, we developed rat antibodies to corticotropin-releasing factor (CRF) to block release of ACTH and related peptides in response to stress. Homologous CRF antibodies have been selected because of the notion that they minimally activate immune cells when injected in vivo. As illustrated in Fig. 4.4, the antibodies can fully neutralize the restraint stress-induced ACTH response without effecting other hormone responses (catecholamines, alpha-MSH, Prolactin). In parallel, the CRF antibody also completely neutralized the increased formation of splenic antibody-secreting cells to SRBC in response to restraint stress (Fig. 4.5). It is not clear from our data whether the stress-related CRF effects on the immune parameters are a function of central secretion of CRF or local production. By using conventional radioimmunoassays, a CRF-like peptide has been shown to circulate in peripheral

---

plasma concentrations of adrenaline and noradrenaline. There plasma catecholamines were determined by use of HPLC, followed by electrochemical detection. Plasma B (corticosterone) was determined fluorimetrically. ACTH, PrL and MSH were measured by radioimmunoassay. Data represent mean and SEM ($n = 4$) and are evaluated by two analyses of variance with Duncan range test for multiple comparison. Significance was defined at the 0.05 level.

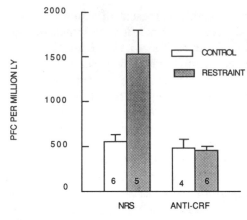

FIG. 4.5. Effect of normal rat serum (NRS) or antiserum to CRF on the plaque-forming response to SRBC in nonstressed rats subjected to restraint stress. Male Wistar rats (160–180 g) were housed and were adapted to experimental conditions as described in the legend of Fig. 4.3. Groups of rats ($n = 6$) were intravenously (0.2 ml) injected with NRS or antiserum to CRF. The same batch of NRS and anti-CRF serum were used as described in the legend of Fig. 4.3. Ninety minutes later rats were exposed to restraint stress of 5-minute duration, followed by immunization with SRBC as described in the legend of Fig. 4.3. Control animals only received immunization with SRBC. Plaque-forming cells (PFC) were determined using splenic cells taken 5 days after immunization as indicated in the legend of Fig. 4.3. The number of plaque-forming cells are expressed as $PFC/10^6$ splenic cells. Data represent mean and SEM of four to six rats and are evaluated by two-way analysis of variance with Duncan range test for multiple comparison. Significance was defined at the 0.05 level.

plasma of the rat (Gibbs & Vale, 1982; Sumitomo et al., 1985). Yet no detectable CRF concentration was found using a nonradiometric CRF assay (IRMA) even after stress exposure or adrenalectomy (Linton et al., 1987), conditions that may be expected to elevate circulating CRF concentrations assuming its source is from the hypothalamus. These data suggest that the RIAs used to detect CRF may cross react with CRF fragments or related molecules that are not detected by the IRMA. CRF receptors have been detected in the mouse spleen, particularly in the marginal zones where macrophages are concentrated (Webster & DeSouza, 1988). Additionally, CRF has been shown to induce POMC peptide production in lymphocytes (Kavelaars, Berkenbosch, Croiset, Ballieux, & Heijnen, 1990; Smith, Morrill, Meyer, & Blalock, 1986), to enhance luminol-induced chemiluminescence signals from rat peritoneal macrophages when costimulated with zymosan (Jiskoot & Berkenbosch, unpublished observations), and to induce IL-1 secretion from rat or human macrophages (Kavelaars et al., 1990). However, these effects occur at CRF concentrations in the nanomolar range, whereas plasma CRF concentrations do not exceed the picomolar range. Thus, although possible, it seems unlikely that CRF-like molecules that circulate in the blood are mediating the modulating effects of acute stress on the immune system. However, it is worth noting that in humans, blood concentrations of authentic CRF have been found in the nanomolar range throughout the third trimester of pregnancy (Campbell et al., 1987; Linton et al., 1987).

A variety of studies have shown that a CRF-like molecule is produced in several peripheral sites (Bruhn, England, Anthony, Gann, & Jackson, 1987; Nieuwenhuijzen-Kruseman, Linton, Lowry, Rees, & Besser, 1982; Petrusz, Merchentaler, Maderdrut, Vigh, & Schultz, 1983). Therefore, it is possible that the effects of acute stress are due to local influences of this hormone within the lymphoid organs. We cannot exclude this possibility. However, by using a sensitive immunocytochemical technique involving well-characterized antibodies to CRF (Berkenbosch, Schipper, Tilders, 1986), we were unable to detect CRF-like immunostaining in the rat lymph nodes or spleen with regard to the lymphoid parenchyma and neuronal innervations (Van der Meer & Berkenbosch, unpublished observations). In view of the correspondent effect of CRF immunoneutralization on the stress-induced ACTH response and the stress-induced humoral response, we advocate the view that the effect of acute stressors are mediated by some of POMC hormones secreted from the pituitary gland. ACTH- and opiate-binding sites have been identified on immune cells (Sibinga & Goldstein, 1988). Moreover, in recent experiments, we have found that the enhanced T cell proliferation in response to restraint stress can be prevented by the opiate-receptor antagonist naloxone. Moreover, our in vitro data and those of others have demonstrated immunomodulatory effects of ACTH and endorphin on immune responses (Berkenbosch,, Heijnen, Croiset, Revers, Ballieux, et al., 1986; Blalock & Smith, 1985). It is worth noting that in our studies, beta-endorphin concentration dependently enhanced the humoral response to the antigen ovalbumin (Berkenbosch, Heijnen, Croiset, Revers, Ballieux, 1986). Preliminary studies indicate that one important mechanism by which endorphin regulate the humoral response is by influencing secretion of soluble factors necessary for the differentiation of B cells in antibody-secreting cells.

CONCLUSIONS AND SPECULATIONS

Based on the described evidence, I propose that POMC-derived peptides may function as signal molecules by which the brain (and/or other organs, such as the placenta and intestine) may regulate immunity. In this role, these peptides appear to be integrated in the overall defense reaction of organisms to stress. The latter reaction appears to be coordinated to a large extent by CRF. In the brain, POMC-derived peptides are involved in regulation of pain perception, whereas in the periphery they may be involved in the boosting of immune responses. These functions may be important in acute social confrontations of mammals such as occurring during the reproductive periods and/or during defense of a position in the social rank order. By boosting immunity during these social confrontations, these peptides may be involved in enhancing the resistance to superficial tissue damage gained during the social confrontation. In this chapter, I avoided discussing the involvement of adrenal glucocorticoids within the context of stress-induced immunomodulation. The role of glucocorticoids in immunoregulation is complex and certainly needs further elucidation. However, it should be noted that ACTH, as part of the POMC precursor, stimulates the adrenal cortex to secrete glucocorticoids. These hormones are considered to be generally immunosuppressive. Thus, part of the POMC precursor can induce immunoinhibitory signals (glucocorticoids) to terminate its own direct immunoenhancing properties. This view is in line with current thoughts of the role of glucocorticoids in the defense to stress as formulated by Munck, Guyer, and Holbrook (1984), stating that glucocorticoids do not protect against the source of stress itself, but rather against the body's normal reaction to stress, preventing those reactions from overshooting and themselves threatening homeostasis.

ACKNOWLEDGMENTS

I thank Dr. C Heijnen for her technical assistance in performing some of the immunological assays, Rob Binnekade for his skillful help in performing the in vivo experiments, and Janet Edmond (Fishberg Research Center, Mount Sinai Medical Center, New York) and Henk Nordsiek for reproducing the figures. This study was supported by the Royal Dutch Academy for Sciences and Arts.

REFERENCES

Axelrod, J., & Reisine, T. D. (1984). Stress hormones: Their interaction and regulation. *Science, 224,* 452–459.

Berkenbosch, F., Heijnen, C. J., Croiset, G., Revers, C., Ballieux, R. E., Binnekade, R., & Tilders, F. J. H. (1986). Endocrine and immunological responses to acute stress. In N. P. Plotnikoff, R. E. Faith, & R. A. Good (Eds.), *Enkephalins and endorphins: Stress and the immune system* (pp. 109–118). New York, London: Plenum Press.

Berkenbosch, F., Oers, van J. W. A. M., Del Rey, A., Tilders, F. J. H., & Beseclovsky, H. O. (1987). Corticotropin-releasing factor producing neurons in the rat activated by interleukin-1. *Science, 238,* 524–526.

Berkenbosch, F., Schipper, J., & Tilders, F. J. H. (1986). Corticotropin-releasing factor immunostaining in the rat spinal cord and medulla oblongata: An unexpected form of cross reactivity with substance P. *Brain Research, 399,* 87–96.

Berkenbosch, F., & Tilders, F. J. H. (1988). Effects of axonal transport blockade on corticotropin releasing factor immunoreactivity in the median eminence of intact and adrenalectomized rats: Relationship between depletion rate and secretory activity. *Brain Research, 442,* 312–317.

Berkenbosch, F., Tilders, F. J. H., & Vermes, I. (1983). Beta-adrenoceptor activation mediates stress-induced secretion of beta-endorphin and related peptides from intermediate but not anterior pituitary. *Nature, 305,* 237–239.

Berkenbosch, F., Vermes, I., Binnekade, R., & Tilders, F. J. H. (1981). Beta-adrenergic stimulation induces an increase of the plasma levels of immunoreactive MSH, endorphin, ACTH and corticosterone. *Life Science, 29,* 2249–2256.

Berkenbosch, F., Vermes, I., & Tilders, F. J. H. (1984). The beta-adrenoceptor blocking drug propranolol prevents secretion of immunoreactive beta-endorphin and alpha-melanocyte stimulating hormone in response to certain stress stimuli. *Endocrinology, 115,* 1051–1059.

Berkenbosch, F., Wolvers, D. A. W., Derijk, R. (1991). Neuroendocrine and immunological mechanisms in stress-induced immunomodulation. *J. Steroid Biochem. Molec. Biol. 40,* 639–647.

Blalock, J., & Smith, E. M. (1985). A complete regulatory loop between the immune and neuroendocrine systems. *Federation Proceedings of the Federal American Society of Experimental Biology, 44,* 108–111.

Brown, M. R., Fisher, L. A., Webb, V., Vale, W., & Rivier, J. (1985). Corticotropin releasing factor: a physiological regulator of adrenal epinephrine secretion. *Brain Research, 238,* 355–357.

Bruhn, T. O., England, W. C., Anthony, E. L. P., Gann, D. S., & Jackson, I. M. D. (1987). Corticotropin-releasing factor in the dog adrenal medulla is secreted in response to hemorrhage. *Endocrinology, 120,* 25–33.

Campbell, E. A., Lintonm, E. A., Wolfe, C. D. A., Scraggs, P. R., Jones, M. T., & Lowry, P. J. (1987). Plasma corticotropin releasing hormone concentrations during pregnancy and parturition. *Clinical Endocrinology and Metabolism, 64,* 1054–1059.

Cannon, W. B., & De La Paz, D. (1911). Emotional stimulation of adrenal secretion. *American Journal of Physiology, 28,* 64–70.

Cannon, J. C., Tatro, J. B., Reichlin, S., & Dinarello, C. A. (1986). Alpha-melanocyte stimulating hormone inhibits immunostimulatory and inflammatory actions of interleukin-1. *Journal of Immunology, 137,* 2232–2236.

Chang, K. J. (1984). Opioid peptides have actions on the immune system. *Trends in Neuroscience, 7,* 234–235.

Coffy, R. G., & Hadden, J. W. (1985). Neurotransmitters, hormones, and cyclic nucleotides in lymphocyte regulation. *Federation Proceedings of the Federal American Society of Experimental Biology, 44,* 122–117.

Cote, T. E., Eskay, R. L., Frey, E. A., Grewe, C. W., Munemera, M., Stoof, J. C., Tsurutak, B., & Kebabian, J. W. (1982). Biochemical and physiological studies of the beta-adrenoceptors and D-2 dopamine receptor in the intermediate lobe of the rat pituitary gland. A review. *Neuroendocrinology, 35,* 217–225.

Croiset, G., Heijnen, C. J., Veldhuis, H. D., De Wied, D., & Ballieux, R. E. (1987). Modulation of the immune response by emotional stress. *Life Science, 40,* 775–782.

Daynes, R. A., Robertson, B. A., Cho, B., Burnham, P. L., & Newton, R. (1987). Alpha-melanocyte-stimulating hormone exhibits target cell selectivity in its capacity to affects interleukin-1 inducible responses in vivo and in vitro. *Journal of Immunology, 139,* 103–109.

Eipper, R. A., & Mains, R. E. (1980). Structure and biosynthesis of pro-adreno-corticotropin/endorphin and related peptides. *Endocrine Review, 1,* 1–25.

Felten, D. L., Felten, S. Y., Carlson, S. L., Olschowka, J. A., & Livnat, S. (1985). Innervation of lymphoid tissue. *Journal of Immunology, 135,* 755s–765s.

Fortier, C. L. (1966). Nervous control of ACTH secretion. In G. Harris & H. Donovan (Eds.), *The pituitary gland* (Vol. 2, pp. 195–234). London: Butterworths.

Gibbs, D. M., & Vale, W. (1982). Presence of corticotropin releasing factor-like immunoreactivity in hypophyseal portal blood. *Endocrinology, 111,* 1418–1420.

Henry, J. P. (1980). Present concept of stress theory. In E. Usdin, R. Kvetnansky, & I. J. Kopin (Eds.), *Catecholamines and stress: Recent advances* (pp. 557–571). New York: Elsevier North-Holland.

Hope, J., & Lowry, P. J. (1981). Pro-opiomelanocortin: The ACTH/LPH common precursor molecule. *Frontiers in Hormone Research, 8,* 44–69.

Johnson, H. M., Smith, E. M., Torres, R. A., & Blalock, J. E. (1982). Regulation of the in vitro antibody response by neuroendocrine hormones. *Proceedings of the National Academy of Sciences USA, 79,* 4171–4174.

Kavelaars, A., Berkenbosch, F., Croiset, G., Ballieux, R. E., & Heijnen, C. J. (1990). Induction of beta-endorphin secretion by lymphocytes after subcutaneous administration of CRF. *Endocrinology, 126,* 759–764.

Keller, S. E., Weiss, J. M., Schleifer, S. J., Miller, N. E., & Stein, M. (1981). Suppression of immunity by stress: Effect of graded series of stressors on lymphocyte stimulation in the rat. *Science, 213,* 1397–1400.

Keller, S. E., Weiss, J. M., Schleiffer, S. J., Miller, N. E., & Stein, M. (1983). Stress-induced suppression of immunity in adrenalectomized rats. *Science, 221,* 1301–1304.

Kvetnansky, R., Sun, C. L., Lake, C. R., Thoa, N., Torda, T., Kopin, I. J. (1978). Effects of handling and forced immobilization on rat plasma levels of epinephrine, norepinephrine and dopamine beta-hydroxylase. *Endocrinology, 103,* 1868–1874.

Kvetnansky, R., Tilders, F. J. H., Van Zoest, I. D., Dobrakovova, M., Berkenbosch, F., Culman, J., Zeman, J., & Smelik, P. G. (1987). Sympatho-adrenal activity facilitates beta-endorphin and alpha-MSH secretion but potentiates ACTH secretion during immobilization stress. *Neuroendocrinology, 45,* 318–324.

Levitzki, A. (1978). Catecholamine receptors. *Reviews of Physiology, Biochemistry and Pharmacology, 82,* 1–26

Linton, E. A., McClean, C., Nieuwenhuyzen-Kruzeman, A. C., Tilders, F. J., Van der Veen, E. A., & Lowry, P. J. (1987). Direct measurements of human plasma corticotropin releasing factor by two-site immunoradiometric assay. *Journal of Clinical Endocrinology and Metabolism, 64,* 1047–1051.

Linton, E. A., Tilders, F. J. H., Hodgkinson, S., Berkenbosch, F., Vermes, I., & Lowry, P. J. (1985). Stress-induced secretion of ACTH in rats is inhibited by administration of antisera to ovine corticotropin releasing factor and vasopressin. *Endocrinology, 116,* 966–970.

Livnat, S., Felten, S. Y., Carlson, S. L., Bellinger, D. L., & Felten, D. L. (1985). Involvement of peripheral and central catecholamines systems in neural-immune interactions. *Journal of Neuroimmunology, 10,* 5–30.

Makara, G. B., Antoni, F. A., Stark, E., & Karteszi, M. (1984). Hypothalamic organization of corticotropin releasing factor (CRF) producing structures. In E. E. Muller & M. McLeod (Eds.), *Neuroendocrine perspectives* (Vol. 3, pp. 71–119). New York: Elsevier Science Publishers.

McCarthy, R., & Kopin, J. (1979). Stress-induced alterations in plasma catecholamines and behavior of rats: Effects of chlorisondamine and bretylium. *Behavior and Neural Biology, 27,* 249–265.

Mueller, R. A., Thoenen, H., & Axelrod, J. (1969). Adrenal tyrosine hydroxylase. Compensatory increase in activity after chemical sympathetectomy. *Science, 163,* 468–469.

Munck, A., Guyer, P. M., & Holbrook, N. J. (1984). Physiological functions of glucocorticoids in stress and their relation to pharmacological actions. *Endocrine reviews, 5,* 25–44.

Nieuwenhuijzen-Kruzeman, A. C., Linton, E. A., Lowry, P. J., Rees, L. H., & Besser, G. M. (1982). Corticotropin-releasing factor immunoreactivity in human gastrointestinal tract. *Lancet, 2,* 1245–1246.

O'Donohue, T. L., & Dorsa, D. M. (1982). The opiomelanotropinergic neuronal and endocrine systems. *Peptides, 3,* 353–395.

Oers, van J. W. A. M., Tilders, F. J. H., & Berkenbosch, F. (1989). Characterization and biological activity of a rat monoclonal antibody to rat/human corticotropin releasing factor. *Endocrinology, 124,* 1239–1246.

Petrusz, P., Merchentaler, I., Maderdrut, J. L., Vigh, S., & Schally, A. V. (1983). Corticotropin-releasing factor (CRF) - like immunoreactivity in the vertebrate pancreas. *Proceedings of the National Academy of Sciences USA, 80,* 1721–1725.

Rivier, C., Rivier, J., & Vale, W. (1982). Inhibition of adrenocorticotropin hormone secretion in the rat by immunoneutralization of corticotropin releasing factor. *Science, 218,* 377–378.

Schipper, J., & Tilders, F. J. H. (1982). Quantification of formaldehyde induced fluorescence and its application in neurobiology. *Brain Research Bulletin, 9,* 69–80.

Schipper, J., Werkman, T. R., & Tilders, F. S. H. (1984). Quantitative immunocy to chemistry of corticotropin releasing factor (CRF). Studies on non-biological models and on hypothalamic tissues of rats after hypophysectomie, adrenalectomy and dexamethasone treatment. *Brain Res, 293,* 111–118.

Sibinga, N. E. S., & Goldstein, A. (1988). Opioid peptides and opioid receptors in cells of the immune system. *Annual Review of Immunology, 6,* 219–249.

Smith, E. M., Morrill, A., Meyer W., III, & Blalock, B. J. (1986). Corticotropin releasing factor induction of leucocyte-derived immunoreactive ACTH and Endorphins. *Nature, 311,* 881–882.

Sumitomo, T., Suda, T., Tozawa, F., Nakagami, Y., Ushiyama, T., Demura, K. H., & Shzuma, K. (1985). Immunoreactive corticotropin releasing factor in rat plasma. *Endocrinology, 1201,* 1391–1395.

Tilders, F. J. H., Berkenbosch, F., & Smelik, P. G. (1982). Adrenergic mechanisms involved in the control of pituitary-adrenal activity in the rat: a beta-adrenergic stimulatory mechanism. *Endocrinology, 110,* 114–120.

Tilders, F. J. H., Berkenbosch, F., & Smelik, P. G. (1985). Control of secretion of peptides related to adrenocorticotropin, melanocyte-stimulating hormone and endorphin. *Frontiers of Hormone Research, 14,* 161–196.

Tilders, F. J. H., Berkenbosch, F., Vermes, I., Linton, E. A., & Smelik, P. G. (1986). CRF and catecholamines: Their place in the central and peripheral regulation of the stress response. *Acta Endocrinologica, Supplementum 276,* 63–75.

Tilders, F. J. H., Tatemoto, T., & Berkenbosch, F. (1984). The intestinal peptide PHI-27 potentiates the action of corticotropin releasing factor on ACTH release from rat pituitary fragments in vitro. *Endocrinology, 115,* 1633–1635.

Vale, W., Rivier, C., Brown, M. R., Spiess, J., Koob, G., Swanson, L., Bilezikjian, L., Bloom, F., & Rivier, J. (1983). Chemical and biological characterization of corticotropin releasing factor. *Recent Progress in Hormone Research, 39,* 245–270.

Vale, W., Spiess, J., Rivier, C., & Rivier, J. (1981). Characterization of a 41-residue ovine hypothalamic peptide that stimulates secretion of corticotropin and beta-endorphin. *Science, 213,* 1394–1397.

Vale, W., Vaughan, J., Smith, M., Yamamoto, G, Rivier, J, & Rivier, C. (1983). Effects of synthetic ovine-corticotropin releasing factor, glucocorticoids, catecholamines, neurohypophysial peptides and other substances on cultures corticotropic cells. *Endocrinology, 113,* 1121–1131.

Verhofstad, A., Steinbusch, H. W. M., Joosten, H. W. J., Penke, B., Varga, J., & Goldstein, M. (1983). Immunocytochemical localization of noradrenaline, adrenaline and serotonin. In J. M. Polak & S. van Noorden (Eds.), *Practical applications in pathology and biology* (pp. 143–168). Wright: Bristol Publishers.

Webster, E. L., & DeSouza, E. D. (1988). Corticotropin-releasing factor receptors in mouse spleen: Identification, autoradiographic localization and regulation by divalent cations and guanine nucleotides. *Endocrinology, 122,* 609–617.

5 Behavioral Responses to Cyclophosphamide in Animals With Autoimmune Disease

Robert Ader
University of Rochester School of Medicine and Dentistry

Lesioning or electrical stimulation of areas within the hypothalamus influence immune responses (e.g., Stein, Schleifer, & Keller, 1981). More recently, it has been found that activation of the immune system can result in electrophysiological changes within the brain (e.g., Besedovsky, Sorkin, Felix, & Haas, 1977). Similarly, immunologic reactivity is altered by the exogenous administration or the endogenous release of hormones and neurotransmitters for which lymphocytes, monocytes, macrophages, and other cells of the immune system bear receptors (e.g., Weigent & Blalock, 1987), and conversely, the response to immunization is associated with the release of hormones and neurotransmitters (e.g., Besedovsky et al., 1983). Behavioral factors, notably "stress" and Pavlovian conditioning that presumably operate via neuroendocrine changes, are also capable of influencing immune responses (Ader & Cohen, 1985; Ader & Felten, Cohen 1991). As with the reciprocal relationship between neural and immune processes and between endocrine and immune processes, there are experimental and clinical data to suggest that the immunologic state of the organism has consequences for behavior (Ader, Grota, Moynihan, & Cohen, 1991; Crnic, 1991; Kurstak, Lipowski, & Morozov, 1987; Schiffer & Hoffman, 1991; Weiner, 1991).

Several behavioral studies have been conducted on strains of mice that spontaneously develop an autoimmune disease that is, in many respects, identical to systemic lupus erythematosus in humans (Theofilopoulos & Dixon, 1985). The most extensively studied model is the New Zealand hybrid (NZB × NZW)F1 mouse. The more susceptible females develop a lethal glomerulonephritis beginning at about 8 months of age. Another lupus-prone strain of mice (MRL) is divided into two congenic inbred substrains. The MRL-lpr/lpr substrain carries the lpr (lymphoproliferative) gene and, in contrast to the (NZB × NZW)F1 mouse, manifests a massive lymphadenopathy and elevated anti-DNA antibody titer relatively early in life (at approximately 12 weeks of age) and shows a 50% mortality at approximately 5–6 months of age. In this strain, females are only slightly more susceptible than males. The MRL +/+ substrain also develops lupus but the disease is delayed; a 50% mortality is seen at approximately 17 months of age in females and 23 months of age in males. The availability of a congenic control strain, the presence of lymphadenopathy, an external marker of disease, and the relatively rapid development of disease are the potential advantages of using MRL mice in behavioral studies.

In an extensive series of studies (Forster & Lal, 1991), it was found that mice with autoimmune disease showed poorer learning of an active avoidance response than healthy, congenic control mice, and that the deficit in performance was associated with the early development of brain reactive antibodies in these animals. This chapter briefly reviews studies from our laboratory on the behavior of lupus-prone (NZB × NZW)F1 and MRL mice in response to immunomodulating and nonimmunomodulating drugs. These experiments indicate that: (a) the immune status of an organism has consequences for its behavior, and (b) such behavior would appear to be adaptive with respect to the immune system.

TASTE AVERSION BEHAVIOR IN LUPUS-PRONE MICE

Capitalizing on the ability to condition an immunosuppressive response (Ader & Cohen, 1975), we found that the development of autoimmune disease in (NZB × NZW)F1 mice could be delayed by treating animals under a partial schedule of pharmacologic reinforcement (Ader & Cohen, 1982). Conditioned stimuli (CSs) that had been paired with the immunosuppressive drug, cyclophosphamide (CY), were substituted for a proportion of the trials on which active drug would have been received in a typical or standard pharmacotherapeutic regimen, that is, a regimen in which drug effects, the unconditioned stimuli (UCSs) invariably follow a reasonably constant complex of CSs. Under a partial schedule of reinforcement, conditioned mice showed a delay in the progression of lupus using a cumulative dose of CY that was not, by itself, sufficient to alter the course of the autoimmune disease. Moreover, conditioned mice repeatedly reexposed to the taste stimulus that had been paired with CY following the termination of active drug therapy survived significantly longer than conditioned animals that received no "medication" (Ader & Cohen, 1985).

It was in the course of these studies that it was first observed that

(NZB × NZW)F1 mice did not display a conditioned taste aversion following the pairing of the taste of saccharin with an ip injection of CY. In a series of experiments (Ader, Grota, & Cohen, 1987), it was established that these lupus-prone mice failed to display a conditioned aversion to a novel taste stimulus previously paired with doses of CY that were effective in inducing taste aversions in normal C57BL/6 or BDF1 mice. Further, it was established that these lupus-prone mice did not have a deficit in learning ability, per se; they were as capable as normal strains of acquiring a conditioned taste aversion based on the pairing of saccharin with the noxious effects of lithium chloride (LiCl).

The immunosuppressive effects of CY prolong the survival of mice with autoimmune disease (Shiraki, Fujiwara, & Tomura, 1984; Smith, Chused, & Steinberg, 1984). Thus, the seemingly poor avoidance behavior of lupus-prone mice when an immunosuppressive drug is used as the UCS was hypothesized to be a reflection of the animal's "recognition" of its dysregulated immune state and/or the immunorestorative effects of CY. More specifically, given the noxious gastrointestinal effects of CY on the one hand, and its immunosuppressive effects on the other, it was hypothesized that the dose of CY and the degree of immunologic dysregulation would interact to influence the acquisition of a conditioned avoidance response based on the pairing of a distinctive taste with an immunosuppressive drug; that is, it would require higher doses of CY — or a greater number of conditioning trials at a constant dose of drug — to condition a taste aversion in lupus-prone mice than in healthy control animals. These predictions were examined in MRL-lpr/lpr and MRL + / + mice.

Our initial results (Ader, Grota, & Cohen, 1987) using chocolate milk (CHOC) as the CS and CY as the UCS were consistent with the prediction of an interaction between CY dose and the progression of autoimmune disease. With the relatively high doses of CY used in our first experiment, there were no differences in the performance of MRL-lpr/lpr and MRL + / + mice on the first test trial following a single conditioning trial, but, as might be expected, extinction was more rapid in the mice with active autoimmune disease. To summarize the results of a series of follow-up studies conducted on animals tested after manifest symptoms of autoimmune disease (lymphadenopathy) appeared in the lpr substrain: Low doses of CY did not induce avoidance responses in either strain; relatively high doses of CY produced aversions to CHOC in both strains; and a moderate dose of CY (100 mg/kg) induced a taste aversion in Mrl + / + animals but no avoidance behavior in the Mrl-lpr/lpr mice. When mice were tested at 10 weeks of age (before the development of palpable lymphadenopathy), there were no substrain differences in taste-aversion behavior.

In a subsequent study (Grota, Ader, & Cohen, 1987), MRL-lpr/lpr mice with manifest symptoms of disease and age-matched MRL $+/+$ mice were conditioned by injections of 50, 100, or 200 mg/kg CY immediately following 1-hour exposures to CHOC. Nonconditioned groups received unpaired presentations of CHOC and CY, and placebo-treated animals were injected with saline following CHOC consumption. A two-bottle preference test that permitted the animals to choose between CHOC and plain water was used to assess the conditioned avoidance response. The drinking behavior of nonconditioned animals confirmed that the decreased consumption of CHOC following conditioning trials was the result of the pairing of CHOC and CY and not a direct effect of CY, per se. Among conditioned animals, neither strain acquired a taste aversion in response to the low dose of CY and both strains displayed avoidance responses to the high dose of CY. At the intermediate dose of CY, however, Mrl-lpr/lpr mice with manifest symptoms of autoimmune disease did not show an aversion to the taste stimulus that had been paired with a dose of CY that was sufficient to induce a taste aversion in Mrl $+/+$ animals. Again, the behavioral difference between MRL-lpr/lpr and MRL $+/+$ mice was related to the degree of active disease because there were no differences when these substrains were tested before the development of external symptoms of their dysregulated immune state.

The possibility that MRL-lpr/lpr mice develop a general impairment of their capacity to acquire conditioned (passive) avoidance responses along with the progression of their autoimmune disease was assessed by comparing the taste-aversion performance of MRL-lpr/lpr and MRL $+/+$ mice when LiCl was used as the UCS and on a conditioned response based on the avoidance of electric shock. We were unable to discriminate between the performance of the lpr and $+/+$ substrains in an initial experiment (Grota et al., 1987) or in a replication involving repeated conditioning trials with doses that ranged from 125 to 500 mg/kg LiCl (Grota, Ader, Moynihan, & Cohen, 1990) whether animals were tested before or after the appearance of manifest lymphadenopathy in the lpr mice. Similarly, we were also unable to discriminate between these substrains in their performance of an electric shock-induced passive avoidance response. Thus, there is no evidence that lupus-prone MRL-lpr/lpr mice have a deficit in their capacity to acquire passive avoidance responses. Nonetheless, mice with manifest symptoms of autoimmune disease do not show an aversion to a taste stimulus previously paired with the noxious and immunosuppressive effects of a dose of CY that is effective in inducing a conditioned response in healthy, control mice. These results confirm previous observations of (NZB × NZW)F1 mice. Considering the congenic nature of the MRL substrains, the observed differences would appear to be related to the immunologic status of the animals.

CONSUMPTION OF CYCLOPHOSPHAMIDE BY
LUPUS-PRONE MICE

Cyclophosphamide has noxious gastrointestinal effects that, in normal animals, usually result in an aversion to flavors with which it has been paired. There are several reasons, therefore, why one would not necessarily expect lupus-prone animals to show a *preference* for a taste stimulus paired with an effective immunosuppressive dose of CY (Ader et al., 1991). However, if the observed differences in taste-aversion conditioning when CY is used as the UCS were due to the immunorestorative effects of CY, MRL-lpr/lpr mice with manifest autoimmune disease might consume more of a CY-laced drinking solution than MRL+/+ mice.

Fluid-deprived MRL-lpr/lpr and MRL+/+ mice, 20 weeks of age, were first provided with a single drinking bottle containing undiluted, homogenized chocolate milk containing 0, 0.2, or 0.4 mg/ml CY. The drinking solution was available for 1-hour per day, 5 days a week, for 3 or 4 weeks. As expected, consumption of the CHOC/CY solution decreased as a function of the concentration of CY. There were no differences between MRL-lpr/lpr and MRL+/+ mice after the first week of exposure to the CY-laced solutions. Subsequently, however, male MRL-lpr/lpr mice with symptoms of disease drank significantly more of the CHOC/CY solution than male MRL+/+ mice. There were no significant strain differences among the females in this experiment. Also, there were no substrain differences in consumption when animals were tested at 10 weeks of age (Grota, Schachtman, Moynihan, Cohen, & Ader, 1989).

Similar results were obtained in a second experiment (Grota et al., 1989) in which exposure to CY-laced drinking solutions began at different ages. In this experiment, however, there were no gender differences. There were no substrain differences when mice were tested prior to the development of manifest lymphadenopathy. Once symptoms of disease were evident (approximately 16–18 weeks), MRL-lpr/lpr mice consumed more of the CHOC/CY solutions than age-matched MRL+/+ mice. The data obtained from lpr and +/+ control mice that received plain, unadulterated CHOC—or the data obtained from the nonconditioned and placebo groups in the taste-aversion experiments (Grota et al., 1987)—provided no evidence that the increased consumption of the CHOC/CY solution by MRL-lpr/lpr relative to MRL+/+ mice was due to an increased sensitivity to or preference for the flavor of chocolate milk—or an increased fluid requirement by Mrl-lpr/lpr mice. These points are also substantiated by additional data that failed to discriminate between the volume of different concentrations of a quinine-laced drinking solution consumed by MRL-lpr/lpr and MRL+/+ mice (Grota, et al., 1990) and by a replication of the differences in the consumption of CY-laced solutions of different dilutions of chocolate milk by nonfluid-deprived MRL-lpr/lpr and MRL + / + mice (Grota, Ader, Moynihan, & Cohen, 1990).

In MRL-lpr/lpr mice with manifest autoimmune disease, the volume of the CHOC/CY solution consumed was sufficient to attenuate lymphadenopathy in both males and females. Consumption of the 0.2 mg/ml CHOC/CY solution prevented the progressive increase in autoantibody titers seen in animals that were provided with plain CHOC. Consumption of the 0.4 mg/ml CY solution by MRL-lpr/lpr mice decreased anti-DNA titer by the end of the first week of testing. MRL-lpr/lpr mice did not display lymphadenopathy at 10 weeks of age when exposure to the CHOC/CY solutions began but, 6 weeks later (2 weeks after the last exposure to CY), lymphoproliferation was evident in 8 of 20 mice that had been provided with plain CHOC but none of the 39 MRL-lpr/lpr mice that drank the CY-laced solutions. Similarly, there was no change in autoantibody titers in mice that drank plain CHOC, whereas there was a significant decrease in autoantibody titers among the MRL-lpr/lpr mice that drank the CHOC/CY solutions.

It should be emphasized that there were no differences in consumption when the Mrl-lpr/lpr and MRL + / + mice with symptoms of autoimmune disease were first exposed to the CY-laced drinking solutions. Strain differences did not appear until the second week of testing, providing no support for the existence of substrain differences in sensory thresholds or neophobic behavior but suggesting, instead, that the increased consumption in the MRL-lpr/lpr mice is a learned response.

DISCUSSION

Cyclophosphamide, a powerful immunosuppressive drug, has noxious gastrointestinal effects and normal animals avoid consuming CY and avoid distinctively flavored solutions that have been associated with the drug. In suppressing immune responses, cyclophosphamide delays the progression of autoimmune disease and lupus-prone mice with manifest symptoms of disease voluntarily drink more of a CY-laced chocolate milk solution than healthy, congenic control mice. They drink sufficient amounts of the CHOC/CY solution to reverse their pre-experimental lymphadenopathy and reduce their elevated autoantibody titers. The difference between MRL-lpr/lpr mice with manifest symptoms of disease and healthy, congenic MRL + / + mice in the voluntary consumption of a CHOC/CY solution was predicted from our findings that mice displaying symptoms of lupus fail to acquire aversions to distinctive taste stimuli that had been paired with doses of CY that were effective in inducing conditioned taste aversions in normal animals or in an asymptomatic congenic control strain. These behaviors in lupus-prone mice with manifest disease are interpreted to be reflections of the animal's ability to "recognize" the immunosuppressive (and immunorestorative) effects of CY. That is, having associated a distinctively flavored drinking solution with the immunosuppressive effects of CY, lupus-prone mice behave in a manner that serves to attenuate their immunologic dysregulation.

Alternative hypotheses to account for these effects need to be considered. The increased consumption of the CY-laced CHOC solution by MRL-lpr/lpr relative to MRL+/+ mice might have been due to an increased sensitivity to or preference for the flavor of chocolate milk—or an increased fluid requirement by MRL-lpr/lpr mice. These substrains did not differ in their consumption of plain chocolate milk (or in their consumption of the plain tap water provided several hours after exposure to the CHOC solutions). Also, similar strain differences in consumption of CHOC/CY solutions were observed in animals that were and were not fluid deprived prior to testing. Further, differences in consumption of the CHOC/CY solution did not occur until the animals had been exposed to the solution for between 1 and 2 weeks. The possibility of sensory differences is not eliminated but is further eroded by the failure to find differences between MRL-lpr/lpr and MRL+/+ mice in their voluntary consumption of nonimmunomodulating and nonpreferred quinine solutions and in passive avoidance behavior when LiCl or electric shock were used as UCSs.

MRL-lpr/lpr mice might be or might become less sensitive to the noxious gastrointestinal effects of CY than MRL+/+ mice. If so, this sensitivity would have to be closely related to the progression of autoimmune disease because there were no substrain differences in taste-aversion conditioning or in consumption of the CHOC/CY solutions prior to the development of manifest symptoms of disease in the lpr substrain. It would also have to be a very finely tuned sensitivity because we have consistently found that only moderate, mid-range doses of CY are effective in discriminating between the lpr and +/+ substrains. Perhaps there are strain differences in response to CY because the effects of CY superimposed upon an existing physiological dysfunction might not be as perceptible to the organism as the effects of CY in healthy animals. The same argument would, of course, apply as well to the noxious effects of LiCl in animals with and without manifest autoimmune disease, but there were no differences between New Zealand or MRL-lpr/lpr mice and control mice when a range of doses of LiCl were used as the UCSs for inducing a taste aversion.

To suggest that the results of these studies implicate behavioral processes, learning, in particular, in the maintenance or restoration of immunocompetence is consistent with an existing literature on the behavioral regulation of a variety of other physiological states. With respect to learned associations between taste stimuli and experimentally induced physiological consequences, distinctively flavored but nonpreferred drinking solutions can become preferred solutions as a result of their association with recovery from illness or the reinstatement of homeostatic balance (e.g., Rozin & Kalat, 1971; Zahorik, Maier, & Pies, 1974). Miller, DiCara, and Wolf (1968) found that salt- or water-loaded diabetes insipidus and normal rats would respond differentially in a maze learning task when reinforced by an injection of antidiuretic hormone as opposed to saline. They hypothesized that, ". . . at least in cases where homeostasis is mediated via the central nervous system, deviations in any direction, if large enough, can function as a drive and the prompt restoration to normal levels by any means can function as a reward" (p. 686). As these investigators noted, sufficiently large deviations from homeostasis may occur only under abnormal circumstances. The dysregulated immune system of animals with autoimmune disease is, by definition, a large deviation from homeostasis. The fact that the spontaneous onset of lupus in genetically predisposed mice can be influenced by conditioned immunosuppressive responses (Ader & Cohen, 1982) suggests that autoimmune disease may constitute an appropriate and particularly interesting model in which to explore the role of learning in the maintenance of homeostasis.

If these data can be viewed in the context of the literature on the behavioral regulation of physiological states and with observations that animals are able to use illness or improved health as cues for adjustments in (consummatory) behavior that restore homeostasis, then the proposed research represents a major extension of such phenomena. The pathophysiology with which we are dealing involves the immune system and, although some behaviorists may take for granted a functional relationship between CNS and immune function, it is not a universally accepted premise. If true, however, this line of research would significantly expand our knowledge of behavioral processes in health and disease by extending the influence of behavior to the regulation of immunologic dysfunctions. In so doing, it would implicate a new set of pathways through which behavioral factors could influence disease susceptibility.

Compelling support for the operation of such a hypothesis would be provided if, relative to healthy animals, lupus-prone mice with manifest symptoms of autoimmune disease acquired a conditioned taste aversion at lower doses of drug (or with fewer conditioning trials) when a novel taste is paired with an UCS that encourages the rapid progression of their autoimmune disorder. And consensual validity for such a finding would be obtained if, relative to healthy animals, symptomatic lupus prone mice consumed *less* of a distinctively flavored solution containing a substance that promoted the development of autoimmune disease.

There is now abundant evidence that the nervous system is capable of receiving information from the immune system. It remains to be determined, however, whether the nervous system is capable of acting upon that information. In the present instance, the source and nature of the cues that signal a dysregulated immune system remain to be determined. Also, it remains to be determined whether the lupus-prone animal is responding to CY-induced changes in immune function, per se, or the effects of CY in normalizing some other specific or nonspecific physiological effect(s) of the autoimmune disease. The data described here suggest that lupus-prone MRL-lpr/lpr mice are *not* responding to their lymphadenopathy or to their elevated autoantibody titers.

Whatever the immediate source of the signals that are motivating the observed changes in behavior, the primary defect of these lupus-prone animals is immunologic. These results thus provide additional evidence for CNS-immune system interactions. Consistent with previous observations, these results also illustrate and extend the role of learning in the regulation of physiological states and raise the interesting possibility that there are circumstances under which behavior can serve an in vivo immunoregulatory function.

ACKNOWLEDGMENT

This chapter constituted part of the Salmon Lecture delivered at the New York Academy of Medicine, December 7, 1989. The author's research was supported by a Research Scientist Award (K3 MH06318) from the National Institute of Mental Health and by Research Grants from the National Institute for Neurological and Communicative Diseases and Stroke (NS22228) and from RJR Nabsico, Inc.

REFERENCES

Ader, R., & Cohen, N. (1975). Behaviorally conditioned immunosuppression. *Psychosomatic Medicine, 37,* 333–340.

Ader, R., & Cohen, N. (1982). Behaviorally conditioned immunosuppression and murine systemic lupus eryrthematosus. *Science, 215,* 1534–1536.

Ader, R., & Cohen, N. (1985). CNS-immune system interactions: Conditioning phenomena. *Behavioral and Brain Sciences, 8,* 379–426.

Ader, R., Felten, D. L., & Cohen, N. (Eds.). (1991). *Psychoneuroimmunology* (2nd ed.). New York: Academic Press.

Ader, R., Grota, L. J., & Cohen, N. (1987). Conditioning phenomena and immune function. *Annals of the New York Academy of Sciences, 496,* 532–544.

Ader, R., Grota, L. J., Moynihan, J. A., & Cohen, N. (1991). Behavioral adaptations in autoimmune disease-susceptible mice. In R. Ader, D. L. Felten, & N. Cohen, (Eds.), *Psychoneuroimmunology* (2nd ed., pp. 685–708). New York: Academic Press.

Besedovsky, H. O., del Rey, A. E., Sorkin, E., DaPrada, M., Burri, R., & Honegger, C.

(1983). The immune response evokes changes in brain noradrenergic neurons. *Science, 221,* 564–566.

Besedovsky, H. O., Sorkin, E., Felix, R., & Haas, H. (1977). Hypothalamic changes during the immune response. *European Journal of Immunology, 7,* 325–328.

Crnic, L. S. (1991). Behavioral consequences of virus infection. In R. Ader, N. Cohen, & D. L. Felten, (Eds.), *Psychoneuroimmunology* (2nd ed., pp. 749–769). New York: Academic Press.

Forster, M. J., & Lal, H. (1991). Autoimmunity and cognitive decline in aging an alzheimer's disease. In R. Ader, D. L. Felten, & N. Cohen, (Eds.), *Psychoneuroimmunology* (2nd ed., pp. 709–748). New York: Academic Press.

Grota, L. J., Ader, R., & Cohen, N. (1987). Taste aversion learning in autoimmune Mrl-lpr/lpr and Mrl+/+ mice. *Brain, Behavior and Immunity, 1,* 238–250.

Grota, L. J., Ader, R., Moynihan, J. A., & Cohen, N. (1990). Voluntary consumption of cyclophosphamide by non-deprived MRL-lpr/lpr and MRL+/+ mice. *Pharmacology, Biochemistry, and Behavior, 37,* 527–530.

Grota, L. J., Schachtman, T., Moynihan, J., Cohen, N., & Ader, R. (1989). Voluntary consumption of cyclophosphamide by Mrl mice. *Brain, Behavior and Immunity, 3,* 263–273.

Kurtstak, E., Lipowski, Z. J., & Morozov, P. V. (1987). *Viruses, immunity, and mental disorders.* New York: Plenum.

Miller, N. E., DiCara, L. V., & Wolf, G. (1968). Homeostasis and reward: T-maze learning induced by manipulating antidiuretic hormone. *American Journal of Physiology, 215,* 684–686.

Rozin, P., & Kalat, J. W. (1971). Specific hungers and poison avoidance as adaptive specializations of learning. *Psychological Review, 78,* 459–486.

Schiffer, R., & Hoffman, S. A. (1991). Behavioral sequelae of autoimmune disease. In R. Ader, D. L. Felten, & N. Cohen, (Eds.), *Psychoneuroimmunology* (2nd ed., pp. 1037–1066). New York: Academic Press.

Shiraki, M., Fujiwara, M., & Tomura, S. (1984). Long term administration of cyclophosphamide in MRL/1 mice: I. The effects on the development of immunological abnormalities and lupus nephritis. *Clinical and Experimental Immunology, 55,* 333–339.

Smith, H. R., Chused, T. M., & Steinberg, A. D. (1984). Cyclophosphamide-induced changes in the MRL-lpr/lpr mouse: Effects upon cellular composition, immune function, and disease. *Clinical Immunology and Immunopathology, 30,* 51–61.

Stein, M., Schleifer, S. J., & Keller, S. E. (1981). Hypothalamic influences on immune responses. In R. Ader (Ed.), *Psychoneuroimmunology* (pp. 429–448). New York: Academic Press.

Theofilopoulos, A. N., & Dixon, F. J. (1985). Murine models of systemic lupus erythematosus. *Advances in Immunology, 37,* 269–390.

Weigent, D. A., & Blalock, J. E. (1987). Interactions between the neuroendocrine and immune systems: Common hormones and receptors. *Immunology Reviews, 100,* 79–108.

Weiner, H. (1991). Social and psychobiological factors in autoimmune disease. In R. Ader, D. L. Felten, & N. Cohen, (Eds.), *Psychoneuroimmunology* (2nd ed., pp. 955–1011). New York: Academic Press.

Zahorik, D. M., Maier, S. F., & Pies, R. W. (1974). Preference for tastes paired with recovery from thiamine deficiency in rats: Appetitive conditioning or learned safety? *Journal of Comparative and Physiological Psychology, 87,* 1083–1091.

6

Depression and Immunity: Central Corticotropin-Releasing Factor Activates the Autonomic Nervous System and Reduces Natural Killer Cell Activity

Michael R. Irwin, M.D.
University of California, San Diego

A number of clinical studies have described relationships between severe life stress, depression, and alterations in cellular immunity. However, few studies have evaluated the physiological mechanisms by which the central nervous system might coordinate immune function. In this chapter, recent data from clinical and preclinical investigations in our laboratory are presented that focus on two primary objectives: (a) to characterize further the relationship between psychological processes and immune function, and (b) to examine the mechanisms by which the central nervous system communicates with immune cells. Using an animal model, central corticotropin-releasing factor has been found to modulate natural killer (NK) cell activity by activation of the sympathetic nervous system.

IMPORTANCE OF NATURAL KILLER CELLS

Evaluation of depression-related changes in natural killer cell activity has been of primary interest in our laboratory for several reasons. First, NK cells are a distinct subpopulation of lymphocytes that are thought to be important in the resistance to viral infections before the immunologic response of other cells can be mounted. Substantial evidence in animals supports the hypothesis that NK cells are involved in the control of experimental herpes simplex virus (HSV) and cytomegalovirus (CMV) infections (Lotzova & Herberman, 1986). For example, an enhanced susceptibility to HSV-1 has been found in mice who are selectively depleted of NK activity and receive HSV-1 simultaneously, but not in mice in which

NK cell depletion is postponed 5 days after the virus inoculation (Habu, Akamatsu, Tamaoki, & Okumura, 1984). Likewise, sensitivity to murine CMV infection increases dramatically in the absence of NK cells; whereas, if cells characteristic of NK cells are transferred, resistance to CMV can occur (Bukowski, Warner, Dennert, & Welsh, 1985). In humans with disorders such as Chediak-Higashi syndrome (Padgett, Reiquam, Henson, & Gorham, 1968), X-linked lymphoproliferative syndrome (Sullivan, Byron, Brewster, & Purtilo, 1980), or chronic fatigue syndrome (Ritz, 1989), positive correlations have been made between sensitivity to viral infections and depressed killer cell functions, although such relationships are not associated with a total loss of killer cells and may merely be coincidental with the underlying disease processes in which other immune abnormalities are also present. However, Biron, Byron, and Sullivan (1989) described a case in whom an extreme susceptibility to herpes virus infections was associated with a complete and specific loss of natural killer cells, killer cell function, and inducible killer cell activity. Together, these data support the contention that natural killer cells are an important immunologic defense against certain of the herpes viruses, but probably not against some other viruses.

REGULATION OF NATURAL KILLER CELLS

The secretion of humoral mediators or lymphokines are involved in the regulation of cell-mediated immune responses including NK activity (Dinarello & Mier, 1987; Hood, Weisman, Wood, & Wilson, 1985). These lymphokines together form a network of regulatory signals that show considerable overlap in patterns of synergism as well as antagonism. For example, the lymphokine interleukin-1 is produced by nearly all immunologic cell types including natural killer cells, T and B lymphocytes, brain astrocytes, microglia, and macrophages (Dinarello, 1986; Libby, Ordovas, Birinyi, Auger, & Dinarello, 1986; Scala, Kuang, Hall, Muchmore, & Oppenheim, 1984). Interleukin-1 serves as an endogenous adjuvant acting as a co-factor during lymphocyte activation (Dinarello & Mier, 1987) inducing the synthesis of other lymphokines and the activation of resting T cells (Kay et al., 1984; Shirakawa et al., 1986). Furthermore, IL-1 acts on natural killer cells to induce the expression of the IL-2 receptor (Lubinski et al., 1988); the binding of IL-2 by its receptor is a crucial step in the activation of the NK cell, predominantly larger granular lymphocytes, to form lymphokine-activated killers that are able to lyse a wide range of targets in a non-major histocompatibility complex restricted manner (Grimm, Mazumder, Zhang, & Rosenberg, 1982; Itoh, Tilten, Kumagai, & Balch, 1985; Kedar & Weiss, 1983; Ortaldo, Mason, & Overton, 1986).

However, in addition to the role of immune response modifiers in modulating natural killer cell activity, recent evidence demonstrates that the central nervous system also is capable of modulating natural killer cells in vivo through either the autonomic nervous system or the neuroendocrine paths.

ADVERSE LIFE EVENTS, DEPRESSION, AND NK CELL ACTIVITY

Decrements in cell-mediated immune function have been found in individuals undergoing severe adverse life events. For example, one of the most severe life events, the death of a spouse (Weiner, 1985), is associated with a suppression of lymphocyte responses to mitogenic stimulation, alterations of T cell subpopulations, and a reduction of natural killer cell activity. Suppression of lymphocyte responses to mitogenic stimulation has been demonstrated in a sample of bereaved men after the death of the spouse as compared to prebereavement baseline values (Schleifer, Keller, Camerino, Thornton, & Stein, 1983). A similar finding of reduced lymphocyte responses has been found in a cross-sectional comparison of bereaved men and women versus age- and gender-matched controls (Bartrop, Lazarus, Luckherst, & Kiloh, 1977). In our investigations of women who are undergoing bereavement, these observations have been extended to other immune parameters such as NK activity and T cell subpopulations, and the potential role of psychological processes in modulating these immune changes has been addressed (Irwin, Daniels, Bloom, Smith, & Weiner, 1987).

In the first study (Irwin et al., 1987), measures of NK activity and T cell numbers were compared among three groups of women: those whose husbands were dying of lung cancer, those whose husbands had recently died, and those whose husbands were in good health. Women who comprised the study population were free of chronic medical disorders and none were tested during the week after an episode of infectious disease. Current changes in the spousal relationship (i.e., the husband's illness or death) and other life experiences were assessed using the Social Readjustment Scale (SRS), and severity of depressive symptoms was rated using the Hamilton Depression Rating Scale (HDRS). Three groups of women were identified on the basis of SRS scores: Women whose husbands were healthy were more likely to be classified within the low SRS groups, whereas women who were anticipating or had experienced the death of their spouse were more likely to be found in the moderate or severe SRS group ($x^2 = 33.7$, $df = 4, 39$, $p < .001$). Age was not significantly different between these three groups. Severity of depressive symptoms was significantly ($p < .05$) greater in the moderate and severe SRS group as compared to that found in the low SRS group.

The immunologic evaluations demonstrated that NK activity expressed in lytic units was significantly ($p < .001$) different between the three groups; the groups with moderate and high SRS scores were found to have significantly ($p < .05$) reduced NK activity as compared to that found in the low SRS subjects (Fig. 6.1). Neither number of T helper cells, T suppressor cells, nor the ratio of T helper to T suppressor cells was significantly different between the three groups.

This cross-sectional study suggested that severity of depressive symptoms might have a role in mediating the reduction of NK activity during bereavement. Depressive symptoms as measured by the HDRS were significantly correlated with a reduction of natural killer cell activity ($r = .28$, $p < .05$). To further evaluate this relationship between depressive symptoms and reduced NK activity, a small longitudinal study was conducted in which a subset of women were followed from pre- to postbereavement, evaluating whether changes in NK activity were related to the actual

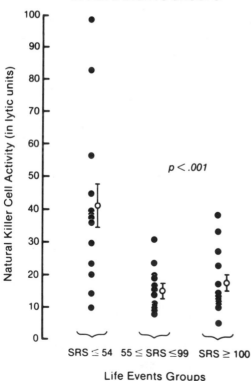

NATURAL KILLER CELL ACTIVITY IN 3 LIFE EVENTS GROUPS

FIG. 6.1. Natural killer cell activity in women with low, moderate, and high Social Readjustment Rating Scale (SRS) scores. Each point represents the individuals mean of multiple measures. (From Irwin, Daniels, Bloom et al., 1987.)

bereavement event or to changes in severity of the depressive symptoms (Irwin, Daniels, Smith, Bloom, & Weiner, 1987). Although NK activity did not significantly change in this sample of women from pre- to postbereavement, differences in the psychological response to the actual death were found between these subjects, and increases in depressive symptoms were correlated ($r = 0.89$, $p < .001$) with decreases in NK activity from pre- to postbereavement. Thus, it appears that psychological responses to the actual death, not merely the death of the spouse, serve to mediate the reduction of NK activity during bereavement.

Clinical depression has been hypothesized to share common neuroimmunologic alterations with the depressive symptoms associated with stressful life events (Irwin, Smith, & Gillin, 1987). For example, depressed patients also show a reduction in natural cytotoxicity, similar to the findings in bereaved women. In a study involving 19 age-matched pairs of men comprised of medication-free, acutely depressed patients and control subjects studied on the same day as the patient, NK activity was significantly ($p < .001$) lower in the patients hospitalized with major depressive disorders than that found in control subjects (Fig. 6.2) (Irwin, Smith, & Gillin, 1987). Together these findings demonstrate a reduction of NK activity both in severe life stress and in depression, although the mechanisms by which central nervous system processes mediate a suppression of NK activity have not yet been fully explored.

ADRENOCORTICAL ACTIVITY AND REDUCED NK ACTIVITY

One efferent pathway by which psychological processes and alterations in the brain during stress might affect immune function including NK activity

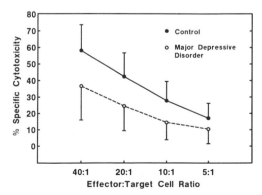

FIG. 6.2. Natural killer cell cytotoxicity in depressed subjects and controls. Each point represents the mean of the percent specific cytotoxicity ± SD ($n = 19$) for each group across the four effector to target cell ratios. (From Irwin Smith, & Gillin, 1987.)

is the activation of the adrenal cortex. Consistent with this hypothesis, extensive experimental evidence has found that *pharmacologic* doses of corticosteroid hormones are capable of reducing the lytic activity of NK cells (Cupps & Fauci, 1982). To test whether *physiologic* increases in plasma cortisol could explain the reduction of cytotoxicity in severe life stress, the relationship between plasma measures of cortisol and NK activity was examined in bereaved women (Irwin, Daniels, Risch, Bloom, & Weiner, 1988). Although bereaved women had reduced NK activity and elevated concentrations of plasma cortisol as compared to the respective mean values found in the controls, anticipatory bereaved subjects had low NK activity but cortisol levels that were similar to the plasma cortisol mean value of the controls (Fig. 6.3). Plasma cortisol was not significantly correlated with reduced NK activity in the total sample or in any of the three groups. These data, as well as those of other clinical (Kronfol & House, 1985; Kronfol, House, Silva, Greden, & Carroll, 1986) and preclinical investigations (Keller, Weiss, Schleifer, Miller & Stein, 1983), suggest that it is unlikely that stress-induced immune suppression is solely mediated by corticosteroid mechanisms and emphasize the need for further studies to clarify the role of other pathways such as the sympathetic nervous system in altering immune responses during stress.

CENTRAL MODULATION OF IMMUNE FUNCTION: ACTION OF CRF

Increased concentrations of corticotropin-releasing factor (CRF) have been found in the cerebrospinal fluid of depressed patients as compared to control subjects (Nemeroff et al., 1984), and the central release of corticotropin releasing factor might have a role in the reduction of NK activity found in depression. In other words, CRF has been postulated to be a physiological central nervous system regulator that integrates biological

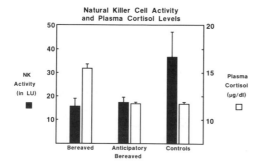

FIG. 6.3.   Natural killer cell activity and plasma cortisol levels in three groups of women: those bereaving the loss of their husbands ($n = 9$), those anticipating his death ($n = 11$), and control subjects. Range shown is mean ± SEM of multiple measures of NK activity and plasma cortisol. (From Irwin, Daniels et al., 1988.)

responses to stress (Axelrod & Reisine, 1984; Taylor & Fishman, 1988), and this neuropeptide is expected to alter not only endocrine function (Vale, Spiess, Rivier, & Rivier, 1981) but also autonomic (Brown et al., 1982) and visceral functions (Lenz, Raedler, Greten, & Brown, 1987) including immune function (Irwin, Britton, & Vale, 1987).

Although the greatest density of CRF immunoreactive cells and fibers are found in the paraventricular nucleus of the hypothalamus (Paull, Scholer, Arimura, Meyers, Chang, & Chang, 1982), immunohistochemical studies have also revealed a wide distribution of CRF throughout the brain (Bloom, Battenberg, Rivier, & Vale, 1982; Olschowka, O'Donohue, Mueller, & Jacobowitz, 1982; Olschowka, O'Donohue, Mueller, & Jacobowitz, 1982; Swanson, Sawchenko, Rivier, & Vale, 1983). Furthermore, CRF receptors have been autoradiographically mapped to a number of other extrahypothalamic structures related to the limbic system and control of the autonomic nervous system (DeSouza, Perrin, Insel, Rivier, Vale, & Kuhar, 1984; Wynn, Hauger, Holmes, Millan, Aguilera, 1984). Thus, in addition to its well-established role as a hypothalamic regulator of the pituitary secretion of adrenocorticotrophic hormone (ACTH) and beta-endorphin (Vale et al., 1981), CRF also acts directly in the central nervous system at extrahypothalamic sites. Correspondingly, studies have shown that exogenous CRF administered to animals induces a number of changes in brain function; intraventricular CRF increases the firing rate of the locus ceruleus (Valentino, Foote, & Aston-Jones, 1983), activates the autonomic nervous system as reflected by increased plasma concentrations of norepinephrine and epinephrine (Fisher, Rivier, Rivier, Spiess, Vale, & Brown, 1982), and produces a pattern of behavioral responses such as decreased feeding and increased locomotor activity (Britton, Koob, & Rivier, 1982; Sherman & Kalin, 1985; Sutton, Koob, LeMoal, Rivier, & Vale, 1982).

In an attempt to understand the central processes involved in the pathogenesis of immune impairment that is associated with depression and stress, we postulated that the central release of CRF might affect immune function, in addition to its regulatory effects on other visceral functions. Consistent with that hypothesis, intraventricular CRF has been found to be involved in the regulation of NK activity in the rat. Our data have demonstrated that central administration of CRF produces a dose-dependent suppression of NK activity that appears specific and independent of direct systemic mechanisms.

Dose Response Profile of Intraventricular CRF

Using doses of CRF that produce behavioral, pituitary, and autonomic actions similar to the responses found in animals subjected to some types of stressors, the effect of intraventricular CRF on rat splenic NK activity has been examined (Irwin, Britton, & Vale, 1987). Measurement of NK activity was carried out 1 hour after intraventricular infusion; a time interval found to result in maximal increases in locomotor activity, in plasma norepinephrine, and in corticosterone levels. Administration of intraventricular CRF under these conditions produced a dose-dependent reduction of NK activity across three CRF doses (0.1, 0.5, 1.0 ug) ($F = 11.4$, $df = 3,74$, $p < .001$) (Fig. 6.4), with the highest dose of intraventricular CRF (1.0 ug) significantly ($p < .05$) decreasing splenic NK activity to $74 \pm 3.1\%$ of the saline-treated group. Although this finding demonstrated that CRF is capable of modulating immune function in vivo, it was not known whether the action of intraventricular CRF was due to a central effect of the neuropeptide or a consequence of CRF being distributed from the brain into the peripheral circulation to act directly on lymphocytes.

Lack of Direct Systemic Action of CRF

To test whether CRF might have a direct peripheral action on NK cells that contributed to the immunosuppressive effect of centrally administered

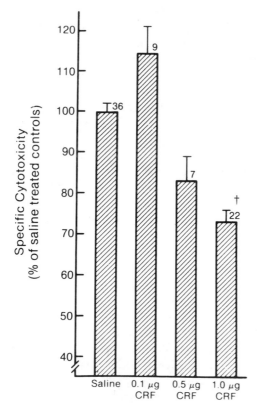

FIG. 6.4. Effect of central administration of CRF on splenic NK cytotoxic activity (expressed as mean percentage ± SEM of saline-treated controls) (+) significantly ($p < .05$) different from saline group. The number of rats in each group is indicated next to the standard error bars. (From Irwin, Britton, Vale, 1987.)

doses, additional experiments were conducted involving the subcutaneous administration of CRF in three doses, 5.0-, 10.0-, and 20.0 ug/kg. Although it is difficult to equate the dose administered peripherally with that given centrally, the lowest systemic dose of 5.0 ug/kg is roughly equivalent per rat to the 1.0 ug ICV-CRF dose and the 20 ug/kg systemic CRF dose represents about 6.0 ug per rat. Thus, if 5.0 ug/kg CRF administered systemically has a similar immunosuppressive effect as that found following central CRF (1.0 ug-ICV), then CRF given centrally might be crossing the blood–brain barrier to act peripherally on the natural killer cell. However, the 5.0 ug/kg dose of CRF administered subcutaneously had no significant effect upon natural killer cell activity. Thus, subcutaneous CRF even in high doses did not appear to significantly alter NK activity.

The potential effect of CRF on lymphocytes was further examined by incubating rat splenic lymphocytes for 1 hour in vitro with CRF at a range of concentrations from 10^{-6} M to 10^{-12} M. Across the range of CRF concentrations, NK activity was similar to the values found in untreated cells, a result demonstrated in three separate experiments. Consistent with the finding of a lack of effect of CRF on NK cells are CRF receptor data; binding of CRF on purified lymphocyte preparations has not been found even though CRF receptors have been identified on monocytes (Webster, Tracey, Jutila, Wolfe, and de Souza, 1990).

Thus, these findings indicate that the direct application of CRF does not acutely reduce NK activity, and further that CRF is unlikely to cross the blood–brain barrier in doses sufficient to alter cytotoxicity. Together, these findings support the hypothesis that the immunosuppressive effect of CRF is centrally mediated and independent of direct systemic mechanisms.

CENTRAL SPECIFICITY OF CRF ACTION

The immunosuppressive effect of centrally administered exogenous CRF may be due to the nonspecific effects of the neuropeptide. To address the specificity of central CRF, the CRF antagonist alpha-helical$_{9-41}$ was coadministered with CRF in a series of experiments. In one set of experiments, the CRF antagonist was administered centrally either alone or in combination with intraventricular CRF. In another group of rats, the antagonist was injected peripherally followed by a central dose of CRF.

In rats that received *intraventricular* CRF and coadministration of the CRF antagonist, values of NK activity were comparable to those observed in saline-treated rats. In contrast, when a *systemic* dose of the antagonist (0.5 mg/kg body weight) was coadministered with intraventricular CRF (1.0 ug), values of NK activity were significantly ($p < .05$) lower than those in saline-treated controls (Fig. 6.5). Thus, central administration of the CRF

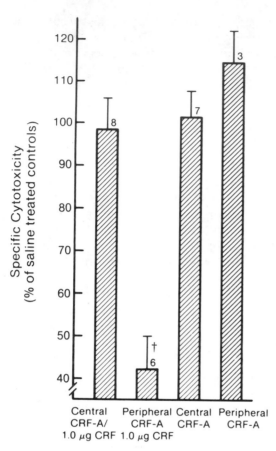

FIG. 6.5. Central antagonism of the effect of intraventricularly administered CRF on NK cytotoxicity (expressed as mean percentage ± SEM of saline-treated controls). Rats were injected either ICV or systemically with the CRF antagonist immediately before central administration of CRF. The number of rats in each group is indicated next to the vertical standard error bars. NK activity in the systemic CRF antagonist/CRF-treated group was significantly ($p < .05$) lower than that in the saline-, antagonist alone, or central antagonist/CRF-treated groups. (From Irwin, Britton, & Vale, 1987.)

antagonist significantly attenuated the action of central CRF, whereas systemic administration of the CRF antagonist failed to alter the suppression of NK activity induced by central CRF. These data have suggested that the action of CRF is a receptor-mediated phenomenon in which CRF binds a specific receptor in the brain to induce a suppression of NK activity.

NEURAL INFLUENCES ON THE IMMUNE RESPONSE: ROLE OF THE AUTONOMIC NERVOUS SYSTEM

Because central administration of CRF produces an acute decrease in splenic NK activity, a preclinical model is available to study the relationship between central processes and immune cells via efferent outflow pathways of either the neuroendocrine or the autonomic nervous systems. In regard to the autonomic nervous system, neuroanatomic studies have suggested that it is likely to serve as a pathway for communication from the brain to cells of the immune system (Livnat, Felten, Carlton, Bellinger, & Felten, 1985). Nervous fibers are distributed throughout the lymphoid tissues including both primary (thymus, bone marrow) (Bulloch & Moore, 1981; Walcott & McLean, 1985) and secondary (spleen, lymph nodes) organs (Livnat et al., 1985; Felten et al., 1988), and are localized in the vasculature and parenchyma of these tissues. Fluorescent histochemical techniques have revealed abundant linear and varicose fibers that branch into areas of lymphocytes in the mouse spleen, and as visualized in recent electromicrograms, terminate on T lymphocytes (Felten, Felten, Bellinger, Carlson, Ackerman, et al., 1988). Thus, regions of lymphoid tissue in which lymphocytes reside receive direct nervous innervation by fibers containing predominantly norepinephrine.

Lymphocytes have receptors that bind monoamines, including norepinephrine, and are thus capable of receiving signals from the sympathetic neurons innervating lymphoid tissue (Hadden, Hadden, & Middleton, 1970; Hall & Goldstein, 1981, 1985). Furthermore, stimulation of lymphocytes by these agonists regulate immune responses, probably via changes in intracellular cyclic AMP (Bourne et al., 1974; Strom, Lundin, & Carpenter, 1977; Watson, 1975). Finally, direct in vitro application of norepinephrine at concentrations of 10^{-6} to 10^{-8} M reduces NK activity and this reduction of NK activity following administration of a beta agonist is antagonized by preincubation with a beta antagonist propranolol (Hellstrand, Hermodsson, & Strannegard, 1985). In summary, the concept has emerged that beta adrenoreceptor binding mediates an inhibition of NK activity.

Autonomic Nervous System Mediation of CRF Suppression

The role of the autonomic nervous system in mediating CRF-induced suppression of NK cytotoxicity was first explored (Irwin, Hauger, Brown, & Britton, 1988) using the peripheral ganglionic blocker chlorisondamine. Chlorisondamine administered to animals who received intraventricular CRF significantly antagonized ($p < .05$) CRF-induced elevations of plasma concentrations of norepinephrine and epinephrine, and completely abolished the immunosuppressive effect of CRF on NK activity (Fig. 6.6). Together these findings suggest that ganglionic blockade is capable of antagonizing the action of central CRF and, second, that autonomic activation is one pathway that communicates the action of CRF in the brain to the immune system.

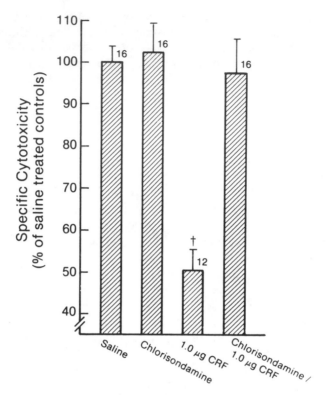

FIG. 6.6.   Effect of ganglionic blockade with chlorisondamine (3 mg/kg IP 60 min before ICV injection) on corticotropin releasing factor (CRF, 1.0 ug ICV)-induced suppression of NK cytotoxicity (expressed as mean percent ± SE of saline-treated controls). (+) Significantly ($p < .001$) different from saline group. Number of rats in each group is indicated next to SE bars. (From Irwin, Hauger et al., 1988.)

NEUROENDOCRINE OUTFLOW AND CRF ACTION

The other major efferent through which CRF might act to suppress NK activity is the pituitary-adrenal axis. To separate the influence of sympathetic activation from the effects due to CRF-induced secretion of ACTH and corticosterone, additional studies have involved the concurrent measurement of NK activity and these neuroendocrine hormones in CRF-treated rats with and without chlorisondamine pretreatment (Irwin, Hauger et al., 1988). Again, although chlorisondamine significantly antagonized CRF suppression of NK activity, it did not significantly attenuate CRF-induced elevations of plasma levels of ACTH and corticosterone. Plasma concentrations of ACTH and corticosterone in rats treated with both CRF and chlorisondamine were comparable to those found in rats treated with CRF alone. Thus, both CRF treatment groups with and without ganglionic blockade demonstrated a significant activation of the pituitary-adrenal axis, whereas only treatment with CRF alone suppressed NK activity. Additional experiments have further suggested that the increased secretion of glucocorticoids does not significantly contribute to CRF suppression of NK cytotoxicity. Intraventricular CRF administered to animals in whom synthesis of corticosterone was blocked pharmacologically by preadministering metyrapone and aminoglutethimide before CRF infusion showed a reduction of NK activity comparable to that in animals who had not undergone similar blockade of glucocorticoid synthesis. Together these data suggest that the immunosuppressive effect of central CRF is dissociated from the activation of the pituitary-adrenal axis.

These data, evaluating the role of the autonomic nervous system and neuroendocrine systems in mediating the effects of CRF, demonstrated that the autonomic nervous system is a salient efferent pathway by which CRF suppresses NK activity; blockade of this outflow completely antagonized the action of CRF. Second, CRF immunosuppression appeared independent of the activation of the pituitary gland. Significant increases of plasma levels of these hormones occurred without necessarily reducing NK activity.

SUMMARY

Clinical studies have clarified that a reduction of immune function is associated with psychological processes in persons undergoing severe, adverse life events. In addition, reduced NK activity is correlated with the severity of depressive symptoms in both stressed persons and depressed patients. Based on our interest in understanding the link between the central nervous system and immune function, our clinical research has been extended to an animal model that involves the central administration of CRF. Intraventricular CRF has been found to reduce NK activity in addition to its abilities to coordinate a pattern of behavioral, pituitary, and autonomic responses similar to those found in animals exposed to some types of stressors. Central action of CRF, together with the finding that ganglionic blockade completely antagonizes the suppression of NK activity induced by CRF, provide direct evidence that changes in the brain are communicated to NK cells via the autonomic nervous system.

ACKNOWLEDGMENTS

This work was partly supported by NIMH grants #MH44275-01, MH30914, the San Diego VA Clinical Research Center on Alcoholism, and a VA Merit Review.

The work described in "Depression and Immunity: Central Corticotropin Releasing Factor Activates the Autonomic Nervous System and Reduces Natural Killer Cell Activity" was done as part of our employment with the federal government and is therefore in the public domain. Parts of this chapter have been previously published.

REFERENCES

Axelrod, J., & Reisine, T. D. (1984). Stress hormones: Their interaction and regulation. *Science, 224,* 452.

Bartrop, R. W., Lazarus, L., Luckherst, E., & Kiloh, L. G. (1977). Depressed lymphocyte function after bereavement. *Lancet, 1,* 834–836.

Biron, C. A., Byron, K. S., & Sullivan, J. L. (1989). Severe herpes virus infections in an adolescent without natural killer cells. *New England Journal of Medicine, 320,* 1732–1735.

Bloom, F. E., Battenberg, E. L., Rivier, J., & Vale, W. (1982). CRF: Immunoreactive neurons and fibers in the rat hypothalamus. *Regulatory Peptides, 4,* 43–48.

Bourne, H. R., Lichtenstein, L. M., Melmon, K., Henney, C. S., Weinstein, Y., & Shearer, G. M. (1974). Modulation of inflammation and immunity by cyclic AMP. *Science, 184,* 19–28.

Britton, K. T., Koob, G. F., & Rivier, J. (1982). ICV-CRF enhanced behavioral effects of novelty. *Life Sciences, 31,* 363–367.

Brown, M. R., Fisher, L. A., Spiess, J., Rivier, C., Rivier, J., & Vale, W. (1982). Corticotropin releasing factor: actions on the sympathetic nervous system and metabolism. *Endocrinology, 111,* 928–931.

Bukowski, J. F., Warner, J. F., Dennert, G., & Welsh, R. M. (1985). Adoptive transfer studies demonstrating the antiviral affect of natural killer cells in vivo. *Journal of Experimental Medicine, 131,* 1531–1538.

Bulloch, K., & Moore, R. Y. (1981). Innervation of the thymus gland by brainstem and spinal cord in the mouse and rat. *American Journal of Anatomy, 162,* 157–166.

Cupps, T. R., & Fauci, A. S. (1982). Corticosteroid-mediated immunoregulation in man. *Immunological Reviews, 65,* 133–155.

DeSouza, E. B., Perrin, M. H., Insel, T. R., Rivier, C., Vale, W., & Kuhar, M. (1984). CRF receptors in rat forebrain: autoradiographic identification. *Science, 224,* 1449–1451.

Dinarello, C. A. (1986). Interleukin-1: amino acid sequences, multiple biological activities and comparison with tumor necrosis factor (cachectin). *Year of Immunology, 2,* 68–89.

Dinarello, C. A., & Mier, J. W. (1987). Medical intelligence: Current concepts: Lymphokines. *New England Journal of Medicine, 317,*(156), 940–945.

Felten, S. Y., Felten, D. C., Bellinger, D. C., Carlson, S. L., Ackerman, K. D., Modden, K. S., Olschowka, J. A., & Livnat, S. (1988). Noradrenergic sympathetic innervation of lymphoid organs. *Progress in Allergy, 43,* 14–36.

Fisher, L. A., Rivier, J., Rivier, C., Spiess, J., Vale, W. W., & Brown, M. R. (1982). CRF: Central effects on mean arterial pressure and heart rate in rats. *Endocrinology, 11,* 2222–2224.

Grimm, E. A., Mazumder, A., Zhang, H. Z., & Rosenberg, S. A. (1982). Lymphokine-activated killer cell phenomenon I. Lysis of natural killer resistant fresh solid tumor cells by interleukin-2 activated autologous human peripheral blood lymphocytes. *Journal of Experimental Medicine, 155,* 1823.

Habu, S., Akamatsu, K., Tamaoki, N., & Okumura, K. (1984). In vivo significance of NK cells on resistance against virus (HSV-1) infections in mice. *Journal of Immunology, 133,* 2743–2747.

Hadden, J. W., Hadden, E. M., & Middleton, E. (1970). Lymphocyte host transformation I. Demonstration of adrenergic receptors in human peripheral lymphocytes. *Journal of Cellular Immunology, 1,* 583–595.

Hall, N. R., & Goldstein, A. L. (1981). Neurotransmitters and the immune system. In R. Ader (Ed.), *Psychoneuroimmunology* (pp. 521–544). New York: Academic Press.

Hall, N. R., & Goldstein, A. L. (1985). Neurotransmitters and host defense. In R. Guillemin, M. Cohn, & T. Melnechuk (Eds.), *Neural modulation of immunity* (pp. 143–154). New York: Raven Press.

Hellstrand, K., Hermodsson, S., & Strannegard, O. (1985). Evidence for a beta-adrenoceptor mediated regulation of human natural killer cells. *Journal of Immunology, 134,* 4095–4099.

Hood, L. E., Weisman, I. L., Wood, H. B., & Wilson, J. H. (1985). *Immunology.* Menlo Park, CA: Benjamin Cummings.

Irwin, M. R., Britton, K. T., & Vale, W. (1987). Central corticotropin releasing factor suppresses natural killer cell activity. *Brain Behavior and Immunity, 1,* 81–87.

Irwin, M., Daniels, M., Bloom, E., Smith, T. L., & Weiner, H. (1987). Life events, depressive symptoms and immune function. *American Journal of Psychiatry, 144,* 437–441.

Irwin, M., Daniels, M., Risch, S. C., Bloom, E., & Weiner, H. (1988). Plasma cortisol and natural killer cell activity during bereavement. *Biological Psychiatry, 24,* 173–178.

Irwin, M. R., Daniels, M., Smith, T. L., Bloom, E., & Weiner, H. (1987). Impaired natural killer cell activity during bereavement. *Brain Behavior and Immunity, 1,* 98–104.

Irwin, M. R., Hauger, R. L., Brown, M. R., & Britton, K. T. (1988). Corticotropin-releasing factor activates the autonomic nervous system and reduces natural cytotoxicity. *American Journal of Physiology: Integrative and Regulatory Mechanisms, 255,* R744–747.

Irwin, M., Smith, T. L., & Gillin, J. C. (1987). Reduced natural killer cytotoxicity in depressed patients. *Life Sciences, 41,* 2127–2133.

Itoh, K., Tilten, B., Kumagai, K., & Balch, C. M. (1985). Leu-11 + lymphocytes with natural killer activity are precursors of recombinant interleukin-2 induced activated killer cells. *Journal of Immunology, 134,* 802.

Kay, J. S., Gillis, S., Mizel, S. B., Shevach, E. M., Malek, T. R., Dinarello, C. A., Lachman, L. B., & Janeway, C. A. (1984). Growth of cloned helper T cell line induced by a monoclonal antibody specific for the antigen receptor: interleukin-1 is required for the expression of the receptors for interleukin-2. *Journal of Immunology, 133,* 1339.

Kedar, E., & Weiss, D. W. (1983). The in vitro generation of effector lymphocytes and their employment in tumor immunotherapy. *Advances in Cancer Research, 38,* 171.

Keller, S., Weiss, J. M., Schleifer, S. J., Miller, N. E., & Stein, M. (1983). Stress-induced suppression of immunity in adrenalectomized rats. *Science, 221,* 1301–1304.

Kronfol, Z., & House, J. D. (1985). Depression, hypothalamic-pituitary adrenocortical activity and lymphocyte function. *Psychopharmacology Bulletin, 21,* 476–478.

Kronfol, Z., House, J. D., Silva, J., Greden, J., & Carroll, B. J. (1986). Depression, urinary free cortisol excretion, and lymphocyte function. *British Journal of Psychiatry, 148,* 70–73.

Lenz, H. J., Raedler, A., Greten, H., & Brown, M. R. (1987). CRF initiates biological action within the brain that are observed in response to stress. *American Journal of Physiology, 252,* 34–39.

Libby, P., Ordovas, J. M., Birinyi, L. K., Auger, K. R., & Dinarello, C. A. (1986). Inducible interleukin-1 gene expression in human vascular smooth muscle cells. *Journal of Clinical Investigation, 78,* 1432–1438.

Livnat, S., Felten, S. J., Carlton, S. L., Bellinger, D. L., & Felten, D. L. (1985). Involvement of peripheral and central catecholamine systems in neural-immune interactions. *Neuroimmunology, 10,* 5–30.

Lotzova, E., & Herberman, R. B. (1986). *Immunobiology of NK cells II.* Boca Raton, FL: CRC Press.

Lubinski, J., Fong, T. C., Babbitt, J. T., Ransone, L., Yodoi, J. J., & Bloom, E. T. (1988). Increased binding of IL-2 and increased IL-2 receptor mRNA synthesis are expressed by an NK-like cell line in response to IL-1. *Journal of Immunology, 140,* 1903-1909.

Nemeroff, C. B., Widerlov, E., Bissette, G., Walleus, H., Karlsson, I., Eklund, K., Kilts, C. D., Loosen, P. T., & Vale, W. (1984). Elevated concentrations of CSF corticotropin-releasing-factor-like immunoreactivity in depressed patients. *Science, 226,* 1342-1344.

Olschowka, J. A., O'Donohue, T. L., Mueller, G. P., & Jacobowitz, D. M. (1982). The distribution of corticotropin releasing factor-like immunoreactivity neurons in rat brain. *Peptides, 3,* 995-1015.

Olschowka, J. A., O'Donohue, T. L., Mueller, G. P., & Jacobowitz, D. M. (1982). Hypothalamic and extrahypothalamic distribution of CRF-like immunoreaction neurons in the rat brain. *Neuroendocrinology, 35,* 305-308.

Ortaldo, J. O., Mason, A., & Overton, R. (1986). Lymphokine-activated killer cells. Analysis of progenitors and effectors. *Journal of Experimental Medicine, 165,* 1193.

Padgett, G. A., Reiquam, C. W., Henson, J. B., & Gorham, J. R. (1968). Comparative studies of susceptibility to infection in the Chediak-Higashi syndrome. *Journal of Pathology and Bacteriology, 95,* 509-522.

Paull, W. K., Scholer, J., Arimura, A., Meyers, C. A., Chang, J. K., & Chang, D. (1982). Immunocytochemical localization of CRF in the ovine hypothalamus. *Peptides i* 3(2):183-191.

Ritz, J. (1989). The role of natural killer cells in immune surveillance. *New England Journal of Medicine, 320,* 1748-1749.

Scala, G., Kuang, Y. D., Hall, R. E., Muchmore, A. V., & Oppenheim, J. J. (1984). Accessory cell function of human B cells I. Production of both interleukin-1-like-activity and an interleukin-1-inhibitory factor (cachectin). *Journal of Experimental Medicine, 159,* 1637-52.

Schleifer, S. J., Keller, S. E., Camerino, M., Thornton, J. C., & Stein, M. M. (1983). Suppression of lymphocyte stimulation following bereavement. *Journal of the American Medical Association, 250,* 374-377.

Sherman, J. E., & Kalin, N. H. (1985). ICV-CRH potently affects behavior without altering antinociceptive responding. *Life Sciences, 39,* 433-441.

Shirakawa, F., Tanaka, Y., Eto, S., Suzuki, H., Yodoi, J., & Yamashita, U. (1986). Effect of interleukin-1 on the expression of interleukin-2 receptor (Tac antigen) on human natural killer cells and natural killer-like cell line (YT cells). *Journal of Immunology, 137,* 551.

Strom, T. D., Lundin, A. P., & Carpenter, C. B. (1977). Role of cyclic nucleotides in lymphocytes activation and function. *Progress in Clinical Immunology, 3,* 115-153.

Sullivan, J. L., Byron, K. S., Brewster, F. E., & Purtilo, D. T. (1980). Deficient natural killer activity in X-linked lymphoproliferative syndrome. *Science, 210,* 535-535.

Sutton, R. E., Koob, G. F., LeMoal, M., Rivier, J., & Vale, W. (1982). Corticotropin releasing factor produces behavioral activation in rats. *Nature, 297,* 331-333.

Swanson, L. W., Sawchenko, P. E., Rivier, J., & Vale, W. W. (1983). The organization of ovine corticotropin releasing factor (CRF). *Neuroendocrinology, 36,* 165-186.

Taylor, A. I., & Fishman, L. M. (1988). Corticotropin releasing hormone. *New England Journal of Medicine, 319,* 213-222.

Vale, W., Spiess, J., Rivier, C., & Rivier, J. (1981). Characterization of a 41-residue ovine hypothalamic peptide that stimulates secretion of corticotropin and beta-endorphin. *Science, 213,* 1394-1397.

Valentino, R. J., Foote, S. L., & Aston-Jones, G. (1983). CRF activates noradrenergic neurons of the locus coeruleus. *Brain Research, 270,* 363-367.

Walcott, B., & McLean, J. R. (1985). Catecholamine containing neurons and lymphoid cells in a lacrimal gland of the pigeon. *Brain Research, 328,*(1) 129-137.

Watson, J. J. (1975). The influence of intracellular levels of cyclic nucleotides on cell proliferation and the induction of antibody synthesis. *Experimental Medicine, 141,* 97–111.

Webster, E. L., Tracey, D. E., Jutila, M. A., Wolfe, S. A., & deSouza, E. B. (1990). Corticotropin-releasing factor receptors in mouse spleen: Identification of receptor-bearing cells as resident macrophages. *Endocrinology, 127,* 440–452.

Weiner, H. (1991). The behavioral biology of stress and psychosomatic medicine. In M. R. Brown, G. F. Koob, C. Rivier (Eds.), *Stress: Neurobiology and Neuroendocrinology* (pp. 23–51). New York: Dekker.

Wynn, P. C., Hauger, R. L., Holmes, M. C., Millan, M. A., Catt, K. J., & Aguilera, G. (1984). Brain and pituitary receptors for corticotropin releasing factor's localization and differential regulation after adrenalectomy. *Peptides, 5,* 1077–1084.

7 Chronic Fatigue Syndrome and Psychoneuroimmunology

Nancy Klimas
Miami Veterans Administration Medical Center;
University of Miami Medical School

Robert Morgan, Fernando Salvato, Flavia Van Riel,
Carrie Millon, and Mary Ann Fletcher
University of Miami Medical School

Chronic fatigue syndrome was defined clinically by a Centers for Disease Control committee only recently (Holmes et al., 1988). Somewhat earlier Straus et al. (1985) employed the term Chronic Epstein-Barr Virus Syndrome to essentially the same disorder. This syndrome is of uncertain etiology—but may have relevance to the field of psychoneuroimmunology. As its immunologic abnormalities are better understood, and the psychosocial and psychoneurologic ramifications described, the possibility of psychoneuroimmunologic pathways in the both the etiology and persistence of this illness should be entertained. Further, behavioral interventions may have a place in treatment.

VIROLOGY

The etiology of chronic fatigue syndrome is not yet established. However, there is support for a role of chronic virus reactivation, particularly herpesviruses, in the clinical symptomatology and chronicity of this syndrome. Reactivation of Epstein-Barr virus and human herpesvirus-6, both ubiquitous viruses with very high prevalence of viral infection in the population, was reported to occur with regularity in chronic fatigue syndrome, and antibodies to these viruses were used as markers for the syndrome (Jones & Straus, 1987; Niederman, Chun-Ren, Kaplan, & Brown, 1988; Straus et al., 1985; Ablashi, et al., 1987).

Following primary infection with a virus of the herpes family, the intact immune system usually fails to eliminate the virus, but can restrict it to a latent state. Persistence of this state requires that some cellular responses must persist and remain vigilant. This long-term memory was demonstrable in T lymphocytes, which exhibited human histocompatibility antigen class I restricted killing and prevented proliferation of Epstein-Barr virus-infected B cells (Jones & Straus, 1987). Nonclass I restricted natural killer cells were shown to contribute to the inhibition of Epstein-Barr virus-induced B cell transformation in vitro (Grazia-Masucci, Bejarano, Masucci, & Klein, 1987). However, this virus in the chronic state has been associated with a wide spectrum of benign to malignant illnesses including nasopharyngeal carcinoma, Burkitt's lymphoma, X-linked lymphoproliferative disorders, and B cell lymphomas that evolve in the settings of primary or secondary immune deficiency states (Epstein & Achong, 1979). A majority of patients with chronic fatigue syndrome were reported to have values for Epstein-Barr virus-specific antibody tests that were different from those of healthy control subjects (Holmes et al., 1987; Jones et al., 1985; Straus et al., 1985; Tobi & Straus, 1985). Frequently, high geometric mean titers of antibodies to both viral capsid antigen and early antigen, and the lack of antibodies to the nuclear antigen (Jones et al., 1985; Straus et al., 1985) were noted. This pattern of elevated Epstein-Barr virus-specific antibodies is suggestive of virus reactivation, rather than primary infection.

The newly recognized human herpesvirus-6 also was reported to infect B cells, but in contrast to the restricted B cell tropism of Epstein-Barr virus, was found to infect T cells in various states of differentiation, megakaryocytes and glioblastoma cells (Lopez, et al., 1988; Lusso et al., 1987; Markhan, 1987). The primary infection in humans probably occurs early in life, and may be associated with roseola infantum, as well as with a mild afebrile illness in adults. A recent report from London noted that the prevalence of anti-human herpesvirus-6 rose to 63% by 11 months of age (Briggs, Fox, & Tedder, 1988). Thus, human herpesvirus-6 may well be a very common infection or co-infection in the population of chronic fatigue syndrome patients, although prevalence studies have been limited due to the lack of widely available serologic testing materials. However, Salahuddin et al. (1986) described, in lymphocyte cultures of cells from patients with human herpesvirus-6, a pathonomonic large granular cell. We noted this cell type in approximately 30% of cultures of lymphocytes from these patients ($n = 58$) (Salvato, Klimas, Ashman, & Fletcher, 1988; Tarsis, Klimas, Baron, Ashman, & Fletcher, 1988).

In addition to Epstein-Barr and human herpesvirus-6, other viruses have been linked to chronic fatigue, including herpes simplex virus (Types 1 and 2), measles, and cytomegalovirus (Holmes et al., 1987). Dual infection with Epstein-Barr virus and Type 2 adenovirus was reported (Okano et al. 1988). More recently, DeFreitas and Hilliard (1990) reported finding evidence of antibody to human T cell leukemia virus, Type II, defined proteins by

Western blot analysis. They also reported evidence for nucleic acids related to this retrovirus in the lymphocytes from chronic fatigue syndrome patients using the technique of polymerase chain reaction. In contrast, we tested serum from 77 patients and found no evidence by either enzyme-linked immunoassay or by Western blot for antibodies to this retrovirus (Klimas, unpublished observation). The preponderance of evidence to date indicates, as with Epstein-Barr and human herpesvirus-6, a lack of correlation between any one of these proposed etiologic agents and the clinical status of the patients. More probable is the hypothesis that reactivation of not one but several viruses is involved in the development of fatigue, myalgia, and the many other clinical symptoms of the syndrome and that this reactivation occurs because of the onset of immunologic dysfunctions. Of course, a possible explanation of the immune abnormalities is that patients with chronic fatigue syndrome are infected with an unknown lymphotropic virus.

IMMUNOLOGY

A typical and common finding in patients who meet the clinical definition has been the presence of immunologic impairment (Caliguri et al. 1987; Klimas, Salvato, Morgan, & Fletcher, 1990; Lloyd, Wakefield, Boughton, & Dwyer, 1989). Depressed cellular immunity as evidenced by poor in vitro lymphocyte response to exogenous stimuli such as the mitogens, phytohemagglutinin, and pokeweed, and by in vivo skin test response to recall antigens was reported in cohorts of chronic fatigue syndrome patients (Klimas et al., 1990; Lloyd et al., 1989). Caliguri et al. (1987) reported a lower number of natural killer (NK) cells as defined by co-expression of surface markers CD56+CD3+ and a decreased function of NK cells in patients with chronic fatigue syndrome. Kibler, Lucas, Hicks, Poulos, and Jones (1985) found diminished in vitro production of gamma interferon and interleukin-2 by in vitro stimulated lymphocytes, as well as diminished NK cell cytotoxicity in 13 patients diagnosed as having Chronic Epstein-Barr Virus Syndrome. However, Borysiewicz et al. (1986) described a normal NK cell activity in their patients, but a reduced specific T cell activity against Epstein-Barr virus. We reported low levels of NK cell activity with a low value of kinetic lytic units per NK cell but a normal to elevated number of effector cells, as measured by the surface expression of CD56 antigen (Klimas et al., 1990; Salvato et al., 1988; Tarsis et al., 1987).

Poor NK cell function may be related to another finding by this laboratory, the impaired ability of lymphocytes from these patients to produce gamma interferon in response to mitogenic stimulation (Klimas et al., 1990). Inability of lymphocytes to produce gamma interferon might represent a cellular exhaustion as a consequence of persistent viral stimulus, a theory that is supported by the elevation of leukocyte 2'5' oligoadenylate synthetase (Straus et al., 1985), an interferon-induced enzyme in lymphocytes of chronic fatigue syndrome patients. In addition to their anti-viral properties, interferons are potent cytokines or immunoregulatory substances. Gamma interferon was reported to enhance both cellular antigen presentation to lymphocytes (Zlotnick, Shimonkewitz, Gefter, Kappler, & Marrack, 1983) and NK cell cytotoxicity (Targan & Stebbing, 1982), as well as to inhibit suppressor T lymphocyte activity (Knop, Stremmer, Neumann, De Maeyer, & Macher, 1982). The lack of gamma interferon production may be responsible for the impaired activation of immunoregulatory circuits, which would, in turn, facilitate the reactivation and progression of viral infections. Gold and co-workers reported the paradoxical finding of decreased gamma interferon but elevated NK cell activity in 24 fatigued patients (Gold et al., 1990). However, in this cohort only 6 met the Centers for Disease Control clinical definition of chronic fatigue syndrome (Holmes et al., 1988).

There have been reports, including ones from this laboratory (Klimas et al., 1990; Salvato et al., 1988; Tarsis et al., 1987), of alterations in the distribution of various T and B cell subsets. In reference to T cell subsets, CD4 (T helper/inducer) and CD8 (T suppressor/cytotoxic), discrepant results have been reported. Straus et al. (1985) reported a statistically higher percentage of CD4 lymphocytes with a normal number of CD8 cells and CD4/CD8 ratio, but Jones et al. (1985) found normal percentages of CD4 and CD8 as well as normal CD4/CD8 ratio. Our laboratory found that most chronic fatigue syndrome subjects studied had a normal number of CD4 cells and an elevation in CD8 (Klimas et al., 1990). These conflicting results among laboratories studying the syndrome may be due to the fluctuation and oscillation in the clinical manifestations of these patients, and the time at which the lymphocytes were obtained. The increase or decrease in a particular subset may represent different stages in the evolution of this syndrome. Results from this laboratory (Klimas et al., 1990; Salvato et al. 1988) indicated an elevation of numbers of several other immunocytes in chronic fatigue syndrome patients. B cells were elevated as were B cells co-expressing the CD5 marker, a subset associated with dysfunctional B cell regulation and with autoimmune disorders (Hayakawa et al., 1984). Increased numbers of T cells expressing the activation marker, CD26 were observed. This subset of T cells is thought to represent activated memory T cells — cells that stimulate B cells to produce antibody in response to antigen. Cells of this phenotype are elevated in multiple sclerosis (Hafler et al., 1985). A portion of the increase in CD8 cells that we observed in these patients was due to an increased number of CD8 cells expressing the Class II antigen marker, a finding confirmed by Levy (1990). The lymphocyte subset of I2 + CD8 + cells has been reported elevated in individuals infected with retroviruses, and may represent cytotoxic T cells (Fletcher et al., 1989). One category that was significantly lower in CFS was a subset of CD4 cells, CD4 + CD45RA +, with the majority of patients having absolute counts greater than 1 *SD* below the mean of healthy controls. Franco et al. (1987) described a decrease in the number of CD4 + CD45RA + lymphocytes in two patients with severe chronic active Epstein Barr virus infection, with one of the patients showing a persistent diminished number of cells despite clinical improvement with the treatment using Interleukin-2. These CD4 cells were identified as the inducer subset, and may activate both T suppressor and T cytotoxic cells (Morimoto, Letvin, Distato, Aldrich, & Schlossman, 1985). Recent publications associated alterations in this subset with a number of clinical entities. A selective depletion of CD4 + CD45RA + cells was noted during the active phases of multiple sclerosis (Rose, Ginsberg, Rothstein, Ledbetter, & Clark, 1988), but not in patients with remissions or inactive multiple sclerosis or other neurological disease (Rose et al., 1985). This particular T cell subset deficiency was also found in systemic lupus erythematosus (Morimoto et al., 1980; Sato et al., 1987) and rheumatoid arthritis (Emery, Gently, Mackay, Muirden, & Rouley, 1987). All of the pathologies just mentioned were postulated to be T cell-mediated autoimmune processes, in which a derangement in immunoregulation was present. A shift in T cell immunoregulatory functions, in part as a consequence of the diminished number of CD4 + CD45RA + lymphocyte, was proposed as a possible etiologic factor in the development of autoimmune diseases (Alpert, Koide, Takada, & Engleman, 1987). Chronic fatigue syndrome patients present also with a pattern of immune dysregulation. A potentially down-regulating subset of T cells, CD4 + CD45RA +, is decreased but total activated T cells, as well as B cells, are increased. The immunoregulatory T cell-produced lymphokine, interleukin-2, is present in abnormally high levels in the serum, as is soluble interleukin-2 receptor, a marker of lymphocyte turnover (Rozovsky, 1990). In fact, Levy (1990) has proposed that the syndrome be renamed, chronic immune activation syndrome. Other immune abnormalities found in these patients included the presence of elevated circulating immune complexes, greater in vitro lymphocyte responses to specific allergens, greater baseline levels of lymphocyte incorporation of tritiated thymidine, and increased numbers of immunoglobulin E-bearing B and T lymphocytes (Olson, Kanaan, Gersuk, Kelley, & Jones, 1986).

Low production of antibody to Epstein Barr nuclear antigen was noted in patients with this syndrome (Miller et al., 1987; Straus, 1988). It was proposed that abnormal levels of this specific antibody might be attributed to a specific defect in antigen recognition by the immune system. Several other alterations in the humoral response of chronic fatigue syndrome patients were described, such as mild immunoglobulin A deficiency (Jones et al., 1985; Straus, 1988), elevated immune complexes, the presence of cold agglutinins, rheumatoid factor, antinuclear antibodies, and false serologic positivity for syphilis (Straus, 1988). These aberrations taken together suggest polyclonal B cell activation, a hypothesis that is supported by the fact that Epstein Barr virus is a potent polyclonal stimulator of B cells (Alpert et al., 1987). B cells are regulated by an intricate balance between T helper and T suppressor lymphocytes as well as by NK cells. The depletion of the CD4+ CD45RA+ lymphocyte subset described above may favor an alteration in B cell regulation.

PSYCHONEUROIMMUNOLOGY AND CHRONIC FATIGUE SYNDROME

Evidence of an association between viral infection and neuropsychiatric disorders is gleaned from studies with schizophrenic, schizoaffective, and affective populations (Allen & Tilkian, 1986; Amsterdam et al., 1986). In each instance, either viral agents, antibodies to viral-like agents or viral-like particles were isolated from the subjects. Of interest are studies that showed that the convalescent periods of viral diseases, such as influenza, were altered by certain premorbid psychoneurotic conditions (Imboden, Canter, & Cluff, 1961). To date, no data exist that define a causal link between Epstein-Barr virus infection and chronic neuropsychiatric impairment. Cognitive impairment in chronic fatigue syndrome patients has been frequently noted but little rigorous research has been done in this area. Jones (1984) reported finding cognitive deficits in 4 of 10 subjects. Specifically, moderate to severe impairment was seen in both long-and short-term memory, mild to moderate deficits were seen in flexible memory, severe impairment was noted in conceptual functions and in the ability to benefit from feedback, and moderate impairment was found in fine motor control. In studies done in Miami, performance was measured on certain of the subscales of the Wechsler Memory Scale, designed to test for severe cognitive difficulties. Chronic fatigue syndrome patients performed poorly. On other subscales, such as the digit-span subtest, subjects performed well above norms (Millon et al., 1989).

That environmental stressors and affective disturbances may modulate immunological functioning is a premise that has received considerable research support (Glaser et al., 1987; Mckinnon, Weisse, Reynolds, Bowles, & Baum, 1989; Schleifer, Keller, Bond, Cohen, & Stein, 1989; Schleifer, Keller, Siris, Davis, & Stein, 1985). That health status is affected by immunologic status is a question rather forcefully answered by the experience over the past decade with human immunodeficiency virus infections

(Antoni et al., 1990). Stress-induced immunosuppression may increase vulnerability to further exogenous immunosuppressants, and perhaps even distinguish those who remain healthy from those who succumb to further deterioration (Bartrop, Luckhurst, Lazarus, Kiloh, & Penny, 1977). Glaser, Kiecolt-Glaser, Speicher, and Holliday (1985) assessed changes in antibody titers to three latent herpesviruses (Epstein-Barr, cytomegalovirus, and herpes simpex) in 49 Epstein-Barr virus seropositive first-year medical students measured at three time points: 1 month before exams, the first day of final exams, and after summer vacation. There were significant changes in the antibody titers to all three herpesviruses across time points, with the lowest levels found in the low stress (third) sample.

Psychosocial factors other than stress have been identified as possible modulators of immune function. Depression, as noted earlier, was associated with impaired immune function, as was depression combined with hostility (Gottschalk, Welch, & Weiss, 1983). Depression in the form of listless, fatigue-like responses was found to be predictive of worse biological status among breast cancer patients (Levy, Herberman, Maluish, Schlien, & Lippman, 1985). Glaser, Kiecolt-Glaser and colleagues reported that loneliness was immunosuppressive for varied immune function measures including NK cell activity, decreased percentages of helper/inducer T lymphocytes, decreased helper/inducer:suppressor/cytotoxic cell ratios, decreased interferon production, poorer T lymphocyte response to mitogen stimulation, and large changes in herpes viruses antibody titers (Glaser et al., 1985; Glaser et al., 1987; Kiecolt-Glaser, Garner, Speicher, Penn & Holliday, 1984). That the commonplace psychosocial factors examined in these studies appeared to modulate immunocompetence is of significance in regard to chronic fatigue syndrome.

A major discussion has focused on the role that psychosocial and psychiatric factors play in the incidence and progression of chronic fatigue syndrome. Straus (1988) reported on a cohort in which many of the subjects had major conflicts with family and public agencies regarding support. His patients consulted numerous physicians and tended to distrust those in the traditional medical field. Amsterdam et al. (1986) observed a constellation of symptoms in their sample: weight loss, sleep disturbances, mood changes, poor concentration, lethargy, and sadness. We have reported evidence of personality pathology and affective distress in a group of 24 chronic fatigue syndrome patients (Millon et al., 1989). In a cohort of 48 patients in Australia studied by Hickie, Lloyd, Wakefield, and Parker (1990), 88% spontaneously reported that neuropsychological and/or psychological difficulties were among their key complaints. Certainly, depressive signs and symptoms and malaise-like fatigue are two of the most commonly noted manifestations of chronic fatigue syndrome (Jones & Straus, 1987; Millon et al., 1989). Most often, chronic fatigue syndrome patients can date the onset of their illness to a certain time, which frequently coincides with an acute infectious illness (Hickie et al., 1989), or to a major life crisis. In the Miami cohort, 2 of the 30 patients were women whose daughters had been murdered (Klimas, unpublished observation).

Formal psychiatric disorders, particularly depression, have been associated with chronic fatigue syndrome. The Centers for Disease Control criteria for diagnosis of the syndrome specifically exclude patients with major depression and other psychiatric diagnoses. This situation has impeded the determination of the role of psychiatric disorders in this syndrome. In large part, the controversy can be reduced to the question: Is the affective disturbance noted in these patients indicative of a reactive depressive state, or does it reflect a predisposing pervasive trait? In other words, is this depression in some way responsible for the onset of symptomatology or does it result from the experience of ill health? Kruesi, Dale, and Straus (1989) interviewed 28 patients in an effort to determine the lifetime rate of psychiatric disorder. Lifetime incidence of depressive disorders was 54%, with major depression in 13 patients. The diagnoses of depression were closely related in time to the onset or course of fatigue. The majority of pre-morbid psychiatric diagnoses were simple phobia. The conclusion reached by Kruesi et al., (1989), that "psychiatric disorders more often preceded the Chronic Fatigue than followed it" (p. 55) was vigorously disputed by Hickie et al., (1990). These latter workers considered that the "high rate of simple phobia reported by Kruesi, et al. (1989) is likely to be the result of the interview method and unlikely to be the of psychopathological significance in patients with Chronic Fatigue Syndrome." Hickie et al., (1990) favor "the hypothesis that the current psychological symptoms of patients with Chronic Fatigue Syndrome are a consequence of the disorder rather than evidence of antecedent vulnerability." However, this dichotomous conflict over which came first, depression or fatigue, may be too simplistic. There may be two types of depression related to chronic fatigue syndrome—predisposing and reactive. There also may be intervening variables that influence the expression of depression in these patients.

PSYCHOIMMUNOLOGIC CORRELATIONS IN CHRONIC FATIGUE SYNDROME

The University of Miami Chronic Fatigue Syndrome research group as well as several other laboratories in the United States and elsewhere are collecting a growing body of evidence that indicates that immunologic abnormalities are a consistent finding in chronic fatigue syndrome patients and that the pattern of immune dysfunction observed is compatible with a chronic viral reactivation syndrome (Klimas et al., 1990). The immunologic pattern seen in chronic fatigue syndrome (T and B lymphocyte activation combined with poor T and B lymphocyte and NK cell function) parallel those described to be associated with psychosocial stressors and affective disorders. Given the data reported by the Miami group and others regarding the frequency of psychological symptoms such as anxiety, tension, depression, and so on, in these patients (Millon et al., 1989), it is clearly desirable to learn the relationship between immune parameters and psychological variables as they relate to the clinical status of patients. However, study designs to test hypotheses regarding the etiology of chronic fatigue syndrome are difficult to devise. Longitudinal data, extending from pre-infection to recovery would be ideal. This design would be difficult, if not impossible, to carry out due to lack of a known high-risk group, and because the symptoms frequently persist for many years. Cross-sectional, correlational studies, although fraught with obvious difficulties in interpretation, are much more easily undertaken. We have done such a study on a group of 24 patients who met the current Centers for Disease Control criteria for the diagnosis of chronic fatigue syndrome (Holmes et al., 1988). Thus, at entry, none of the patients had a history of a medical or psychiatric diagnosis that would have made them ineligible for the chronic fatigue syndrome classification. In fact, as the study proceeded, 4 of the subjects scored sufficiently high on the clinical syndromes scale of the Millon Clinical Multiaxial Inventory (MCMI-II, Millon, 1987) to warrant a diagnosis of a major depression. By this same instrument, 13 had pathological levels of anxiety, 12 had dysthymia, and 10 had somatoform disorder.

METHODS

Comprehensive immunologic evaluation included flow cytometric analysis of T, B, and NK cell subsets (Fletcher et al., 1989), lymphocyte proliferation in response to the mitogens with phytohemagglutinin and pokeweed mitogen (Fletcher, Baron, Ashman, Fischl, & Klimas, 1987), and NK cell cytotoxicity against a tumor cell target, K562 (Baron, Klimas, Fischl, & Fletcher, 1985). In addition, the patients underwent neuropsychological testing. Affective distress was measured using the Profile of Mood States (POMS; McNair, Lorr, & Droppleman, 1971). Axis II, personality style, and Axis I, clinical syndromes, data were obtained using the MCMI-II (Millon, 1987). The interviewer-administered Hamilton Rating Scale of Depression (HAM-D) was used (Hamilton, 1960). Cognitive function was assessed using the Folstein Mini-mental State Exam (Folstein, Folstein, & McHugh, 1975) and the Wechsler Memory Scale (WMS; Wechsler & Stone, 1973). The Pearson Product Moment correlations presented in the tables are abstracted from a larger set of correlations between immunologic and psychological measures. All correlations were carefully examined for the influence of distributional abnormalities, using both nonparametric (Spearman Rank Order correlations) and graphical techniques. Only those correlations with a probability level less that 0.05, by both Spearman and Pearson, are listed.

RESULTS

As shown in Table 7.1, increased depression, as measured by the HAM-D subscale, correlated positively with increased proliferative response to the B and T cell stimulant, pokeweed mitogen, but with no other immunologic markers. The POMS depression subscale correlated, also positively, only with number of B cells. The POMS subscales, anger and tension, correlated with decreased NK cell cytotoxicity. Tension also correlated but positively with elevated numbers of CD8 cell that expressed the Class II marker, I2. Cells of this subset have been reported variously to be naive cells (Salazar-Gonzales et al., 1987) or activated suppressor cells (Horowitz, Linker-Israeli, Gray, & Lemoine, 1987). Fatigue was related to increases in NK cell number. Lymphocyte response to the T cell mitogen, phytohemagglutinin, was inversely related to vigor (Table 7.1).

The MCMI, Axis 2, analysis revealed immune correlations with personality style subscales, BCPP 1 through 8 (Table 7.2). Natural killer cell cytotoxicity decreased with increasing avoidant and self-defeating styles. Numbers or percentage of NK cells had a positive correlation with dependent, self-defeating, and schzioid scales. Lymphocyte subset correlations included positive B cell relationships with the avoidant and the

TABLE 7.1
Correlations of Immune Variables With HAM-D and POMS

Measure	Scale	Immune Measures	Correlations Pearson Coefficients (Probability)
HAM-D	Total score	Pokeweed mitogen response	0.49 (0.018)
POMS	Depression	B cells, number	0.47 (0.021)
POMS	Anger	Natural killer cell function	−0.47 (0.022)
POMS	Fatigue	Natural killer cells, number	0.47 (0.020)
POMS	Tension	Natural killer cell function	−0.46 (0.024)
		CD8+12+ cells, number	0.57 (0.004)
POMS	Vigor	Phytohemagglutinin response	−0.51 (0.013)
		Pokeweed mitogen response	−0.43 (0.038)

TABLE 7.2
Correlations of Immune Variables With MCMI-II, AXIS 2 (Personality Styles)

Measure	Scale	Immune Measures	Correlations Pearson Coefficients (Probability)
BCPP1	Schizoid	B cells, percent	0.41 (0.048)
		Natural killer cells, percent	0.42 (0.040)
BCPP2	Avoidant	Natural killer cell function	−0.45 (0.028)
		B cells, number	0.45 (0.026)
BCPP3	Dependent	Activated T memory cells, number (CD2+CD26+)	−0.41 (0.048)
		Memory T cells, number (CD4+CD29+)	−0.43 (0.036)
BCPP6A	Anti-social	CD4 cells, number	0.50 (0.013)
		Memory T cells, number (CD4+CD29+)	0.45 (0.027)
		Activated T memory cells (CD2+CD26+)	0.52 (0.010)
BCPP6B	Sadistic	CD4 cells, number	0.43 (0.037)
		Memory T cells, number (CD4+CD29+)	0.43 (0.035)
		Activated memory T cells, number (CD2+CD26)	0.56 (0.005)
BCPP8A	Passive–Agressive	CD4 cells, number	0.41 (0.044)
		B cells, number	0.57 (0.004)
PCPP8B	Self-defeating	Natural killer cell, function	−0.55 (0.006)

passive–aggressive pattern. Absolute CD4 counts increased with increasing passive–aggressive, antisocial, and sadistic style of personalities. The CD4 subset of memory cells, CD4+CD29+, increased with increasing passive–aggressive, anti-social, and sadistic scores, and activated memory cells, CD2+CD26+, with anti-social and sadistic scales. Both memory cells and activated memory cells were inversely related to scores on the dependent scale. No correlations with immune markers were observed with the severe personality disorders, schizotypical, borderline, and paranoid.

Axis 1 subscales also showed correlations with immunologic measures (Table 7.3). Response to pokeweed mitogen increased with heightened anxiety, somatoform, dysthymia, drug dependence, and alcohol dependence. Natural killer cell function decreased with elevated dysthymic disorder.

Lymphocyte subsets also correlated with the Axis 1 subscales, with B cell number increasing with increased scores on the anxiety, dysthymia, major depression, and drug and alcohol dependency subscales. Changes in T cell regulatory subsets were evidenced by increasing numbers of T helper cells, CD4, seen with elevations in drug and alcohol dependency. Memory T cells

TABLE 7.3
Correlations of Immune Variables With MCMI-II, AXIS I (Clinical Syndromes)

Measure	Scale	Immune Measures	Correlations Pearson Coefficients (Probability)
BCSA	Anxiety	Pokeweed mitogen response	0.55 (0.006)
		B cells, number	0.42 (0.040)
BCSH	Somatoform	Pokeweed mitogen response	0.57 (0.004)
BCSN	Bipolar-manic	Memory T cells, number (CD4+CD29+)	0.43 (0.036)
		Activated memory T cells, number (CD2+CD26+)	0.42 (0.042)
BCSD	Disthymia	B cells, number	−0.44 (0.034)
		Natural killer cell, function	−0.42 (0.040)
BCSB	Drug dependence	Pokeweed mitogen response	0.53 (0.009)
		B cells, number	0.46 (0.023)
		CD4 cells, number	0.46 (0.22)
BCST	Alcohol dependence	Pokeweed mitogen response	0.49 (0.019)
		B cells, number	0.52 (0.009)
		CD4 cells, number	0.53 (0.007)
		Memory T cells, number (CD4+CD29+)	0.47 (0.021)
		Activated T cells, number (CD2+CD26+)	0.60 (0.002)
BSSCC	Major depression	B cell, number	0.51 (0.010)

and activated memory cells increased along with bipolar-manic, and alcohol dependence scores. There were no significant correlations with thought disorder or delusional disorder in this population.

Cognitive function also showed correlations, with pokeweed mitogen response and B cell number decreasing with poorer Folstein scores. In contrast, CD4 cell percentage, and numbers of the CD45RA+ subset of CD4 as well as the CD26+ subset of T cells increased with increased scores in visual reproduction.

In conclusion, this cross-sectional study has demonstrated some provocative interactions between a broad panel of immune markers and markers of psychological distress, psychiatric clinical states, and cognitive markers. Because a large number of correlations were examined, some caution is necessary in interpreting these results. Hopefully, however, they provide some clues that will facilitate efforts to answer the "chicken or the egg" puzzle of chronic fatigue syndrome. First, the study indicates that the syndrome is unlikely to be simply a clinical manifestation of depression. Only a small minority of the study group were depressed and there were few correlations of depression with immunologic markers. Additionally, it does suggest a rather strong positive relationship between those immunologic parameters that are markers of activated T and B cells and several affective and personality measures. Interestingly, all significant correlations of the pokeweed mitogen response were positive except for an inversely relationship to vigor. In contrast, all significant correlations of NK cell function were negative. The data lend support to the efforts to develop behavioral cognitive stress management interventions in this disorder. The results of the study suggest that more comprehensive and longitudinal investigations of the psychoneuroimmuology of chronic fatigue syndrome are warranted.

REFERENCES

Ablashi, D. V., Salahuddin, S. Z., Josephs, S. F., Imam, F., Lusso, P., Gallo, R. C., Hung, C., Lemp, J., & Markham, P. D. (1987). HBLV (or HHV-6) in human cell lines [Letter]. *Nature, 329,* 207.

Allen, A. D., & Tilkian, S. M. (1986). Depression correlated with cellular immunity in systemic immunodeficient Epstein-Barr virus syndrome. *Journal of Clinical Psychiatry, 47*(3), 133–135.

Alpert, D., Koide, J., Takada, S., & Engleman, E. G. (1987). T cell regulatory disturbances in the rheumatic diseases. *Rheumatic Disease Clinics of North America, 13*(3), 431–445.

Amsterdam, J. D., Henle, W., Winokur, A., Wolkowitz, O. M., Pickar, D., & Paul, S. M. (1986). Serum antibodies to Epstein-Barr virus in patients with major depressive disorder. *American Journal of Psychology, 143,* 1593–1596.

Antoni, M. H., Schneiderman, N., Fletcher, M. A., Goldstein, D., Ironson, G., & LaPerriere, A. (1990). Psychoneuroimmunology and HIV-1. *Journal of Consulting and Clinical Psychology, 58,* 38–49.

Baron, G. C., Klimas, N. G., Fischl, M. A., & Fletcher, M. A. (1985). Decreased natural cell mediated cytotoxicity per effector cell in the acquired immunodeficiency syndrome. *Diagnostic Immunology, 3,* 197–204.

Bartrop, R. W., Luckhurst, E., Lazarus, L., Kiloh, L. G., & Penny, R. (1977). Depressed lymphocyte function after bereavement. *Lancet, 1*(8016), 834–836.

Borysiewicz, L. K., Haworth, S. J., Cohen, J., Mundin, J., Rickinson, A., & Sisson, J. G. (1986). Epstein-Barr virus-specific immune defects in patients with persistent symptoms following infectious mononeucleosis. *Quarterly Journal of Medicine, 58,* 111–121.

Briggs, M., Fox, J., & Tedder, R. S. (1988). Age prevelance of antibody to human herpes virus-6 [letter]. *Lancet, 331,* 1058–1060.

Caliguri, M., Murray, C., Buchwald, C., Levine, H., Cheney, P., Peterson, D., Komaroff, A. L., & Ritz, J. (1987). Phenotypic and functional deficiency of natural killer cells in patients with chronic fatigue syndrome. *Journal of Immunology, 139,* 3306–3313.

DeFreitas, E., & Hilliard, B. (1990, November) *Association of an HTLVII-like virus with CFIDS.* Paper presented at Chronic Fatigue and Immune Dysfunction Syndrome. The CFIDS Association 1990 Research Conference, Charlotte, NC.

Emery, P., Gently, K. C., Mackay, I. R., Muirden, K. D., & Rowley, M. (1987). Deficiency of the suppressor inducer subset of T lymphocytes in rheumatoid arthritis. *Arthritis and Rheumatism, 30,* 849–856.

Epstein, M. A., & Achong, B. G. (1979). *The Epstein-Barr virus.* New York: Springer-Verlag.

Fletcher, M. A., Azen, S., Adelsberg, B., Gjerset, G. Hassett, J., Kaplan, J., Niland, J., Odom-Maryon, T., Parker, J., Stites, D., Mosley, J., & the Transfusion Safety Study Group (1989). Immunophenotyping in a multicenter study: The Transfusion Safety Study experience. *Clinical Immunology and Immunopathology, 52,* 38–47.

Fletcher, M. A., Baron, G. C., Ashman, M. R., Fischl, M. A., & Klimas, N. G. (1987). The use of whole blood methods in assessment of immune parameters in immunodeficiency states. *Diagnostic Immunology, 5,* 69–81.

Folstein, M. F., Folstein, S. E., & McHugh, P. R. (1975). Minimental state. *Journal of Psychiatric Research, 12,* 189–198.

Franco, K., Kawa-Ha, K., Doi, S., Yumura, K., Murata, M., Ishihara, S., Tawa, A., & Yabuuchi, H. (1987). Remarkable depression of CD4+2H4+ T cells in severe chronic active Epstein-Barr virus infection. *Scandinavian Journal of Immunology, 26,* 769–773.

Glaser, R., Kiecolt-Glaser, J., Speicher, C. E., & Holliday, J. E. (1985). Stress, loneliness, and changes in herpes virus latency. *Journal of Behavioral Medicine, 8,* 249–256.

Glaser, R., Rice, J., Sheridan J., Fertel, R., Stout, J. C., Speicher, C., Pinsky, D., Kotur, M., Post, A., Beck, M., & Kiecolt-Glaser, J. K. (1987). Stress-related immune supression: Health implications. *Brain, Behavior and Immunity, 1,* 7–20.

Gold, D., Bowden, R., Sixbey, J., Riggs, R., Caton, W., Ashley, R., Obrigewitch, R., & Corey, L. (1990). Chronic fatigue: A prospective clinical and virological study. *Journal of the American Medical Association, 264,* 48–53.

Gottschalk, L. A., Welch, W. D., & Weiss, J. (1983). Vulnerability and immune response. An overview. *Psychotheraphy and Psychosomatics, 39*(1), 23–35.

Grazia-Masucci, M., Bejarano, M. T., Masucci, G., & Klein, E. (1987). Large granular lymphocytes inhibit the in vitro growth of autologus Epstein-Barr virus infected B cells. *Cellular Immunology, 76,* 311–321.

Hafler, D. H., Fox, D. A., Manning, M. E., Schlossman, S. F., Reinherz, E. L., & Weiner, H. L. (1985). In vivo activated T lymphocytes in the peripheral blood and cerebrospinal fluid of patients with Multiple Sclerosis. *New England Journal of Medicine, 312,* 1405–1411.

Hamilton, M. (1960). A rating scale for depression. *Journal of Neurological and Neurosurgical Psychiatry, 23,* 56–62.

Hayakawa, K., Hardy, R. R., Honda, M., Herzenberg, L. A., Steinberg, A. D., & Herzenberg, L. A. (1984). Ly-1 B cells: Functionally distinct lymphocytes that secrete IgM autoantibodies. *Proceedings of the National Academy of Science, USA, 81*(8), 2494–2498.

Hickie, I., Lloyd, A., Wakefield, D., & Parker, G. (1990). The psychiatric status of patients with the Chronic Fatigue Syndrome. *British Journal of Psychiatry, 156,* 534–540.

Holmes, G. P., Kaplan, J. E., Stewart, J. A., Hunt, B., Pinsky, P. F., & Schonberger, L. B. (1987). A cluster of patients with a chronic mononeucleosis-like syndrome. *Journal of the American Medical Association, 257,* 2297–2302.

Holmes, G. P., Kaplan, J. E., Komarott, A., Schonberger, L. B., Straus, S., Jones, J., Dubois, R., Chowers, I., Feldman-Weiss, V., Michaeli, Y., Ben Chertrit, E., Shalit, M., & Knobler, H. (1988) Chronic fatigue syndrome: A working case definition. *Annals of Internal Medicine, 108,* 387–389.

Horowitz, D., Linker-Israeli, L., Gray, D., & Lemoine, C. (1987). Functional properties of CD8 positive lymphocyte subsets in systemic lupus erythematosus. *Journal of Rheumatology. Supplement 13,* 49–52.

Imboden, J. B., Canter, A., & Cluff, L. E. (1961). Convalescence from influenza: Psychological parameters. *Archives of Internal Medicine, 108,* 115–121.

Jones, J. F. (1984, November). Untitled conference, Le Chateau Champlain, Montreal, Canada.

Jones, J. F., Ray, C. G., Minnich, L. L., Hicks, M. J., Kibler, R., & Locus, D. O. (1985). Evidence for active Epstein-Barr virus infection in patients with persistent, unexplained illnesses: Elevated anti-early, antigen-antibodies. *Annals of Internal Medicine, 102,* 1–7.

Jones, J., & Straus, S. (1987). Chronic Epstein-Barr virus infections. *Annual Review of Medicine, 38,* 195–209.

Kibler, R., Lucas, D., Hicks, M. J., Poulos, B. T., & Jones, J. F. (1985). Immune function in chronic active Epstein-Barr virus infection. *Journal of Clinical Immunology, 5,* 46–54.

Kiecolt-Glaser, J. K., Garner, W., Speicher, C., Penn, G. M., Holliday, & J. (1984). Psychosocial modifiers of immunocompetence in medical students. *Journal of Psychosomatic Medicine, 46*(1), 7-14.

Klimas, N. G., Salvato, F., Morgan, R., & Fletcher, M. A. (1990). Immunologic abnormalities in chronic fatigue syndrome. *Journal of Clinical Microbiology, 28*(6), 1403-1410.

Knop, J., Stremmer, R., Neumann, C., De Maeyer, E., & Macher, E. (1982). Interferon inhibits the suppressor T cell response of delayed hypersensitivity. *Nature, 296,* 757-759.

Kruesi, M. J. P., Dale, J., & Strauss, S. E. (1989). Psychiatric diagnoses in patients who have chronic fatigue syndrome. *Journal of Clinical Psychiatry, 50,* 53-56.

Levy, S. M., Herberman, R. B., Maluish, A. M., Schlien, B. M., & Lippman, M. (1985). Prognostic risk assessment in primary breast cancer by behavioral and immunological parameters. *Health Psychology, 4*(2), 99-113.

Levy, J. A. (1990, November). *CIAS: Reflections on a hyperactive immune state.* Paper presented at Chronic Fatigue and Immune Dysfunction Syndrome. The CFIDS Association 1990 Research Conference, Charlotte, NC.

Lloyd, A. R., Wakefield, D., Boughton, C. R. & Dwyer, J. M. (1989). Immunologic abnormalities in the chronic fatigue syndrome. *The Medical Journal of Australia, 151,* 122-124.

Lopez, C., Pellet, P., Stewart, J., Goldsmith, C., Sanderlin, K., Black, J., Warfield, D., & Feorino, D. (1988). Characteristics of human herpes virus-6. *Journal of Infectious Diseases, 157,* 1271-1273.

Lusso, P., Salahuddin, S. Z., Ablashi, D. V., Gallo, R. C., di Marzo, V., & Markham, P. D. (1987). Diverse tropism of human B-lymphotropic virus (human herpesvirus-6). *Lancet, 2,* 743-744.

McKinnon, W., Weisse, C. S., Reynolds, C. P., Bowles, C. A., & Baum. A. (1989). Chronic stress, leukocyte subpopulations and humoral response to latent viruses. *Health Psychology, 8*(4), 389-402.

McNair, D. M., Lorr, M., & Droppleman, S. (1971). *Profile of mood states.* San Diego, CA: Educational and Industrial Testing Service.

Miller, G., Grogan, E., Rowe, D., Rooney, C., Heston, L., Eastman, R., Andiman, W., Neiderman, J. Lenoir, G., & Henle, W. (1987). Selective lack of antibody to a component of EB nuclear antigen in patients with chronic active Epstein-Barr virus infection. *Journal of Infectious Diseases, 156*(1), 26-35.

Millon, T. (1987). *Millon Clinical Multiaxial Inventory II: Manual for the MCMI-II.* Minneapolis: National Computer Systems.

Millon, C., Salvato, F., Blaney, N., Morgan, R., Mantero-Antienza, R., Klimas, N. G., & Fletcher, M. A. (1989). A psychological assessment of chronic fatigue syndrome/chronic Epstein-Barr virus patients. *Psychology and Health, 3,* 131-141.

Morimoto, C., Letvin, N. L., Distato, J. A., Aldrich, W. R., & Schlossman, S. F. (1985). The isolation and characterization of the human suppressor inducer T cell subset. *Journal of Immunology, 134,* 1508-1512.

Morimoto, C., Reinherz, E. L., Schlossman, S. F., Schur, P. H., Mills, J. A., & Steinberg, A. D. (1980). Alternatives in immunoregulatory T cell subsets in active systemic lupus erythmatosus. *Journal of Clinical Investigation, 66,* 1171-1177.

Niederman, J. C., Chun-Ren, L., Kaplan, M. H., & Brown, N. A. (1988). Clinical and Serological features of human herpes virus-6 infection in three adults. *Lancet,* 817-819.

Okano, M., Thiele, G. M., Davis, J. R., Nauseef, W. M., Mitros, F., & Purtilo, D. T. (1988). Adenovirus Type-2 in a patient with Lethal Hemorrhagic Colonic Ulcers and Chronic Active Epstein-Barr virus infection. *Annals of Internal Medicine, 108,* 693-699.

Olson, G., Kanaan, M. N., Gersuk, G. M., Kelley, L. M., & Jones, J. F. (1986). Correlation between allergy and persistent Epstein-Barr infections in chronic-active Epstein-Barr virus-infected patients. *Journal of Allergy Clinical Immunology, 78,* 308-314.

Palmblad, J., Blömbäck, M., Edberg, N., Froberg, J., & Karlsson, C., (1977). Experimentally induced stress in man: Effects on blood coagulation and fibronolylisis. *Journal of Psychosomatic Research, 21,* 87–92.

Reinherz, E. L., Kung, P. C., Goldstein, G., & Schlossman, S. F. (1979). A monoclonal antibody with selective reactivity with functionally mature human thymocytes and all peripheral human T cells. *Journal of Immunology, 123*(3), 1312–1317.

Rose, L. M., Ginsberg, A. H., Rothstein, T. L., Ledbetter, J. A., & Clark, E. A. (1985). Selective loss of a subset of T helper cells in active multiple sclerosis. *Proceedings of the National Academy of Science, USA, 82,* 7389–7393.

Rose, L. M., Ginsberg, A. H., Rothstein, T. L., Ledbetter, J. A., & Clark, E. A. (1988). Fluctuations of CD4+ T cell subsets in remitting-relapsing multiple sclerosis. *Annals of Neurolology, 24,* 192–199.

Rozovsky, I. (1990, November) *Levels of lymphokines, soluble receptors and IL-2 inhibitors in sera from CFIDS patients.* Paper presented at Chronic Fatigue and Immune Dysfunction Syndrome. The CFIDS Association 1990 Research Conference, Charlotte, NC.

Salahuddin, S. Z., Ablashi, D. V., Markham, P. D., Josephs, S. F., Sturzenegger, S., Kaplan, M., Halligan, G., Biberfeld, P., Wong-Staal, F., & Kramarsky, B. (1986). Isolation of a new virus, HBLV, in patients with lymphoproliferative disorders. *Science, 234,* 596–601.

Salazar-Gonzales, J., Moody, D., Giorgi, J., Martinez-Maza, O., Mitsuyasu, R., & Fahey, J. (1987). Reduced ecto-5' nucleosidase activity and enhanced OFT 10 and HLA/DR expression on CD 8 (T suppressor/cytotoxic) lymphocyte in the acquired immune deficiency syndrome: Evidence of CD8 cell immaturity. *Journal of Immunology, 135,* 1778–1785.

Salvato, F., Klimas, N., Ashman, M., & Fletcher, M. A. (1988). Immune dysfunction among chronic fatigue syndrome patients with evidence of Epstein-Barr virus reactivation. *Journal of Clinical Cancer Research, 7,* 89.

Sato, K., Miyasaka, N., Yamaoka, K., Okuda, M., Yata, J., & Nishioka, K. (1987). Quantitative defect of CD4+2H4+ cells in systemic lupus erythematosus and Sjörgren's syndrome. *Arthritis Rheumatism, 30*(12), 1407–11.

Schleifer, S. J., Keller, S., Bond, R., Cohen, J., & Stein, M. (1989). Major depressive disorder and immunity: role of age, sex, severity and hospitalization. *Archives of General Psychiatry, 46,* 81–87.

Schleifer, S. J., Keller, S. E., Siris, S. G., Davis, K. L., & Stein, M. (1985). Depression and immunity lymphocyte function in ambulatory depressed patients, hospitalized schizophrenic patients, and patients hospitalized for hernionaphy. *Archives of General Psychiatry, 42,* 129–133.

Straus, S. E. (1988). The chronic mononucleosis syndrome. *Journal of Infectious Diseases, 157*(3), 405–412.

Straus, S. E., Tosato, G., Armstrong, G., Lawley, T., Preble, O. T., Henle, W., Davey, R., Pearson, G., Epstein, J., Brus, I., & Blaese, R. M. (1985). Persisting illness and fatigue in adults with evidence of Epstein-Barr virus infection. *Annals of Internal Medicine, 102,* 7–16.

Targan, S., & Stebbing, N. (1982). In vitro interactions of purified cloned human interferons on NK cells enhanced activation. *Journal of Immunology, 129,* 934–935.

Tarsis, S., Klimas, N., Baron, G., Ashman, M., & Fletcher, M. A. (1987). *Immunological considerations in chronic Epstein-Barr virus syndrome.* Paper presented at the Medical Laboratory Immunology Conference, Williamsburg, VA.

Tedder, R. S., Briggs, M., Cameron, C. H., Honess, R., Robertson, D., & Whittle, H. (1987). A novel lymphotropic herpes virus [letter]. *Lancet, 2,* 390–392.

Tobi, M., & Straus, S. E. (1985). Chronic Epstein-Barr virus disease: A workshop held by the National Institute of Allergy and Infectious Diseases. *Annals of Internal Medicine, 103,* 951–953.

Tosato, G., Straus, S., Henle, W., Pike, S. E., & Blaese, R. M. (1985). Characteristic T cell dysfunction in patients with chronic active Epstein-Barr virus infection (chronic infectious mononucleosis). *Journal of Immunology, 134*(5), 3082–3088.

Wechsler, D., & Stone, C. P. (1973). *Manual for the Wechsler Memory Scale.* New York: The Psychological Corporation.

Zlotnick, A., Shimonkewitz, P., Gefter, M. L., Kappler, J., & Marrack, P. (1983). Characterization of the gamma-interferon mediated induction of antigen-presenting ability in P388 D1 cells. *Journal of Immunology, 131*(6), 2814–2820.

8
Psychoneuroimmunology and Stress Responses in HIV-1 Seropositive and At-Risk Seronegative Gay Men

Michael H. Antoni
Neil Schneiderman
Arthur LaPerriere
Lilly Bourguignon
Mary Ann Fletcher
University of Miami

A recently released briefing by the National Academy of Sciences (1989) reviewing behavioral influences on endocrine and immune function highlighted the importance of studying the effects of psychosocial stressors on immune functioning among individuals with well-defined immunologic abnormalities in order to ascertain the biological significance of affective distress and behavioral arousal. Among other things this report stressed the need for future work to:

1. collect adequate baseline immunologic information from which to assess stressor-induced changes,
2. employ age- and gender-matched control groups and to carefully assess (and covary) the potential influence of medications on immune function,
3. examine the role of neural, neuroendocrine, and neuropeptide mediation of stressor-induced immunomodulation by studying not only the peripheral levels of these substances but also the nature of their ligand-like interaction with lymphocyte receptors (e.g., beta-2 adrenergic receptors),
4. evaluate the role of the host's immunological structural integrity when testing the effects of behavioral and neuroendocrine changes on immune function,
5. employ flourescence-activated cell sorting procedures to isolate specific lymphocyte subsets (e.g., helper-inducer cells) in tissue culture in order to examine which stressor-associated ligands they

respond to separately and how such ligands synergize (e.g., cortisol and epinephrine) in their immunomodulatory actions,

6. study the effects of such stressor-related ligands on lymphokine production and the regulation of lymphocyte post-receptor activity (e.g., gene expression), and

7. to demonstrate the biological significance of stressor-related immune changes by documenting changes in health outcomes (e.g., emergence of symptoms)concurrently with or subsequent to immunomodulation.

In addressing several of these issues, this chapter briefly reviews the human psychoneuroimmunologic literature with respect to assessment, population, and paradigmatic issues. Specifically, we highlight the importance of concurrent measurement of psychological, neuroendocrine/neuropeptide, and immunological responses; the inclusion of populations who are likely to be clinically impacted by small changes in immune status; and the use of designs that examine changes in responses to acute, potent, and externally valid stressors among subjects who are not displaying physical symptoms that might thwart efforts to establish temporality between psychoneuroimmunologic phenomena and health status. We present two studies that feature several of these qualities — one involving psychoneuroimmunologic changes from pre- to postbereavement among grieving spouses and another examining similar variables during the periods preceding and following HIV-1 antibody status notification among gay men. The second of these studies, conducted in our laboratory, is discussed in terms of the discordance and asynchronism among psychological, neuroendocrine, and immunological responses among HIV-1 infected gay men in comparison to their seronegative counterparts. Recommendations for future work include expanded assessment protocols (at the cytokine, lymphocyte receptor, and second messenger levels), repeated-measurement designs utilizing standardized stressors with special attention to the examination of the time course of psychoneuroimmunologic responsivity (latency and recovery times), and the study of populations spanning the spectrum of HIV-1 infection (asymptomatic and symptomatic stages) who might differ in the degree to which immunomodulation affects clinical status.

RESEARCH ISSUES

Paradigmatic Issues

A good deal of contemporary human psychoneuroimmunologic (PNI) research can be classified into two broad domains; those studies focusing on the immunologic effects or correlates of acute stressors (*stressor* studies), and those associating stress responses or distress states with immunologic status (*stress response/state* studies). The former approach has been used to investigate the consequences of medical school examinations (Glaser et al., 1987), sleep deprivation (Palmblad, Petrini, Wasserman, & Akerstedt, 1979), and death of a spouse (Irwin, Daniels, Smith, Bloom, & Weiner, 1987). The latter approach has focused mostly on previously well-adjusted individuals experiencing prolonged periods of distress (Kiecolt-Glaser, Fisher et al., 1987; McKinnon, Weisse, Reynolds, Bowles, & Baum, 1989), or clinically depressed patients (Schleifer, Keller, Siris, Davis, & Stein, 1985) with some work also looking at other affective distress states (e.g., panic disorders; Surman et al., 1986). Interestingly, there has been little work to date examining human PNI responses to acute laboratory stressors and hence little is known regarding the time course of responsivity among these types of variables.

Population Issues

Overall, the populations typically studied in *stressor* designs have been healthy, young and geriatric ones ranging from medical school students (Glaser et al., 1987) to nursing home residents (Kiecolt-Glaser et al., 1985). These studies have provided some generality for PNI relationships across wide age ranges and have offered preliminary support for the efficacy of stress management interventions in modulating immune function. One line of PNI *stress response/state* studies has focused on individuals who are manifesting psychiatric levels of affective symptomatology (e.g., major depressive disorder; Schleifer et al., 1985), independent of the role of transient or chronic environmental stressors. Another paradigm looks at healthy people who are subjected to chronic life-threatening (e.g., threat of exposure to unknown levels of radiation; McKinnon et al., 1989) or interpersonal stressors (e.g., caring for a family member with Alzheimer's disease; Kiecolt-Glaser, Glaser, & Dyer et al., 1987; or enduring marital distress and divorce; Kiecolt-Glaser, Fisher et al., 1987). These studies have done much to enhance our understanding of important psychoimmunologic relationships. Our laboratory has examined similar relationships in populations who are likely to be clinically affected by small, but statistically significant changes in immune functioning (i.e., HIV-1 infected gay males; Ironson et al., 1990).

Assessment Issues

The types of data collected in PNI studies vary widely. Often, broad concurrent assessments of affective distress and markers of cell-mediated immunity (e.g., lymphocyte proliferative responses to mitogens) comprise the balance of measures collected. In such psychoimmunologic investigations, correlations are ascertained among these variables and little attention is paid to the examination of physiological–biochemical (e.g., corticosteroids) or psychological (e.g., cognitive interpretations of stressor stimuli and perceived coping resources available) mediators. The empirical studies that have drawn support for psychoimmunologic relationships have suggested that stressors or stress states that are characterized by a perceived loss of personal control are associated with the greatest decrements in immune functioning (e.g., natural killer cell cytotoxicity; Shavit & Martin, 1987), although not all psychoimmunologic findings have been supportive of such associations. The supportive findings reveal that psychosocial factors contribute, at best, approximately 25% of the variance in immunologic measures suggesting that a good deal of measurement error and extraneous variables have been left to vary unsystematically in these investigations (see Kiecolt-Glaser & Glaser, 1988, for a review of these issues). Relevant exclusion criteria (e.g., drug and alcohol abuse) could be used to reduce these problems and repeated measurements of potential biobehavioral immunomodulatory confounds (e.g., sleep, physical activity, and nutritional changes) across observation periods could identify important covariates to be employed in statistical analyses.

In addition to the assessment of control variables, it is important to collect data on putative mediators of psychoimmune relationships. Neuroimmunologic studies, based largely on animal models of stress (usually uncontrollable stressors), have produced some data suggesting that several hypothalamic-pituitary adrenocortical (HPAC) and sympathoadrenomedullary (SAM) system products may modulate immune functioning. In that the rationale for most psychoimmunologic investigations rests on the assumption that stressors or distress states relate to immune functioning through changes in CNS (e.g., hypothalamic electrical activity, Besedovsky et al., 1983), autonomic (e.g., increased release of catecholamines from sympathetic terminals to target organs such as the thymus; Felten, Felten, Carlson, Olschawka, & Livnat, 1985), neuroendocrine (e.g., elevations in plasma cortisol concentrations; Calabrese, Kling, & Gold, 1987; Cupps & Fauci, 1982), and/or neuropeptide (e.g., beta-endorphin levels; Brummitt, Sharp, Gekker, Keane, & Peterson, 1988; Sibinga & Goldstein, 1988) events/agents, it is striking that so few human studies have attempted to ascertain such changes across the periods comprising their observation windows. As such we are left with a voluminous animal literature linking stressors to immunologic outcomes by way of neuromediators and a lack of human studies that are able to say the same. Although some animal studies have actually focused on the issue of the "clinical relevance" of observed immunologic changes (e.g., tumor growth and mortality rates as consequences of uncontrollable stressor-induced immunosuppression; Riley, 1981; Visintainer, Volpicelli, & Seligman, 1982), there remains a paucity of similar designs employed with humans.

Another critical assessment issue concerns the quantification of the psychological (i.e., cognitive/affective) distress response to environmental stimuli and its association with changes in neuromediators on the one hand and immunological outcomes on the other. Some psychoendocrine research has suggested that affective distress states such as clinical depression and anxiety disorders (e.g., panic disorder, generalized anxiety disorder) are associated with elevations in peripheral cortisol and catecholamine levels, measured basally and during acute episodes, as well as with alterations in the homeostatic mechanisms that control the chronic resting levels of these substances (see Winters, Ironson, & Schneiderman, 1990, for review). In the case of one affective phenomenon tied to an actual or relived environmental crisis—posttraumatic stress disorder (PTSD)—some investigators have noted a dissociation between overt signs of affective distress (anxiety and depression) and urinary cortisol, norepinephrine (NE), and epinephrine (E) levels (Mason, Giller, Kosten, Ostroff, & Podd, 1986). These investigators collected, on average, four urine samples at 2-week intervals following hospitalization and noted that compared to patients with major depressive disorder, bipolar I:manics, and undifferentiated schizophrenics, the DSM-III-classified PTSD patients showed lower mean cortisol values despite displaying nearly double the urinary catecholamine (NE and E) levels found in any of these comparison groups. The findings were independent of any demographic or medication differences among groups and suggested that SAM and HPAC products may not covary in parallel with distress states in all populations. Other work has observed decreased urinary-free cortisol, increased plasma cortisol, blunted adrenocorticotropic hormone (ACTH) responses to corticotropin-releasing hormone (CRH) challenge, and elevated urinary NE and E levels in PTSD patients (see Winters et al., 1990, for review). The psychoendocrine literature then appears to offer important, although inconclusive, data on the relationship between psychosocial stressors or distress responses/states and neuroendocrine events. The bulk of the empirical data has been collected on individuals manifesting psychiatric levels of affective distress and, as such, it is difficult to tease out the role of environmental stressors from the dysregulated neuroendocrine responses that are secondary to the psychiatric disorder.

One paradigm has been used to study the degree to which urinary levels of cortisol, NE and E are associated with symptoms of PTSD in individuals experiencing chronic stress but not diagnosed with the disorder (e.g., Davidson & Baum, 1986). In one study from this laboratory, residents of Three Mile Island (TMI)—the site of a nuclear reactor accident—showed catecholamine and cortisol levels that were higher than those of a comparison group, on samples collected more than 1 year after the accident (Schaeffer & Baum, 1984). Follow-up work indicated that as late as 58 months after the reactor accident the TMI sample continued to show higher cortisol and NE levels compared to controls and evidenced positive correlations between PTSD symptom levels (as measured by the Impact of Events Scale; Horowitz, Wilner, & Alvarez, 1979) and cortisol, NE and E. These findings are important because they suggest (a) the presence of potentially immunomodulatory physiologic changes in normal functioning individuals undergoing chronic stress and PTSD-like symptoms, and (b) that qualitatively similar affective distress responses may be characterized by a different physiological pattern in psychiatric versus nonpsychiatric populations. Perhaps of most interest to the current discussion is the finding that these TMI residents also show decrements in total T lymphocyte, total macrophage, and CD4 cell numbers (McKinnon et al., 1989).

Other psychosocial factors have been associated with changes in both stress hormone levels (e.g., glucocorticoid elevations) and cellular immunomodulation (e.g., natural killer [NK] cell activity, and proliferative responses to phytohemagglutinin [PHA] and/or concanavalin A [Con A]) in humans including loneliness (Kiecolt-Glaser, Ricker et al., 1984), marital disruption (Kiecolt-Glaser, Fisher, Ogrocki, et al., 1987), and poor social support networks (Levy, Herberman, Lippman, & d'Angelo, 1987). However, few studies have concurrently assessed psychoneuroimmunologic variables among populations likely to be clinically impacted by small changes in immune function. Moreover, there has been a distinct lack of paradigms that feature repeated assessments before and after the onset or manipulation of acute, potent and externally valid field stressors in individuals who are on the one hand totally asymptomatic and on the other hand likely to be affected by small changes in immunity. Such designs would enhance external validity at the same time as minimizing the role of historical confounds and elucidating the precise temporal relationships among response measures (i.e., internal validity).

ACUTE STRESSORS AND PSYCHONEUROIMMUNOLOGY

Bereavement

One of the most widely studied stressors in the PNI literature is conjugal bereavement (Bartrop, Lazarus, Luckhurst, Kiloh, & Penny, 1977; Calabrese et al., 1987; Irwin, Daniels, & Weiner, 1987). This line of work has included assessments of both phenotypic (T lymphocyte subpopulations) and functional (lymphocyte proliferative and NK cytotoxic responses) immune markers as well as psychological factors such as life events and severity of depressive symptoms among bereaving spouses. This is also one of the few examples of human PNI research in which psychological, neuroendocrine (plasma cortisol), and immunologic variables have been measured concurrently before and after the onset of an acute and potent field stressor (e.g., Irwin, Daniels, Risch, Bloom, & Weiner, 1988). To the credit of this last investigatory team, the populations of surviving spouses studied were required to be free of both chronic medical conditions and acute infections at study entry thus increasing the likelihood that changes in the PNI variables were stressor-induced and generalizable to other healthy populations experiencing crises of a similar magnitude. The likelihood, however, that the amount of immunomodulation observed in this and other bereavement studies is predictive of health outcomes or the often cited increased mortality rate among the recently bereaved is yet to be demonstrated. As such it is possible that bereavement-associated immunologic changes may have little clinical impact on the populations studied to date. It may be of future interest to examine similar variables in those bereaved individuals who are likely to manifest health changes as a consequence of small changes in immune status. For instance, asymptomatic HIV-1 infected persons who are anticipating the death of a lover or spouse might evidence the emergence of opportunistic infections such as pneumocystis carinii pneumonia in a relatively short period following the loss event. The bereavement PNI paradigm applied to this group might yield valuable information for treatment design as well as elucidating psychoneuroimmunologic mechanisms underlying health and disease course.

HIV-1 Antibody Testing and Serostatus Notification

Our laboratory has examined the effects of acute psychosocial stressors on psychological, neuroendocrine, and immunologic markers among asymptomatic HIV-1 infected and at-risk, but seronegative, gay men using repeated measurements collected before and after the onset of the stressors. Regarding the assessment issues mentioned previously, we have included a broad array of psychological (affective and cognitive distress) and immunological (phenotypic, mitogen responsivity, cytotoxic activity, and cytokine production) outcome/response measures as well as some putative physiological (plasma cortisol and B-endorphin) and psychological (cognitive coping strategies, locus of control, and social support) mediators. In addition, we have employed exclusion criteria (e.g., recent non-HIV viral infection, alcohol and recreational drug abuse, antihistamine and steroid use, participation in potentially immunomodulatory treatment regimens) and repeated measurements of biobehavioral variables (e.g., weeknight sleep duration, strenuous physical activity, high-risk sexual activity frequency, serum albumin concentration, extraneous environmental stressors [hassles]) to minimize or statistically control sources of error variance in outcome measures. Our paradigm consists of enrolling gay males, ignorant of their HIV-1 antibody status and free of any HIV-1 related symptoms, into a protocol in which they are tested for and notified of their serostatus while being concurrently exposed to one of several behavioral stress management conditions (aerobic exercise, relaxation training, assessment-only control) in a randomized experimental design.

The measurements noted previously are made at multiple time points in the 5-week periods preceding and following notification of antibody status. We have reasoned that because all of these individuals have, for one reason or another, previously avoided undergoing the antibody test, the decision to join this study would likely function as a potent stressor in and of itself (Antoni et al., 1990). The data collected in the first 5-week observation period (preceding serostatus notification) might reflect the initial decision to enter the study and any resolution (or exacerbation) of such anticipatory phenomena (e.g., anxiety) over the subsequent weeks. The second acute stressor that this design presents for study—most likely the more potent of the two—is the actual notification of antibody status. We have assessed both the immediate impact of this news and changes occurring in the subsequent 5-week period to examine the magnitude and duration of stressor-related PNI responses. Three additional design features in this paradigm are noteworthy: (a) all subjects are asymptomatic and therefore not likely to be "responding" to their symptoms; (b) some subjects receive distressing and others receive relieving information allowing us to test the specificity of the host responses to the notification event; and (c) some subjects are infected (subclinically) with the virus, whereas others are not, thereby allowing us to assess the generalizability of PNI relationships in those with intact and compromised immune systems. The third point is salient with regard to the population issue mentioned previously. Individuals infected with HIV-1, although still asymptomatic, have been shown to have decrements in several phenotypic and functional immune indices and some work suggests that uninfected members of AIDS risk groups (e.g., healthy homosexual males) have abnormal numbers of certain lymphocyte subpopulations (DeMartini et al., 1988; Nicholson et al., 1986). Moreover, it has been empirically demonstrated that the emergence of opportunistic infections such as *pneumocystis carinii* pneumonia are preceded (in a 6–11 month period) by changes in certain T lymphocyte subsets (e.g., helper/inducer counts) in HIV-1 infected men (DeMartini et al., 1988). As such, it is likely that small changes in immune status may have clinical implications for the populations studied in our lab.

A recent review of studies documenting psychological responses to HIV-1 antibody testing (Jacobsen, Perry, & Hirsch, 1990) raised several methodological concerns in this line of work including (a) lack of knowledge concerning subjects' distress states prior to antibody testing, (b) determining the appropriate psychological variables to study and measures to assess them (e.g., many affective distress measures are designed for psychiatric populations and would be inappropriate for assessing distress changes in newly diagnosed, previously healthy functioning individuals), (c) the possibility that prior AIDS-related experiences (e.g., engaging in unsafe sexual behaviors or having a lover die of AIDS) may influence the subject's response to seropositivity notification, (d) the "interactions" between HIV-1 associated symptoms and signs of affective distress and the inability of psychometric devices to distinguish between infection-mediated organic signs and those attributable to reactive depression, and (e) confounding the effects of notification with ongoing counseling efforts, especially when the latter are dispensed unsystematically. In that these methodological concerns are likely to compromise our ability to ascertain stressor-induced psychological changes, the investigation of PNI relationships in this type of design also needs to address such issues. To do so our lab has studied the impact of antibody testing with (a) multiple pre- and postnotification measurement points; (b) assessment devices designed for nonpsychiatric populations; (c) measurement of prenotification life stressors, sexual behaviors, and predicted serostatus; (d) asymptomatic samples of at-risk gay males not previously tested; and (e) comparisons of individuals receiving pre- and postnotification intervention with those in a non-intervention control group.

We have reported that upon entering a study in which they were tested for and notified of their antibody status, gay males showed impaired proliferative responses to PHA and pokeweed mitogen (PWM), despite the fact that they were all shown to be seronegative (Ironson et al., 1990). Five weeks later, but before learning of their seronegativity, these individuals showed a recovery of mitogen responsiveness to the level of laboratory controls. These findings suggested that the decision to enter a study in which serostatus would be definitively identified was operating as a potent acute stressor with immunological effects. To further investigate this hypothesis we examined changes in plasma cortisol, denial coping strategies, intrusive thoughts related to AIDS risk, and several markers of affective distress (anxiety, depression, confusion) in an expanded sample of HIV-1 seronegative gay males across similar time points (Antoni et al., 1990). Results indicated that (a) these individuals showed the same pattern of changes in proliferative responses to PHA and PWM that we had observed in the smaller sample, (b) they had significant elevations in plasma cortisol (relative to resting levels for age-equivalent males; Meyerhoff, Oleshansky, & Mougey, 1988) at study entry that were positively correlated with affective distress markers, and (c) their cortisol values receded to normal levels across a subsequent 5-week period in conjunction with the

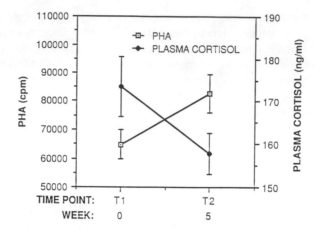

FIG. 8.1.   Mean (±SEM) lymphocyte proliferative responses to phytohemagglutinin (PHA) and plasma cortisol values at baseline (T1) and 5 weeks later (T2) among HIV-1 seronegative gay men.

recovery period observed for mitogen responsivity (see Fig. 8.1 and 8.2). Importantly, the immunologic and neuroendocrine patterns observed were independent of differences in predicted serostatus at baseline and unrelated to changes in HIV-1 related symptoms, extraneous stressful life events, high-risk sexual behavior frequency, sleep, physical activity levels, aerobic fitness, or albumin concentrations across the study period.

Viewing the decision to enter the study as a psychosocial stressor, we reasoned that the ability to deny or distract oneself from the magnitude and

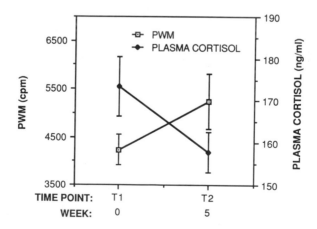

FIG. 8.2.   Mean (±SEM) lymphocyte proliferative responses to pokeweed mitogen (PWM) and plasma cortisol values at baseline (T1) and 5 weeks later (T2) among HIV-1 seronegative gay men.

ramifications of such a stressor might buffer its short-term deleterious immunological effects. Analyses of individual differences indicated that higher baseline cortisol concentrations and lower denial coping strategy scores were associated with the greatest impairment in PHA responses at study entry. These findings suggested that a dispositional denial tendency, which might shield at-risk individuals from ruminating about their perceived risk of infectivity, contributes to transient impairments in mitogen responsivity. Using a situational measure of stressor-specific disturbing cognitions – the Impact of Events Scale (Horowitz et al., 1979) – these dispositional denial scores were found to be positively correlated with the active avoidance of AIDS risk-related thoughts at multiple time points before and after serostatus notification for this group (Antoni et al., 1990). Some have suggested that the use of denial strategies may help to minimize perceived stress and thereby facilitate coping (Cohen & Lazarus, 1973), although others restrict this benefit to the "primary appraisal" stage of stressor interaction (Mullen & Suls, 1982). Interestingly, some work has found the use of denial defenses to be inversely related to chronic urinary corticosteroid levels (Mason et al., 1986) as well as with suppressed corticosteroid responses to acute stressors (Mason, 1975), thereby suggesting a potential role of neuroendocrine mediation in this phenomenon. In summary, we have observed significant neuroendocrine and immunologic changes in healthy seronegative gay males exposed to a potent psychosocial stressor and identified individual difference variables that may interact with this stressor in affecting immune functioning.

In contrast to the patterns of change in PNI variables noted in our seronegative subjects, we found that over the 5-week prenotification period, individuals who were ultimately shown to be seropositive displayed no such change in mitogen responsivity despite the fact that they evidenced a greater degree of affective distress (anxiety, depression, and intrusive thoughts) than their seronegative counterparts at each time point. Moreover, we observed that although the seropositive group reported increases in anxiety, depression, and intrusive thoughts in response to antibody status notification – at elevations comparable to psychiatric outpatients – they showed virtually no change in mitogen responsivity pre- to postnotification (Ironson et al., 1990). Other psychoimmunologic studies have provided evidence for decrements in lymphocyte proliferative responses to mitogens such as PHA or Con A among healthy individuals experiencing acute examination stress (Halvorsen & Vassend, 1987; Kiecolt-Glaser, Garner et al., 1984; Workman & LaVia, 1987), among bereaving males pre- to postdeath of spouse (Irwin, Daniels, & Weiner, 1987), and in patients suffering from major depressive disorder (Schleifer et al., 1984). Impaired mitogen responses have also been correlated with severity of depressive symptoms (Irwin, Daniels, & Weiner, 1987) and degree of intrusiveness of stressor-related thoughts (using the IES; Workman & LaVia, 1987) suggesting that individual differences in psychological distress responses also impact this index of cell-mediated immunity. Given this literature we were surprised at the absence of a PHA response change in our seropositives who (a) were exposed to a potent psychosocial stressor, and (b) were displaying clinical elevations on several distress markers characterizing anxiety, depression, confusion, and intrusive thoughts.

We next examined the nature of this disparity by assessing concurrently measured psychological distress, plasma cortisol, and mitogen responsivity changes in the periods preceding and following serostatus notification in expanded samples of seropositive and seronegative gay males. This design allowed us to study the correlates and effects of the two stressors previously mentioned: (a) the decision to enter the study; and (b) serostatus notification. Importantly, the seropositive and seronegative groups showed no differences in age, ethnicity, education, or income nor any differences in recent stressful events. The groups were also similar in terms of weeknight sleep, serum albumin, aerobic fitness, strenuous physical activity levels, and high-risk sexual activities at baseline and there were no significant changes in any of these variables across the study period. We assessed between-serostatus group differences in PNI variables at the time of the first stressor and in response to the second as well as intercorrelations among measures within the HIV-1 infected group. Results converged on a pattern of discordance and asynchronism among distress, neuroendocrine, and immunologic response measures in seropositives as compared to seronegatives who showed significant psychoimmunologic associations and synchronous movement (Antoni, Schneiderman, Klimas et al., 1991).

Regarding the asynchrony observed in seropositives, we noted that despite displaying marked increases in several psychosocial distress markers (state anxiety, depression, confusion, and intrusive thoughts) pre- to postnotification, these individuals showed significant decrements in cortisol over this period (see Fig. 8.3). In contrast, the seronegative comparison group showed parallel decreases in both distress and cortisol over an identical observation period—consonant with the relief of a negative antibody test. We reasoned that the asynchronism between psychological and endocrine response measures across this acute stressor period in seropositives, might explain, in part, the psychoimmunologic dissociation previously documented for this group (Ironson et al., 1990).

We next evaluated the role of individual differences in PNI variables within the seropositive group. Among seropositives, plasma cortisol concentrations were negatively correlated with psychological distress and positively correlated with lymphocyte responses to PHA when these measures were assessed basally and in response to serostatus notification. This "reversed" pattern of psychoendocrine and endocrine-immune associations

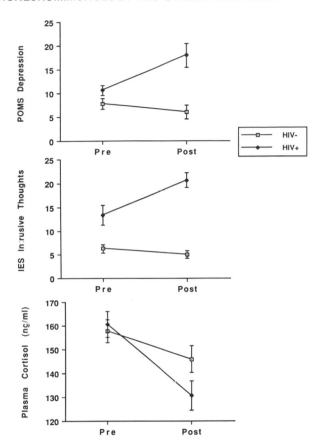

FIG. 8.3.   Mean (±SEM) pre and postnotification Profile of Mood States (POMS) depression and Impact of Events Scale (IES) intrusive thoughts scores and plasma cortisol concentrations among HIV-1 seronegative and seropositive gay men.

was in opposition to the positive distress-cortisol and negative cortisol-PHA correlations found in their seronegative counterparts and could not be explained by individual differences in perceived risk of infectivity (predicted serostatus) prior to notification or extraneous environmental stressors within the seropositive group. The fact that this atypical pattern was (a) evident in seropositives before and after notification but at neither set of time points in seronegatives, (b) independent of negative life events experienced in the subjects' environments, and (c) unrelated to predicted serostatus, suggest that the phenomenon is not a stress-induced one but more likely determined by the presence of HIV-1.

Others have provided evidence suggesting similar disparities between HIV-1 seropositive and seronegative men. For instance, perceived lympha-denopathy-positive status among HIV-1 seropositive males with and without later physical confirmation of lymphadenopathy was associated with a greater degree of depressed affect but not with differences in CD4/CD8 cell ratios (Ostrow et al., 1986). In contrast, perceived lympha-denopathy-positive status was associated with both greater depression and lower CD4/CD8 ratios in a seronegative group of lymphadenopathy-positive and negative men. These investigators came to the conclusion that the "modest" effects of psychological stressors on immune functioning will be difficult to document until we can "factor out" the larger contribution of the viral infection itself.

Although there is as yet no reliable procedure available for assessing the precise amount of "viral burden or load" that an infected host is enduring, some have attempted to classify the severity of the infection on the basis of immunologic (CD4, CD4/CD8 ratios) cell counts (Zolla-Pazner et al., 1987)—this index being presumably related to the number of CD8 cells produced in response to the viral infection and inversely related to the number of CD4 targets destroyed by HIV-1. To explore the degree to which severity of the viral infection contributed to our atypical pattern of findings, we dichotomized our seropositive sample into those with CD4 counts above and below the group median (713 cells/mm^3) and compared the two resulting subgroups on psychological, neuroendocrine, and immune response measures. There were no subgroup differences on any measure at either prenotification time point nor the magnitude of change scores between time points between these two groups. We repeated these analyses using the Zolla-Pazner (Z-P) scale as the classification criterion. Again we found no differences in raw scores or change scores between Z-P Scale 1 and 2 seropositive subjects. These two sets of findings suggested that the presence but not severity of HIV-1 infection determines the unique pattern of response values noted in this study. Such conclusions are, however, limited by the fact that the "severity" criteria employed in this study (median CD4 counts and the Zolla-Pazner et al. scale) are somewhat gross and are likely to have more clinical utility than research precision. A more precise marker of the infection process (e.g., B$_2$-microglobulin; Fahey et al., 1990) may have elucidated the role of HIV-1 infection severity in the phenomena noted in this study.

In view of the fact that the atypical pattern of PNI relationships evident in this asymptomatic seropositive sample could not be explained by individual differences in perceived risk or infection severity as operationa-lized herein, we have begun to examine possible mechanisms that might account for these findings. Some possibilities that we have considered include a neurotropic effect of HIV-1 perhaps affecting (a) the availability of HPAC neuropeptides (CRH, ACTH) and regulation in long and short HPAC feedback loops (Falkenbach, St. Klauke, Michels, Hunold, & Schifferdecker, 1989; Lewi et al., 1989) with consequent alterations in the production of these substances in stressful circumstances, or (b) the responsivity of the autonomic nervous system (Cohen & Laudenslager, in press) with secondary effects on HPAC potentiation (Axelrod & Reisine, 1984). Importantly, however, the only empirical evidence to date suggesting neuroendocrine abnormalities in HIV-1 infected populations has been restricted to samples of AIDS patients where the likelihood is high that adrenal dysfunctions are directly caused by opportunistic infections (e.g., cytomegalovirus) of the adrenals and neoplasms (Kaposi's sarcoma) or the treatments utilized in their treatment (Aron, 1989). We are unaware of any work that indicates that asymptomatic HIV-1 seropositive individuals show such endocrine changes, however. Especially relevant to the atypical endocrine-immunologic relationships noted in the present sample of infected individuals, HIV-1 may compromise neuroendocrine target availability by depleting helper cell (CD4 cells) numbers below some critical threshold (e.g., 700 cells/mm^3), by inducing a state of corticosteroid resistance in mononuclear cells (Balotta et al., 1989), or by altering lymphocyte intracellular (nuclear) phenomena necessary for incorporating steroid ligands.

An alternative explanation for the apparently counterintuitive neuroendocrine patterns previously noted may lie in the nature of the measurement protocol — specifically, the timing of neuroendocrine samples relative to the notification stressor. In that the first postnotification cortisol value is obtained 72 hours after the fact, it is conceivable that the magnitude of the cortisol concentration at this point is reflective of a rebound effect rather than an initial response. As such, initial cortisol "responses" — at the time of notification — may actually be manifest as a sharp increase followed by a greater decrease. A separate issue concerns the temporal relationship between neuroendocrine and immunologic responses. Specifically, different response latencies for cortisol and mitogen responsivity — a likely scenario — complicate the evaluation of intersystem relationships and would limit the degree to which concurrent measurement designs (such as the present one) can address this issue.

PNI Mechanism Studies

Our ongoing work examines potential mechanisms underlying our previous findings while attending to these methodological concerns by assessing basal levels (to assess chronic stress effects) and stress responsivity (to assess acute stressor effects) across multiple response channels including cognitive/affective, autonomic, neuroendocrine, neuropeptide, cytokine, and functional immune response systems. These phenomena are being studied in asymptomatic seropositive and matched-seronegative gay males, seropositives with lymphadenopathy, and a group of matched nonrisk group members. We are using a standardized laboratory task (speech stressor) in order to maximize control over extraneous sources of variance, to establish extensive pre- and post-stressor baseline information, and to assess the time course of stressor reactivity in systems that as yet remain unstudied. We are also examining the role of structural differences and changes in lymphocytes isolated from members of these groups in order to evaluate further the dissociation among response measures previously noted. Specifically, we plan to quantify lymphocyte receptors (e.g., number and affinity) for stressor-associated ligands (e.g., ACTH, epinephrine), as well as membrane changes and postreceptor activities (calcium influx and second messenger changes) following in-vitro stimulation with these ligands in seropositive and seronegative groups. Through a series of systematic in-vivo and in-vitro tests, this research program will allow us to explore the location(s) of intersystem dysregulation(s) (i.e., psychoendocrine, neuroimmune) that might account for the disparities in PNI relationships between our seronegative and seropositive men (see Table 8.1).

Physiological Reactivity

Other laboratories have provided structural (e.g., lymphocyte receptors; Plaut, 1987, for review) and functional (e.g., infusion studies; Crary et al.,

TABLE 8.1
Paradigms Used to Examine the Mechanisms of Differential PNI Relationships in HIV+ and HIV− Men in Our Lab (E = epinephrine, NE = norepinephrine, ACTH = adrenocorticotropin hormone, C = cortisol)

System Interaction	Laboratory Paradigm	Ligands	Parameters
Psychoendocrine	in-vivo physiological reactivity to standardized stressor	E, NE, ACTH, C	magnitude and recovery of response
Neuroimmune: Within lymphocyte	receptor characterization for stressor-associated ligands	E, NE, ACTH	number, affinity, down-regulation
	membrane permeability	E, NE, ACTH, C	membrane fluidity, capping response
	postmembrane studies	E, NE, ACTH, C	exogenous CA^{++} influx, endogenous Ca^{++} release, 2nd messenger activities
Neuroimmune: Immune function	in-vitro dose-response effects of ligands on cell-mediated immune function	E, NE, ACTH, C	mitogen (PHA, PWM)-induced cytokine production and blastogenic responses

1983) evidence for the immunomodulatory effects of several neuroendo-crines and neuropeptides (E, NE, ACTH, and cortisol) that are often associated with an organism's response to stressors (McCabe & Schneider-man, 1985). However, little is known regarding the responsivity or immu-nomodulatory effects of these agents under conditions of both acute and chronic stress within immunologically intact hosts, and nothing is known about these effects in HIV-1 infected individuals. We are currently assessing cardiovascular (heart rate, blood pressure, cardiac output, total peripheral resistance, sympathetic drive on the myocardium, cardiac vagal tone), neuroendocrine (ACTH, cortisol, E, NE), and immunologic (interleukin-1 [IL-1], IL-2, gamma-interferon levels; proliferative responses to PHA and PWM; NK cell cytotoxicity) measures at rest and in response to a standardized speech stressor. This protocol utilizes several procedures that have been developed by our lab in conjunction with other major centers for the study of psychophysiologic reactivity in hypertensive populations (Nagel et al., 1989; Tischenkel et al., 1989). We are especially interested in examining differences in the magnitude and recovery of neuroendocrine and immunologic responses to the speech stressor among HIV-1 seronega-tives, asymptomatic seropositives, and those seropositives with lymphade-nopathy.

Lymphocyte Isolate Studies

Recent advances in the understanding of lymphocyte architecture and intracellular functioning have permitted the study of interactions between stressor-associated ligands and individual immune cells. Lymphocytes are the primary cellular repositories for immune responsiveness. During normal immune function, specific binding between a lymphocyte surface receptor and ligand (e.g., lymphokines, mitogens, and stressor-associated ligands) initiates a cascade of biochemical processes that produce intracellular signals including membrane-cytoskeleton interactions, calcium (Ca^{++}) influxes, activation of phospholipase C by GTP-binding protein(s) and inositol triphosphate (IP_3)-induced internal CA^{++} release. This transmem-brane signaling process ultimately causes a change in the behavior of lymphocytes—for example, receptor redistribution (so-called patching/capping), secretion of lymphokines and antibodies, cell motility, cell–cell recognition, or initiation of cell division (Bourguignon & Bourguignon, 1984).

We are hypothesizing that some dysregulation of signal transducing pathways may occur during ligand-induced lymphocyte activation in HIV-1 infected individuals. Such a dysregulation might contribute to the psy-choimmunological dissociations previously observed in our early stage seropositive subjects. Specifically, we are attempting to identify certain important cellular components in signal transducing pathways (e.g., receptor activation, Ca^{++} influxes, activation of phospholipase C by GTP-binding protein(s) measured by IP_3 production, and IP_3-induced internal Ca^{++} release) that may be responsible for abnormal functioning of lymphocytes infected by HIV-1.

Receptor Studies. Because the majority of the molecules on the surface of mammalian cells have not been well characterized, studies of the surface antigens and their functional interrelationships in normal lymphocytes and virus-infected lymphocytes are of great importance. We plan to first identify various lymphocyte surface receptors (e.g., IL-1, IL-2, and G-IFN receptors; ACTH and beta-adrenergic binding sites) and then compare the biochemical properties of those receptors (receptor numbers, ligand binding affinity, biosynthesis of the receptors, down-regulation of the receptor-ligand complexes) on peripheral lymphocytes isolated via cell-sorting techniques. We intend to compare such data collected from samples of sociodemographically matched HIV-1 seronegative, seropositive-asymptomatic, and seropositive-lymphadenopathy classified gay males. The results of these proposed experiments should help us to identify the possible changes of lymphocyte surface receptors that may occur during HIV-1 infection.

Postreceptor Studies. We are also investigating the effects of these ligands on lymphocyte membrane organization and postmembrane activities. Membrane organization effects are assessed with membrane fluidity studies and capping response studies. Ligand-induced postmembrane activities are of key interest to our lab. Intracellular Ca^{++} is known to play an important role in lymphocyte activation by transmitting signals (e.g., via lymphokines, mitogens, and stress-associated ligands) from the cell surface molecules to the intracellular components responsible for producing the functional response(s) including hormone receptor exposure, c-myc gene expression, and DNA synthesis (Bourguignon, Jy, Majercik, & Bourguignon, 1988). However, at the present time, it is still not clear whether the intracellular Ca^{++} increases that occur following the addition of external ligands is derived from intracellular or extracellular sources. At least two subcellular structures have been suggested to play a crucial role in regulating intracellular Ca^{++} concentration: the plasma membrane (with Ca^{++} influx and efflux components); and a vesicular, intracellular IP_3-sensitive Ca^{++} store that releases Ca^{++} into the cytosol (Jy, Fregien, Bourguignon, & Bourguignon, 1989; see Fig. 8.4). The entry of extracellular Ca^{++} into lymphocytes appears to occur via activation of receptor-operated (not voltage-dependent) Ca^{++} channels (Muallem, Schoeffield, Pandol, & Sachs, 1985). We are now planning to measure intracellular Ca^{++} activity during various ligand-induced signal transducing events in peripheral

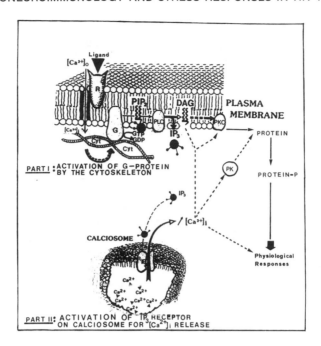

FIG. 8.4.   Model of Receptor-Mediated Signal Transduction. First, the binding of a ligand (e.g., mitogens, lymphokines, lectins, antibodies against specific surface molecules and antigens) to a plasma membrane receptor (R) induces an increase in Ca^{2+} influx that is required for the onset of cytoskeletal function. The Ca^{2+}-activated cytoskeleton (Cyt) will subsequently bind to and activate the membrane-associated GTP-binding proteins (G-proteins) (consisting of α, β & τ subunits) (as shown in Part I). The cytoskeleton-activated G-proteins (Giα) will then activate phospholipase C (PLC) that degrades phosphatidylinositol-4, 5-bisphosphate (PIP$_2$) to yield diacylglycerol (DAG) and inositol-triphosphate (IP$_3$). IP$_3$ will subsequently bind to the IP$_3$ receptor on internal Ca^{2+} storage sites (calciosomes) and induce internal Ca^{2+} release (as shown in Part II). In the presence of Ca^{2+}, DAG will stimulate protein kinase C (PKC) activity. The elevated intracellular Ca^{2+} (from either internal Ca^{2+} release or Ca^{2+} influx) will also activate other protein kinases (PK) that, in turn, phosphorylate their specific cellular substrates required for various physiological responses such as receptor capping, cell adhesion, secretion and proliferation.

lymphocytes isolated from each group of individuals previously mentioned. The results of these experiments should allow us to detect the possible dysfunction of receptor-mediated Ca^{++} mobilization that may occur in lymphocytes infected by HIV-1.

Recent studies also indicate that certain substances such as Con A, anti-Ig antibodies, and lymphokines induce phosphoinositide (PI) turnover in lymphoid cells (Suchard, Lo, & Bourguignon, 1988). Furthermore, this ligand-induced PI turnover can be potentiated by an activator of guanine nucleotide binding proteins (G-proteins), and depressed by an inhibitor of G-protein (e.g., pertussis toxin) (Bijsterbosch, Meade, Turner, & Klaus,

1985). Therefore, it is suggested that a G-protein may be involved in ligand-induced activation of lymphocytes. All G-proteins are heterotrimers consisting of alpha, beta, and theta subunits. The beta and theta subunits are closely associated and may participate in anchoring the subunit to the membrane. The αi subunit contains the binding site for GTP and exhibits GTPase activity. Studies have established that a family of similar G-proteins (Gsα, 45,000 kDa; Giα, 41,000 kDa; Gtα, 39,000 kDa, and Goα, 39,000 kDa) exist in all eukaryotic cells (Bourguignon, Walker, & Huang, 1990). It is now clear that these G-proteins are involved in transmembrane signal transduction as well as a number of other membrane-associated cellular activities. In particular, Gi is known to be involved in the activation of phospholipase C (PLC) that degrades all three phosphoinositides (PI, PIP, PIP$_2$) yielding diacylglycerol plus three inositol phosphates-inositol monophosphate (IP), inositol-4, 5-bisphosphate (IP$_2$), and inositol-1, 4, 5-triphosphate (IP$_3$) (Lochrie & Simon, 1988). These PLC-generated molecules have recently been recognized as important intracellular messengers for the initiation of a variety of cellular responses (Itoh et al., 1988). For example, diacylglycerol stimulates protein kinase C activity (Nishizuka, 1988). Protein phosphorylation by this enzyme appears to induce a wide range of cellular events, including cell shape changes, granule secretion, and the phosphorylation of certain membrane proteins as well as cytoskeletal proteins (Bourguignon, Walker, & Bourguignon, 1985). IP$_3$ is believed to be responsible for inducing intracellular Ca^{++} release that also triggers a number of subsequent cellular responses (Bourguignon, Field, & Bourguignon, 1985). We intend to explore second messenger systems such as G-protein and subsequent PLC activity during ligand-induced lymphocyte activation using peripheral lymphocytes isolated from members of the study groups. The results of these experiments should also help us to detect dysfunction in second messenger systems during HIV-infection.

Neuroimmune Functional Studies

The lymphocyte isolate studies have been designed to evaluate the degree to which the atypical PNI patterns observed in our seropositives can be attributed to abnormalities in the lymphocyte's processing of stressor-associated neuroendocrine signals. This model should yield important information about the basic mechanisms underlying neuroendocrine–lymphocyte interactions in both seronegative and seropositive hosts. A final component of our research program examines the effects of varying doses of stressor-associated neuroendocrines (E, NE, ACTH, cortisol) on proliferative responses to PHA and PWM using a whole blood assay procedure (Fletcher, Baron, Ashman, Fischl, & Klimas, 1987). Here we quantify the effects of five doses of ligand on responses to both mitogens and compare these graded effects between matched HIV-1 seronegative and seropositive men. We also evaluate the dose-response relationship between these neuroendocrines and mitogen-induced IL-2 production between these groups of individuals. These studies should provide information on the shape of the functions (e.g., linear, quadratic) describing neuroendocrine effects on mitogen responsivity in populations (seropositive and seronegative) previously shown to display patterns suggestive of a divergence in such relationships (Antoni et al., 1991).

As indicated in Table 8.1, the various paradigms employed in our lab are designed to systematically investigate the nature of the divergent PNI patterns that we have observed in our HIV-1 seronegative and seropositive gay men. A dysfunction at the psychoendocrine level of intersystem communication (e.g., over or underreactivity of neuroendocrine response to stressor) will be detectable with the reactivity paradigm, whereas a dysfunction at the neuroimmune level could be ascertained in the lymphocyte isolate and/or dose-response functional studies. Beyond the identification and localization of such dysfunction(s), these experiments may provide information with implications for other PNI work.

Summary

We have presented some contemporary assessment, population, and paradigmatic issues relevant to PNI research with an emphasis on their implications for human studies of stressor-associated phenomena. Previous work from our lab, focusing on the affective, neuroendocrine, and immunologic effects of a potent field stressor are discussed in light of these issues. Finally, our ongoing programmatic study of the mechanisms underlying differential PNI relationships in HIV-1 seropositive and seronegative men is outlined. We stress the importance of assessing multiple levels of stress responsivity during exposure to both chronic and acute field and laboratory stressors with in-vivo and in-vitro models using populations who are likely to differ in the degree to which immunomodulation affects clinical status. The findings emerging from these studies may provide important information concerning the generalizability of previously documented PNI relationships to the study of HIV-1 infected individuals and other immunocompromised populations.

REFERENCES

Antoni, M., H., August, S., LaPerriere, A., Baggett, H. L., Klimas, N., Ironson, G., Schneiderman, N., & Fletcher, M. A. (1990). Psychological and neuroendocrine measures related to functional immune changes in anticipation of HIV-1 serostatus notification. *Psychosomatic Medicine, 52,* 496–510.

Antoni, M. H., Schneiderman, N., Klimas, N., LaPerriere, A., Ironson, G., & Fletcher, M. A. (1991). Disparities in psychosocial, neuroendocrine, and immunologic patterns in asymptomatic HIV-1 seropositive and seronegative gay men. *Biological Psychiatry, 29*, 1023–1041.

Aron, D. C. (1989). Endocrine complications of the Acquired Immunodeficiency Syndrome. *Archives of Internal Medicine, 149*, 330–333.

Axelrod, J., & Reisine, T. (1984). Stress hormones: Their interaction and regulation. *Science, 224*, 452–459.

Balotta, C., Vago, T., Bevilacqua, M., Galli, M., Norbiato, G., & Moroni, M. (1989). *HIV induces glucocorticoid resistance in mononuclear cells.* Paper presented at the fifth International Conference on AIDS, Montreal.

Bartrop, R., Lazarus, L., Luckhurst, E., Kiloh, L., & Penny, R. (1977). Depressed lymphocyte function after bereavement. *Lancet, 1*, 834–836.

Besedovsky, H., del Rey, A., Sorkin, E., DaPrada, M., Burri, R., & Honegger, C. (1983). The immune response evokes changes in brain noradrenergic neurons. *Science, 221*, 564–565.

Bijsterbosch, M. K., Meade, C. J., Turner, G. A., & Klaus, G. B. (1985). B lymphocyte receptors and polyphosphoinositide degradation. *Cell, 41*, 999–1006.

Bourguignon, L. Y. W., & Bourguignon, J. (1984). Capping and the cytoskeleton. *International Review of Cytology, 87*, 195.

Bourguignon, L. Y. W., Field, S., & Bourguignon, G. J. (1985). Phosphoregulation of A tropomyosin-like (30 KD) protein during platelet activation. *Journal of Cell Biochemistry, 29*, 19–30.

Bourguignon, L. Y. W., Jy, W., Majercik, M. H., & Bourguignon, G. J. (1988). Lymphocyte activation and capping of hormone receptors. *Journal of Cell Biochemistry, 37*, 131–150.

Bourguignon, L. Y. W., Walker, G., & Bourguignon, G. J. (1985). Phorbol ester-induced phosphoregulation of A transmembrane glycoprotein CGP (80) in human blood platelets. *Journal of Biology and Chemistry, 260*, 11775–11780.

Bourguignon, L. Y. W., Walker, G., & Huang, H. S. (1990). Interactions between a lymphoma membrane-associated GTP-binding protein and the cytoskeleton during receptor patching and capping. *Journal of Immunology, 144*, 2242–2252.

Brummitt, C., Sharp, B., Gekker, G., Keane, W., & Peterson, P. (1988). Modulatory effects of β-endorphin on interferon-γ production by cultured peripheral blood mononuclear cells: Heterogeneity among donors and the influence of culture medium. *Brain, Behavior, and Immunity, 2*, 187–197.

Calabrese, J., Kling, M., & Gold, P. (1987). Alterations in immunocompetence during stress, bereavement, and depression: Focus on neuroendocrine regulation. *American Journal of Psychiatry, 144*, 1123–1134.

Cohen, F., & Lazarus, R. (1973). Active coping processes, coping dispositions, and recovery from surgery. *Psychosomatic Medicine, 35*, 375–389.

Cohen, J., & Laudenslager, M. (in press). Autonomic nervous system involvement in patients with human immunodeficiency virus infection. *Neurology.*

Crary, B., Borysenko, M., Sutherland, D., Kutz, I., Borysenko, J., & Benson, H. (1983). Decrease in mitogen responsiveness of mononuclear cells from peripheral blood after epinephrine administration in humans. *Journal of Immunology, 130*, 694–697.

Cupps, T., & Fauci, A. (1982). Corticosteroid-mediated immunoregulation in man. *Immunology Review, 65*, 133–155.

Davidson, L., & Baum, A. (1986). Chronic stress and posttraumatic stress disorders. *Journal of Consulting and Clinical Psychology, 54*(3), 303–308.

DeMartini, R. M., Turner, R. R., Formenti, S. C., Boone, D. C., Bishop, P. C., Levine, A. M., & Parker, J. W. (1988). Peripheral blood mononuclear cell abnormalities and their relationship to clinical course in homosexual men with HIV infection. *Clinical Immunology and Immunopathology, 30*, 258–271.

Fahey, J., Taylor, J., Detels, R., Hofmann, B., Melemed, R., Nishanian, P., & Giorgi, J. (1990). The prognostic value of cellular and serologic markers in infection with human immunodeficiency virus type 1. *New England Journal of Medicine, 322,* 166–172.

Falkenbach, A., St. Klauke, B., Michels, P., Hunold, E., & Schifferdecker, P. (1989). *Deficiency of glucocorticoids in AIDS.* Paper presented at the fifth International Conference on AIDS, Montreal.

Felten, D., Felten, S., Carlson, S., Olschawka, J., & Livnat, S. (1985). Noradrenergic and peptidergic innervation of lymphoid tissue. *Journal of Immunology, 135*(Suppl 2), 755s–765s.

Fletcher, M. A., Baron, G., Ashman, M., Fischl, M., & Klimas, N. (1987). Use of whole blood methods in assessment of immune parameters in immunodeficiency states. *Diagnostic and Clinical Immunology, 5,* 69–81.

Glaser, R., Rice, J., Sheridan, J., Fertel, R., Stout, J., Speicher, C., Pinsky, D., Kotur, M., Post, A., Beck, M., & Kiecolt-Glaser, J. (1987). Stress-related immune suppression: Health implications. *Brain, Behavior, and Immunity, 1,* 7–20.

Halvorsen, R., & Vassend, O. (1987). Effects of examination stress on some cellular immunity functions. *Journal of Psychosomatic Research, 31*(6), 693–701.

Horowitz, M., Wilner, N., & Alvarez, W. (1979). Impact of event scale: A measure of subjective stress. *Psychosomatic Medicine, 41*(3), 209–218.

Ironson, G., LaPerriere, A., Antoni, M., O'Hearn, P., Schneiderman, N., Klimas, N., & Fletcher, M. A. (1990). Changes in immune and psychological measures as a function of anticipation and reaction to news of HIV-1 antibody status. *Psychosomatic Medicine, 52,* 247–270.

Irwin, M., Daniels, M., & Weiner, H. (1987). Immune and neuroendocrine changes during bereavement. *Psychiatric Clinic of North America, 10,* 449–465.

Irwin, M., Daniels, M., Risch, S., Bloom, E., & Weiner, H. (1988). Plasma cortisol and natural killer cell activity during bereavement. *Biological Psychiatry, 24,* 173–178.

Irwin, M., Daniels, M., Smith, T., Bloom, E., & Weiner, H. (1987). Impaired natural killer cell activity during bereavement. *Brain, Behavior, and Immunity, 1,* 98–104.

Itoh, H., Toyama, R., Kozasa, T., Tsukamoto, T., Matsuoka, M., & Kaziro, Y. (1988). Presence of three distinct molecular species of C_{Ti} protein α subunit. *Journal of Biology and Chemistry, 263,* 6656–6664.

Jacobsen, P., Perry, S., & Hirsch, D. (1990). Behavioral and psychological responses to HIV antibody testing. *Journal of Consulting and Clinical Psychology, 58*(1), 31–37.

Jy, W., Fregien, N., Bourguignon, G. J., & Bourguignon, L. Y. W. (1989). Role of Ca^{2+} in the regulation of hormone receptor exposure during lymphocyte activation. *Biochemistry and Biophysics Acta, 983,* 153–160.

Kiecolt-Glaser, J., & Glaser, R. (1988). Methodological issues in behavioral immunology research with humans. *Brain, Behavior, and Immunity, 2,* 67–78.

Kiecolt-Glaser, J., Fisher, L., Ogrocki, P., Stout, J., Speicher, C., & Glaser, R. (1987). Marital quality, marital disruption, and immune function. *Psychosomatic Medicine, 49,* 13–34.

Kiecolt-Glaser, J., Garner, W., Speicher, C., Penn, G. M., Holliday, J., & Glaser, R. (1984). Psychosocial modifiers of immunocompetence in medical students. *Psychosomatic Medicine, 46,* 7–14.

Kiecolt-Glaser, J., Glaser, R., Dyer, C., Shuttleworth, E., Ogrocki, P., & Speicher, C. (1987). Chronic stress and immunity in family caregivers of Alzheimer's disease victims. *Psychosomatic Medicine, 49,* 523–535.

Kiecolt-Glaser, J., Glaser, R., Williger, D., Stout, J., Messick, G., Shepard, S., Ricker, D., Romisher, S. C., Briner, W., Bonnell, G., & Donnerberg R. (1985). Psychosocial enhancement of immunocompetence in a geriatric population. *Health Psychology, 4,* 25–41.

Kiecolt-Glaser, J., Ricker, D., George, J., Messicak, G., Speicher, C., Garner, W., & Glaser, R. (1984). Urinary cortisol levels, cellular immunocompetency, and loneliness in psychiatric inpatients. *Psychosomatic Medicine, 46,* 15-23.

Levy, S., Herberman, R., Lippman, M., & d'Angelo, T. (1987). Correlation of stress factors with sustained depression of natural killer cell activity and predicted prognosis in patients with breast cancer. *Journal of Clinical Oncology, 5,* 348-353.

Lewi, D., Acetturi, C., Sader, H., Dias, R., Kater, C., & Motta, P. (1989). *Reduced cortisol production and adrenal necrosis in patients with AIDS.* Paper presented at the fifth International Conference on AIDS, Montreal.

Lochrie, M. M., & Simon, M. I. (1988). G protein multiplicity in eukaryotic signal transduction systems. *Biochemistry, 27,* 4957-4965.

Mason, J. (1975). Clinical psychophysiology: Psychoendocrine mechanisms. In M. Reiser (Ed.), *American handbook of psychiatry* (Vol. 4, pp. 553-582). New York: Basic Books.

Mason, J., Giller, E., Kosten, T., Ostroff, R., & Podd, L. (1986). Urinary free-cortisol levels in posttraumatic stress disorder patients. *Journal of Nervous and Mental Disease, 174*(3), 145-149.

McCabe, P. M., & Schneiderman, N. (1985). Psychophysiologic reactions to stress. In N. Schneiderman & J. T. Tapp (Eds.), *Behavioral medicine: The biopsychosocial approach* (pp. 99-131). Hillsdale, NJ: Lawrence Erlbaum Associates.

McKinnon, W., Weisse, C., Reynolds, C., Bowles, C., & Baum, A. (1989). Chronic stress, leukocyte subpopulations, and humoral response to latent viruses. *Health Psychology, 8*(4), 389-402.

Meyerhoff, J., Oleshansky, M., & Mougey, E. (1988). Psychologic stress increases plasma levels of prolactin, cortisol, and POMC-derived peptides in man. *Psychosomatic Medicine, 50,* 295-303.

Muallem, S., Schoeffield, M., Pandol, S., & Sachs, G. (1985). Inositol triphosphate modification of ion transport in rough endoplasmic reticulum. *Proceedings of the National Academy of Science, 82,* 4433-4437.

Mullen, B., & Suls, J. (1982). The effectiveness of attention and rejection as coping styles: A meta-analysis of temporal differences. *Journal of Psychosomatic Research, 26,* 43-49.

Nagel, J., Shyu, L., Reddy, S., Hurwitz, B., McCabe, P., & Schneiderman, N. (1989). New signal processing techniques for improved precision of noninvasive impedance cardiography. *Annals of Biomedical Engineering, 17,* 517-534.

National Academy of Sciences. (1989). *Research briefing: Behavioral influences on the endocrine and immune systems.* Washington, DC: National Academy Press.

Nicholson, J., Echenberg, D., Jones, B., Jaffe, H., Feorino, P., & McDougal, J. (1986). T-cytotoxic/suppressor cell phenotypes in a group of asymptomatic homosexual men with and without exposure to HTLV III/LAV. *Clinical Immunology and Immunopathology, 40,* 505-514.

Nishizuka, Y. (1988). The molecular heterogeneity of protein kinase C and its implications for cellular regulation. *Nature* (London), *334,* 661-665.

Ostrow, D., Joseph, J., Monjan, A., Kessler, R., Emmons, C., Phair, J., Fox, R., Kingsley, L., Dudley, J., Chmiel, J., & VanRaden, M. (1986). Psychosocial aspects of AIDS risk. *Psychopharmacology Bulletin, 22*(3), 678-683.

Palmblad, J., Petrini, B., Wasserman, J., & Akerstedt, T. (1979). Lymphocyte and granulocyte reactions during sleep deprivation. *Psychosomatic Medicine, 41,* 273-278.

Plaut, M. (1987). Lymphocyte hormone receptors. *Annual Review of Immunology, 5,* 621-669.

Riley, V. (1981). Psychoneuroendocrine influences on immunocompetence and neoplasia. *Science, 212,* 1100-1109.

Schaeffer, M., & Baum, A. (1984). Adrenal cortical response to stress at Three Mile Island. *Psychosomatic Medicine, 46,* 227-237.

Schleifer, S., Keller, S., Meyerson, A., Raskin, M., Davis, K., & Stein, M. (1984). Lymphocyte function in major depressive disorder. *Archives of General Psychiatry, 41,* 484–486.

Schleifer, S., Keller, S., Siris, S., Davis, K., & Stein, M. (1985). Depression and immunity: Lymphocyte function in ambulatory depressed patients, hospitalized schizophrenic patients, and patients hospitalized for herniorrhaphy. *Archives of General Psychiatry, 42,* 129–133.

Shavit, Y., & Martin, F. (1987). Opiates, stress, and immunity: Animal studies. *Annals of Behavioral Medicine, 9,* 11–15.

Sibinga, N., & Goldstein, A. (1988). Opioid peptides and opioid receptors in cells of the immune system. *Annual Review of Immunology, 6,* 219–249.

Suchard, S. J., Lo, H. K., & Bourguignon, L. Y. W. (1988). Isolation of Thy-1 cAMP and analysis of their phospholipid composition in mouse T-lymphoma cells. *Journal of Cell Physiology, 134,* 67–77.

Surman, O., Williams, J., Sheehan, D., Strom, T., Jones K., & Coleman, J. (1986). Immunological response to stress in agoraphobia and panic attacks. *Biological Psychiatry, 21,* 768–774.

Tischenkel, N., Saab, P., Schneiderman, N., Nelesen, R., DeCarlo-Pasin, R., Goldstein, D., Spitzer, S., Woo-Ming, R., & Weidler, D. (1989). Cardiovascular and neurohumoral responses to behavioral challenge as a function of race and sex. *Health Psychology, 8*(5), 503–524.

Visintainer, M., Volpicelli, J., & Seligman, M. (1982). Tumor rejection in rats after inescapable or escapable shock. *Science, 216* (4544), 437–439.

Winters, R., Ironson, G., & Schneiderman, N. (1990). The neurobiology of anxiety. In R. Rosenman, & D. Byrne (Eds.), *Anxiety and the heart* (pp. 187–210). Washington, DC: Hemisphere.

Workman, E., & LaVia, M. (1987). T-lymphocyte polyclonal proliferation: Effects of stress and stress response style on medical students taking National Board Examinations. *Clinical Immunology & Immunopathology, 43,* 308–313.

Zolla-Pazner, S., DesJarlais, D., Friedman, S., Spira, T., Marmor, M., Holzman, R., Mildvan, D., Yancovitz, S., Mathur-Wagh, U., Garber, J., El-Sadr, W., Cohen, H., Smith, D., Kalyanaraman, V., Kaplan, J., & Fishbein, D. (1987). *Nonrandom development of immunologic abnormalities after infection with human immunodeficiency virus: Implications for immunologic classification of the disease.* Proceedings of the National Academy of Sciences (USA), *84,* 5404–5408.

Clinical Significance of Psychoneuroimmunology: Prediction of Cancer Outcomes

9

Sandra M. Levy
University of Pittsburgh School of Medicine
Pittsburgh Cancer Institute

Dawn C. Roberts
University of Iowa

Most psychological studies that assess immunological components implicitly use these measures in one of two ways. In the first, an immunological measure may be used as an indicator of a psychological process. The primary goal of these studies is to draw inferences about psychological constructs or theories. In the second, an immunological measure may be used to explain the relation between a psychological process and a physical health outome. The goal of this second class of studies is to specify the mechanism of disease initiation or progression.

Distinction of these two classes is important because it guides research questions and methodologies, and directs overall progress within the field of psychoneuroimmunology. For instance, a common research strategy within psychoneuroimmunology is to establish covariation between psychological and immunological measures. However, establishing covariation does not necessarily advance the goal of the first class of studies (Cacioppo & Tassinary, 1990) nor does it automatically achieve the purposes of the second class of studies. The aim of the former additionally requires the delineation of immunological (and possibly other physiological system) patterns in the search for invariant relationships with psychological processes (Cacioppo & Tassinary, 1990). Likewise, the aim of the latter group of studies additionally requires demonstration of clinical as well as statistical significance of psychoimmunological covariation by predicting health outcomes. It is important, however, to note that these aims are not mutually exclusive, and indeed, investigations that strive to meet both goals likely will make stronger advances toward knowledge in the field.

It is the purpose of this chapter to discuss the use of immunological

165

measures in accordance with the goal of the second class of studies noted here, using cancer progression as the health outcome of interest. First, we briefly note conceptual and practical issues in the design of such investigations. Then, we provide examples of these issues with a review of our work in the area.

PSYCHONEUROIMMUNOLOGY AS A MECHANISM OF CANCER OUTCOME

A brief summary of steps in a research program of which the goal is to demonstrate a psychoimmunological mechanism of disease progression is listed in Table 9.1. These steps are not intended to be an exhaustive list, nor do they necessarily represent procedures for determining other disease processes such as etiology or initiation.

Practical issues in the application of these steps to predict cancer outcomes include: (a) selection of subjects for study, (b) selection of psychological, immunological, and disease outcome variables, and (c) timing of assessment.

Selection of Subjects

In attempting to understand initially the role of psychological processes in disease progression, it makes sense to study cancers in which such variables

TABLE 9.1
Overview of Steps Toward Establishing a Psychoneuroimmunological
Mechanism of Disease Progression

Demonstrate covariation between psychological factors of interest and immunological parameters relevant to disease progression. (Are psychological and immunological processes associated in subjects with this disease?)

Rule out alternative explanations of covariation through potentially confounding or coincidental variables through statistical (e.g., regression) or design (e.g., experimental manipulation) considerations. (Is this association the result of an artifactual influence?)

Identify degree of specificity of covariation. (What other psychological processes in addition to the one of interest relate to the immunological variables of interest?)

Specify differential immunological/physiological patterning for psychological factor of interest, if necessary. (What is the invariant relationship?)

Demonstrate presence of psychoimmunological relationship across time within subjects. (What is the longitudinal course of this association?)

Docuent serial, predictive associations between psychological factors, immunological patterns, and disease changes. (Do these factors interact in their influence on disease progression?)

Replicate and determine limits of psychoimmunological mediation. (What is the generalizability of these findings? For whom and under what conditions does this mediation hold?)

---

are most likely to play a substantial part. In other words, cancers in which biological factors do not account for total outcome variance may be those in which psychoimmunological mediation is strongest. Tumor site and stage are two examples. Very early or very advanced tumors, as well as cancers with a particularly virulent cell histopathology (e.g., lung or pancreatic cancer) rarely deviate from their expected course, and thus would be less likely to be influenced by any host characteristic, including psychological ones. Also, if there is a wide range of outcome across individuals despite similar disease characteristics and treatments, this variation may be due to some as yet unmeasured individual difference, such as psychological factors. Finally, mediation will be most easily (and perhaps only) demonstrated in cancers with previously documented susceptibility to neurological, endocrinological, or immunological influences (e.g., immunotherapy is an effective treatment). Examples include breast cancer and melanoma, which are susceptible to hormonal and immune responses (Hersey, Edwards, & McCarthy, 1980; Shimakowara, Imamura, Ymanaka, Ishii, & Kikuchi, 1982) and cervical cancer, for which a viral precipitating agent has been identified (Meisels & Morin, 1981).

Selection of Variables

Psychological Variables. Psychological variables will largely be determined by the particular theoretical interests of the investigators, although selection of these variables may be guided by previously established associations with immunological processes in animals or healthy individuals (e.g., uncontrollable stressors) or by previously established associations with disease outcomes (e.g., supressed emotional expression, depression). Articulated examples of the role that psychological processes play in cancer progression include learned helplessness/depression (Levy, 1985; Levy & Wise, 1988), Type C behavior (Temoshok, 1987), repressive coping style (Antoni & Goodkin, 1988), "fighting spirit" (Greer & Watson, 1987), and cancer-prone personality (Grossarth-Maticek, Eysenck, & Vetter, 1988). In addition to the selection of variables by theoretical guidance, methodological issues (e.g., self-report, interviewer-rated, or observational measures) may also be considered (see Temoshok & Heller, 1984, for a review).

Immunological Variables. As noted previously, selection of immunological variables for study may be guided by previously demonstrated associations with psychological variables (e.g., mitogen proliferation), although the most important consideration should be a previously demonstrated association with disease progression. For instance, natural killer (NK) cell activity (Whiteside & Herberman, 1989), lymphocyte proliferation to phytohemagglutinin (Burford-Mason, Gyte, & Watkins, 1989), and even peripheral lymphocyte counts (DiSaia, Morrow, Hill, & Mittelstaedt, 1978) have been demonstrated to have prognostic relevance for human cancer patients. In addition to these nonspecific immune defenses, tumor-specific antigens may affect tumor control (Doherty, Knowles, & Wettstein, 1984). Many functional assays require information about the number of peripheral cells and about functioning of other cell subsets before results may be interpreted from an immunological standpoint. However, increasing the number of immunological variables that are assessed will also lead to Type I inferential errors unless corrected.

Disease Outcomes. Cancer "outcomes" may include identification of a cancerous predisposition, cancer initiation, cancer severity (size of tumor, nodal status), recurrence (or disease-free interval), and death (or survival time). For the purposes of this chapter, the latter three outcomes are of interest, and it is possible that each outcome may be the result of its own specific mechanism. Although severity is usually assessed at diagnosis, time to final assessment of disease outcome typically requires at least 5 years.

Studies using recurrence and survival as endpoints have been criticized for their presumed promotion of self-blame and subsequently poorer emotional adjustment on the part of the patient. However, the empirical relation between self-blame and adjustment in these patients is unclear (Roberts, Harvey, & Andersen, 1988), and beliefs about blame may be modified to less threatening forms while remaining consistent with the existing literature (Cella, 1990). Alternatives to purely biological outcomes that weight survival time by quality of life have been suggested (Gelber & Goldhirsch, 1986; Kaplan, 1989). This excellent idea, however, may diminish independence between predictors and outcome.

Additional Variables. Other variables that may potentially confound associations between psychological variables and immunity include demographic characteristics (age, gender), disease characteristics, diurnal timing, alcohol and caffeine intake, nutrition, body mass, medication use, general health status, smoking, sleep, physical activity, menstrual cycle day, and so on (Kiecolt-Glaser & Glaser, 1988). In addition to those already listed, variables that may confound an association with disease outcomes include cancer risk factors, delay in seeking a diagnosis, and treatment or diagnostic procedures (Fox, 1978; Hersey et al., 1980; Teasdale, Hughes, Whitehead, & Newcombe, 1979). The importance of these variables may be diminished by excluding subjects with particular characteristics from the sample, by including subjects within a restricted range of a particular characteristic, or by using a within-subject design.

Timing of Assessment(s)

One of the most difficult aspects of designing investigations to determine a psychoimmunological mechanism of disease progression is the timing of psychological and immunological assessments. The low incidence of any particular type of cancer thwarts most attempts to predict the onset of cancer in the general population, although assessment of identified individuals with a precancerous condition may offer stronger predictive power (DeCosse, 1983). Thus, the strategy of predicting disease progression rather than initiation is preferred.

In predicting disease progression, individuals are often assessed relatively soon after diagnosis, to mitigate unknown or differential immunological or psychological effects of treatment. A problem with this strategy is that discovery of the biological presence of cancer occurs at approximately the same time as the imposing stressor of learning of (or suspecting) one's diagnosis of cancer, thereby producing indistinguishable disease effects and psychological stress effects on immunity. One solution has been to assess subjects over a time period when psychological factors change, but disease factors remain stable (Roberts, Andersen, Anderson, & Lubaroff, 1990).

Further opportunities for study may include individuals who have already received treatment and are at risk for recurrence. Traditionally, cancer treatments have been thought to impose alterations in immunity not only during, but for an extended period following termination of treatment (Penn, 1982; Zoller, Heumann, Betzler, Stimmel, & Matzku, 1989), leading to the assumption that immunological assessment may be meaningful only if conducted prior to treatment. Recently, however, there have been indications that at least one measure of immunological functioning, NK cell activity, was not affected by administration of chemotherapy and/or radiotherapy (Levy, Herberman, Lippman, & d'Angelo, 1987), suggesting that immunological assessments may be included with psychological assessments following treatment.

Finally, demonstration of the effects of psychological variables on disease progression among patients with advanced disease (Levy, Lee, Bagley, & Lippman, 1988; Spiegel, Bloom, Kraemer, & Gottheil, 1989), pushes investigators toward a search for the mechanism of this association. While behavioral mediators (treatment compliance, nutrition, sleep, physician interaction) may be assessed, immunological mediators may be uninterpretable, due to highly individualized treatments and variable tumor growth or metastases.

TOWARD AN EMPIRICAL DEMONSTRATION

Taking into account these issues, a series of investigations with breast cancer patients and a preliminary investigation with uterine cancer patients have been conducted. The aim of these studies was to test the hypothesis that psychological processes (specifically, depression that is the consequence of a helpless coping style and poor quality of social support) influence the progression of cancer through alterations in immunological functioning. In summary, these research programs attempt to clarify "how psychological variables interact with biological processes in the . . . early progression of cancer," the question articulated in a recent cancer research agenda (Andersen, Beck, Ouelette-Kobasa, Revenson, & Temoshok, 1989, p. 754).

The first step in this series of investigations was to document an association between psychological processes and tumor-relevant immunity within a sample of subjects with cancer (Levy, Herberman, Maluish, Schlien, & Lippman, 1985). Sixty-three women with early stage breast cancer were psychologically and immunologically assessed after surgery, but before pathology findings were known. Natural killer cell activity predicted concurrent measures of disease progression, with higher activity associated with fewer lymph nodes positive for malignant cells. Regression analyses additionally revealed that psychosocial factors (adjustment to illness, self-reported fatigue, and social support) accounted for 51% of the variance in NK cell activity. Patients who were rated as well adjusted to their illness, who reported receiving low support from their environment, and who expressed symptoms of fatigue tended to have lower immunological functioning. Thus, associations between psychological variables and immunity and between psychological variables and early disease status were demonstrated.

These initial findings were replicated and extended in a subsequent investigation with 120 early stage breast cancer patients (Levy, Herberman, Whiteside, et al., 1990). Assessment procedures were similar to the first investigation, but included finer grained measurement of the psychological variables of interest and of potentially confounding physiological and behavioral (e.g., sleep quality) variables. Perceived social support again emerged as an important predictor of NK cell activity, accounting for a greater portion of variance in immunological functioning than tumor characteristics (estrogen receptor status) and other disease relevant variables. However, disease status at assessment was not predicted by either immunological or psychological variables.

A similarly designed investigation was also conducted with early stage uterine cancer patients. Roberts and Andersen (1990) psychologically and immunologically assessed 68 women prior to treatment. Higher self-reported emotional distress, particularly depression, was significantly associated with higher white blood cell and lymphocyte counts, after accounting for variance due to disease factors. Disease status at diagnosis was not predicted by either immunological or psychological variables, a finding that may have been affected by the relatively coarse nature of immunological assessment.

Although replication of these findings supported the covariation of psychological factors and immunity in a sample with disease, failure to support consistently an association with concurrent measures of disease progression leads to examination of the ultimate effect on future progression, a question that was not addressed. The next step, therefore, was to demonstrate continued psychoimmunological covariation across time. Levy et al. (1987) followed the initial sample of patients and reassessed them 3 months later. As hypothesized, NK cell activity (at diagnosis), in addition to adjustment to illness, fatigue, and perceived social support (at either diagnosis or at repeat assessment) significantly predicted natural killer cell activity at reassessment. Further, this measure of immunological functioning was associated with disease progression, as measured by nodal status.

In addition to these replications, a stronger test of covariation between psychological and immunological processes would increase the generalizability and improve the internal validity of the previous research findings. Therefore, the focus of the next investigation was a manipulation of psychological variables of interest (Levy, Herberman, Rodin, & Seligman, 1990). It was hypothesized that an intervention that targeted the symptoms of depression, fatigue, and helplessness would also improve immunological functioning in cancer patients at risk for disease recurrence. Thirty colon cancer and malignant melanoma patients were randomized to an 8-week course of individually administered cognitive-behavioral therapy versus standard medical care following initial surgical treatment. Patients were psychosocially and immunologically assessed pre-randomization, mid-treatment, and posttreatment. In general, results showed that treated individuals showed a significant increase in NK cell number, and a trend toward significantly higher NK cell activity. In fact, NK values for the control group significantly decreased from pre- to post treatment. Parallel changes occurred in the psychosocial measures. Thus, the association between psychological and immunological processes was again supported. The clinical implications of this covariation were heightened because subjects were without detectable cancer, but at high risk for recurrence.

The latest step in approaching an answer to the question of psychoimmunologic mediation of cancer progression was the attempt to prospectively predict the endpoints of recurrence and death. The breast cancer subjects from the first investigation were followed for a minimum of 5 years (Levy, Herberman, Lippman, d'Angelo, & Lee, 1990). Using causal path modeling, NK cell activity (at diagnosis and at repeated assessments) strongly predicted probability of recurrence, and psychosocial factors (emotional distress and social support) predicted the rate of progression. Overall, these findings suggest the presence of both immunological and psychological influences on disease progression, although an interactive or mediational influence was not established.

Likewise, the initial uterine cancer sample was followed for at least 5 years, with similar findings (Roberts & Andersen, 1990). The probability of recurrence was not predicted by immunological or psychological variables. However, higher levels of self-reported emotional distress at diagnosis predicted a lowered probability of survival as well as shorter survival time. These associations remained even after accounting for the influence of other established prognostic indicators (e.g., stage, cell histopathology). The covariation between emotional distress and disease progression was documented, although serial linkages indicating direct psychoneuroimmunologic mediation of cancer progression could not be supported. Taken together, this series of studies suggests indirect support for psychoimmunological mediation of disease progression, and supports efforts toward continued, refined investigation. However, it also demonstrates the difficulty in establishing the clinical significance of psychoimmunological covariation within a complex model of disease progression. In light of these findings, it continues to be important to stress that biological factors (tumor type, site, stage, and biological treatments) are the major determinants of cancer progression and outcome. Until the conditions outlined in this chapter are empirically documented, the impact of a psychoimmunological mechanism on cancer progression remains a question awaiting answer.

REFERENCES

Andersen, B. L., Beck, G., Ouelette-Kobasa, S., Revenson, T. A., & Temoshok, L. (1989). Directions for a psychology research agenda in cancer. *Health Psychology, 8, 753-760.*

Antoni, M. H., & Goodkin, K. (1988). Life stress and moderator variables in the promotion of cervical neoplasia. I: Personality facets. *Journal of Psychosomatic Research, 32, 327-338.*

Burford-Mason, A., Gyte, G. M., & Watkins, S. M. (1989). Phytohaemagglutinin responsiveness of peripheral lymphocytes and survival in patients with primary breast cancer. *Breast Cancer Research and Treatment, 13, 243-250.*

Cacioppo, J. T., & Tassinary, L. G. (1990). Inferring psychological significance from physiological signals. *American Psychologist, 45, 16-28.*

Cella, D. F. (1990). Health promotion in oncology: A cancer wellness doctrine. *Journal of Psychosocial Oncology, 8, 17-31.*

DeCosse, J. J. (1983). Precancer: An overview. *Cancer Surveys, 2, 347-357.*

DiSaia, P. J., Morrow, C. P., Hill, A., & Mittelstaedt, L. (1978). Immune competence an survival in patients with advanced cervical cancer: Peripheral lymphocyte counts. *International Journal of Radiation Oncology, Biology, and Physics, 4, 449-451.*

Doherty, P., Knowles, B., Wettstein, P. (1984). Immunological surveillance of tumors in the context of major histocompatibility complex restriction of T cell function. *Advances in Cancer Research, 42, 1-65.*

Fox, B. H. (1978). Premorbid psychological factors as related to cancer incidence. *Journal of Behavioral Medicine, 1, 45-133.*

Gelber, R. D., & Goldhirsch, A. (1986). A new endpoint for the assessment of adjuvant therapy in postmenopausal women with operable breast cancer. *Journal of Clinical Oncology, 4, 1772–1779.*

Greer, S., & Watson, M. (1987). Mental adjustment to cancer: Its measurement and prognostic importance. *Cancer Surveys, 6, 439–453.*

Grossarth-Maticek, R., Eysenck, H. J., & Vetter, H. (1988). Personality type, smoking habit and their interaction as predictors of cancer and coronary heart disease. *Personality and Individual Differences, 9, 479–495.*

Hersey, P., Edwards, A., & McCarthy, W. H. (1980). Tumour-related changes in natural killer cell activity in melanoma patients: Influence of stage of disease, tumour thickness, and age of patients. *International Journal of Cancer, 25, 187–194.*

Kaplan, R. M. (1989). Health outcome models for policy analysis. *Health Psychology, 8, 723–735.*

Kiecolt-Glaser, J. K., & Glaser, R. (1988). Methodological issues in behavioral immunology research with humans. *Brain, Behavior, and Immunity, 2, 67–78.*

Levy, S. M. (1985). *Behavior and cancer.* San Francisco: Jossey-Bass.

Levy, S. M., Herberman, R. B., Lippman, M., & d'Angelo, T. (1987). Correlation of stress factors with sustained depression of natural killer cell activity and predicted prognosis in patients with breast cancer. *Journal of Clinical Oncology, 5, 348–353.*

Levy, S. M., Herberman, R. B., Lippman, M., d'Angelo, T., & Lee, J. (1990). *Immunological and psychosocial predictors of disease recurrence in patients with early stage breast cancer.* Manuscript submitted for publication.

Levy, S. M., Herberman, R. B., Maluish, A. M., Schlien, B., & Lippman, M. (1985). Prognostic risk assessment in primary breast cancer by behavioral and immunological parameters. *Health Psychology, 4, 99–113.*

Levy, S. M., Herberman, R. B., Rodin, J., & Seligman, M. (1990). Psychological and immunological effects of a randomized psychosocial treatment trial for colon cancer and malignant melanoma patients. In H. Balner & Y. van Rood (Eds.), *Conceptual and methodological issues in cancer psychotherapy intervention studies* (pp. 75–88). Amsterdam: Swets & Zeitlinger.

Levy, S. M., Herberman, R. B., Whiteside, T., Sanzo, K., Lee, J., & Kirkwood, J. (1990). Perceived social support and tumor estrogen/progesterone receptor status as predictors of natural killer cell activity in breast cancer patients. *Psychosomatic Medicine, 52, 73–85.*

Levy, S. M., Lee, J., Bagley, C., & Lippman, M. (1988). Survival hazards analysis in first recurrent breast cancer patients: Seven-year follow-up. *Psychosomatic Medicine, 50, 520–528.*

Levy, S. M., & Wise, B. D. (1988). Psychosocial risk factors and cancer progression. In C. L. Cooper (Ed.), *Stress and breast cancer* (pp. 77–96). Chichester: Wiley.

Meisels, A., & Morin, C. (1981). Human papillomavirus and cancer of the uterine cervix. *Gynecologic Oncology, 12, s111–s123.*

Penn, I. (1982). Mechanisms of therapy-induced malignancies. *Cancer Surveys, 1, 763–782.*

Roberts, D. C., & Andersen, B. L. (1990). *Emotional distress, immunological parameters, and disease outcomes among cancer patients.* Unpublished manuscript, University of Iowa, Iowa City.

Roberts, D. C., Andersen, B. L., Anderson, B. A., & Lubaroff, D. M. (1990). *Course of psychological distress and cellular immunity at cancer diagnosis.* Unpublished doctoral dissertation, University of Iowa, Iowa City.

Roberts (Turnquist), D. C., Harvey, J. H., & Andersen, B. L. (1988). Attributions and adjustment to life-threatening illness. *British Journal of Clinical Psychology, 27, 55–65.*

Shimakowara, I., Imamura, M., Yamanaka, N., Ishii, Y., & Kikuchi, K. (1982). Identification of lymphocyte subpopulations in human breast cancer tissues and its significance. *Cancer, 49, 1456–1464.*

Spiegel, D., Bloom, J. R., Kraemer, H. C., & Gottheil, E. (1989). Effect of psychosocial treatment on survival of patients with metastatic breast cancer. *Lancet, 2, 888-891.*

Teasdale, C., Hughes, L. E., Whitehead, R. H., & Newcombe, R. G. (1979). Factors affecting pretreatment immune competence in cancer patients. *Cancer Immunology and Immunotherapy, 6, 89-99.*

Temoshok, L. (1987). Personality, coping style, emotion and cancer: Towards an integrative model. *Cancer Surveys, 6, 545-567.*

Temoshok, L., & Heller, B. W. (1984). On comparing apples, oranges and fruit salad: A methodological overview of medical outcome studies in psychosocial oncology. In C. L. Cooper (Ed.), *Psychosocial stress and cancer* (pp. 231-260). Chichester: Wiley.

Whiteside, T., & Herberman, R. B. (1989). The role of natural killer cells in human disease. *Clinical Immunology and Immunopathology, 53, 1-23.*

Zoller, M., Heumann, U., Betzler, M., Stimmel, H., & Matzku, S. (1989). Depression of nonadaptive immunity after surgical stress: Influence on metastatic spread. *Invasive Metastases, 9, 46-68.*

10

Interactive Models of Reactivity: The Relationship Between Hostility and Potentially Pathogenic Physiological Responses to Social Stressors

Edward C. Suarez
Redford B. Williams, Jr
Duke University Medical Center

The influence of behaviors on the development and progression of coronary heart disease (CHD) is thought to involve both psychosocial and physiological processes. For example, high blood pressure, high serum cholesterol, and cigarette smoking, considered to be risk factors for CHD, are each affected by behavior. One avenue of research has attempted to determine the direct effects of coronary-prone behaviors on physiological responses to environmental stimuli. It has been hypothesized that the link between coronary-prone behaviors and CHD involves excessive or prolonged hyperactivation of the sympathetic nervous system (SNS; Krantz & Manuck, 1984). It is believed that pronounced and recurrent activation of the SNS by particular behavioral stimuli can precipitate endothelial injury, and thus promote atherosclerotic plaque build-up (Ross & Glomset, 1973). Animal studies (Manuck, Muldoon, Kaplan, Adams, & Polefrone, 1989) have indicated that behaviorally induced cardiovascular (CV) hyperactivity is significantly positively associated with degree of intimal damage and severity of coronary artery disease (CAD). Although there is a paucity of evidence suggesting a direct link between behaviorally induced CV changes and CHD in man, results from two longitudinal studies have indicated that the cold pressor test (Keys, Taylor, Blackburn, Brozck, Anderson, & Somonson, 1971) and changes in posture (Sparrow, Tifft, Rosner, & Weiss, 1984) evoke diastolic blood pressure (DBP) responses that are positively associated with risk of CHD. Consistent with the notion of hyperresponsitivity as a contributing factor for CHD, some studies (Corse, Manuck, Cantwell, Giordani, & Matthews, 1982; Dembroski, MacDougall, & Lushene, 1979) have shown that cardiac patients, relative to noncoronary

175

patient controls, respond with greater physiological increases to behavioral stressors.

In addition to the hypothesized role of CV hyperreactivity in precipitating and initiating the progression of atherosclerosis, neuroendocrine responses to behavioral stressors have also been linked to the pathogenic process. For example, catecholamines are known to mediate both CV activation and lipid mobilization (Havel & Goldstein, 1959). The latter action could contribute to acceleration of the atherosclerotic process by increasing serum cholesterol. Corticosteroids,on the other hand, have been positively associated with the development of atherosclerosis, elevated serum lipids, and increased proportions of dead and injured endothelial cells (see Henry, 1983).

Thus, the link between behavioral attributes and CHD could involve excessive neuroendocrine and cardiovascular responses to behavioral stimulation. The primary aim of this chapter is to review new evidence for a link between behaviors that are risk engendering, specifically hostility and anger, and potentially pathogenic physiological responses to behavioral stressors. In addition to excessive SNS reactivity, we present preliminary evidence to indicate that persons displaying coronary-prone behaviors may also be at increased risk by virtue of deficient parasympathetic antagonism of the effects of SNS activation of the CV system. These new findings are used to develop an interactional approach to the study of physiological reactivity.

THE TYPE A PATTERN, CHD, AND REACTIVITY

One behavioral attribute that has been implicated in CHD pathogenesis is the multidimensional Type A behavior pattern (TABP). The link between the Type A pattern and CHD was first documented in the Western Collaborative Group Study (WCGS; Rosenman et al., 1975), where it was shown that Type A persons, relative to Type B persons, were at twice the risk for CHD. Because the increased risk of CHD associated with the Type A pattern was independent of standard risk factors, such as smoking, serum cholesterol, and hypertension, researchers have attempted to understand physiological mechanisms linking Type A to CHD. This latter observation directly contributed to research on the link between TABP and stress-induced cardiovascular and neurohormonal responses. In three decades of research on Type A behavior, journals have published numerous studies aimed at examining potential reactivity differences between Type A and B subjects. In a large number of these psychophysiological studies, researchers employed common laboratory stressors (sometimes with monetary incentives for performing well), to see if greater physiological responses occurred in Type A subjects. Subjects were asked to participate in tasks such as mental arithmetic, the Stroop color word task, cold pressor, solvable anagrams, physical stressors, and speech stressor while cardiovascular and neurohormonal responses were assessed. In a small percentage of studies, interpersonal challenge in the form of harassment was used to elicit physiological response differences between Type A and B subjects. Although the large number of studies prohibits specific description of findings, results from a recent meta-analytic study (Harbin, 1989) suggest that the Type A pattern is moderately associated with greater stress-induced systolic blood pressure (SBP) and heart rate (HR) changes.

THE ROLE OF HOSTILITY AND ANGER IN CHD

Although the first 20 years of research produced findings that confirmed the increased risk of CHD associated with Type A (Review Panel, 1981), recent failures in a growing number of epidemiological studies (for review see Williams, 1987b) have raised some questions as to the extent that the global Type A pattern is coronary-prone. For example, in the Multiple Risk Factor Intervention Trial (MRFIT; Dembroski, MacDougall, Costa, & Crandits, 1989), Structured Interview (SI)-derived Type A scores failed to predict CHD incidence. Surprisingly, in one study (Ragland & Brand, 1988) of participants who survived a clinically confirmed myocardial infarction primary event, Type B subjects, relative to Type A subjects, died at a substantially higher rate. In several angiography studies (Williams, 1987a), SI-derived Type A scores have also failed to correlate with severity of CAD. The failure of global Type A to predict CHD endpoints has led researchers to re-examine the concept of coronary-prone behaviors and to suggest the possibility that only particular components of the global TABP may be "toxic" (e.g., coronary-prone), and thus constitute greater risk for developing CHD. A recent test of this hypothesis using prospective data from the MRFIT (Dembroski et al., 1989) indicated that although the global TABP and its paralinguistic components (e.g., loudness, explosiveness, rapid speech) were not related to CHD incidence, a clinical rating of hostility was positively and significantly associated with incidence of CHD. Consistent with the MRFIT results, Hecker, Chesney, Black, and Frautschi (1989) showed that, in a case-control study of participants in the WCGS, hostility was the strongest predictor of CHD.

The role of hostility in the development of CHD has also received support from studies that have assessed hostility via self-report scales, such as the Cook and Medley Hostility (Ho) scale (Cook & Medley, 1954) and the Buss–Durkee Hostility Inventory (BDHI, Buss & Durkee, 1957). In three prospective studies (Barefoot, Dahlstrom, Williams, 1983; Barefoot, Williams, Dahlstrom, & Dodge, 1987; Shekelle, Gale, Ostfeld, & Paul,1983), Ho scores have significantly predicted CHD incidence and total mortality. Although three other studies (Hearn, Murray, Luepker, 1989; Leon, Finn, Bailey, Murray, 1988; McCranie, Watkins, Brandsma, Sisson, 1986) have failed to confirm this association, results from these studies must be interpreted with caution due to methodological problems, such as inappropriate testing conditions (Williams, 1987a). Ho scores, as well as scores derived from the BDHI, have also been positively associated with severity of CAD (Siegman, Dembroski, & Ringel, 1987; Williams et al., 1980). In light of these positive findings suggesting that hostility is an important dimension of coronary-prone behaviors, researchers have begun to focus their efforts on determining the degree of association between hostility and behaviorally induced physiological reactivity.

Similar to the Type A-reactivity hypothesis, it is believed that the hostility-related risk of CHD may be associated, in part, with stress-induced physiological hyperreactivity. As we see here, however, using appropriately challenging tasks that elicit anger and anger-related emotional states is essential in testing this hypothesis.

HOSTILITY AND REACTIVITY: AN INTERACTIVE PROCESS

Early studies examining the link between hostility and physiological arousal produced mixed results and for the most part, used samples of Type A and B subjects. For example, in a study of young Type A and B males, Dembroski, MacDougall, Shields, Petitto, and Lushene (1978) showed that SI-derived ratings of potential for hostility were positively and significantly related to stress-induced CV changes. Glass, Lake, Contrada, Kehoe, and Erlanger (1983), however, found a negative relationship between potential for hostility and cardiovascular responses to laboratory challenges. More recent studies (Sallis, Johnson, Treverron, Kaplan, & Hovell, 1987; Smith & Houston, 1987) that have assessed hostility via the Ho scale and the BDHI have also failed to document a consistent positive relationship between hostility and stress-induced reactivity.

Although several explanations may account for the inconsistency of the results described here, we propose that the failure to replicate is largely due to the type of stressors used to evoke hostility-related physiological responses. Given the interpersonal nature of hostility (Averill, 1982), it seems likely that only tasks that are socially and interpersonally challenging, and thus more likely to invoke hostility-related emotions and behaviors, would be successful in documenting a relationship between behaviorally induced reactivity and hostility. It is conceivable that hostility and anger may have little or no impact on physiological responses in the absence of anger inducement. Given that the arousal of anger or anger-related states is not a salient characteristic of commonly used laboratory challenges, such as mental arithmetic or cold pressor, the failure of prior studies to document hostility-related reactivity is not surprising.

In light of the preliminary evidence and the hypothesized role of interpersonal stressors in moderating the hostility-reactivity link, we conducted a study to directly assess the effect of task characteristics on the relationship between Ho scores and CV reactivity. In our first study (Suarez & Williams, 1989), we manipulated the degree of interpersonal challenge by having two conditions, one in which subjects participated in a solvable anagram task with a monetary incentive and another in which subjects participated in the same task but were also harassed by a confederate. Participants in this study were young males (aged 18–24) selected for having a negative family history of CHD and Ho scores in the upper or lower quartile (e.g., above 24 or below 14) of their respective distribution.

Consistent with our hypothesis, results indicated that hostility and reactivity were positively related but only in the harassment condition. High Ho subjects, relative to low Ho subjects who were harassed, evidenced significantly greater cardiovascular increases during the anagrams with harassment and poorer recovery. Additional comparisons between harassed and nonharassed low Ho groups indicated that harassment failed to evoke significant differences in CV responses. As predicted, in the nonharassment condition, we failed to detect CV differences between high and low Ho subjects.

We next explored the possibility that CV changes were associated with increased anger and irritation states. Similar to the two-factor model proposed by Manuck et al. (1989), we hypothesized that the CV hyperreactivity observed in high Ho subjects would be positively associated with negative affects, specifically anger and irritation. Results showed that in high Ho subjects, self-reported ratings of anger and irritation were positively and significantly associated with CV changes to task ($rs > .50$). In contrast, for low Ho men, these correlations were not significant. Additional analyses confirmed that the best predictor of task-related changes was the interactions between negative affects (e.g., anger, irritation) and Ho group. This indicates that hostile individuals who become angry and irritated to the harassment are physiologically most reactive.

Finally, we examined the relationships between dimensions of hostility and CV changes as a function of the harassment condition (Suarez & Williams, 1990). Recent evidence (Siegman et al., 1987) has suggested that the BDHI expression of anger scores are positively associated with severity of coronary artery disease (CAD), whereas the BDHI experience of anger scores are negatively associated with CAD severity. It seems likely, therefore, that the expression of anger, relative to the experience of anger, would be more strongly and positively associated with CV responses to harassment.

We derived the two dimensions of hostility by performing a factor analysis on the following scales: hostility, neuroticism, and agreeableness from the NEO-Personality Inventory (Costa & McRae, 1985), expression and experience of anger factors from BDHI, and anger-out and anger-in from the Anger Expression scale (AX; Spielberger, et al., 1985). Consistent with results from previous studies (Costa, McCrae, & Dembroski, 1989; Musante, MacDougall, Dembroski, & Costa, 1989) a two-factor model emerged. Factor 1, representing *antagonistic hostility,* was defined by positive loadings on both anger-out and expression of anger and a negative loading for agreeableness. A second factor representing *neurotic hostility* was defined by positive loadings on anger-in, neuroticism, and the experience of anger.

Analysis of the data revealed that high scores on the antagonistic factor predicted harassment-induced SBP and FBF changes during task and poorer SBP recovery. Surprisingly, high scores on the neurotic factor also predicted increased FBF changes to harassment. Correlational analyses between self-reported affect ratings and reactivity scores showed that, for subjects with high scores on either the antagonistic or neurotic hostility factor, CV changes were positively and significantly correlated with self-reported ratings of negative affects. These results confirmed our hypothesis that antagonistic hostility is a better predictor of behaviorally induced reactivity.

In our most recent work we have replicated and extended the above set of findings to include the association of Ho scores to harassment-induced CV responses in young women (Suarez, Williams, Harlan, & Peoples, 1990), as well as harassment-induced neuroendocrine changes in young men (Suarez, Williams, Harlan, People, Kuhn, & Schanberg, 1990). Results from the study (Suarez, Williams, Harlan, & Peoples, 1990) of high and low Ho women showed a significant Ho group by condition interaction for SBP and marginally significant for DBP. Post-hoc analysis revealed that harassed high Ho women, relative to low Ho women, exhibited significantly greater SBP and DBP changes during task and poorer SBP recovery. In contrast to our men's study, however, harassment induced greater CV responses in the low Ho women.

Preliminary analysis of the young men's neuroendocrine data has indicated that in comparisons to all other groups, harassed high Ho men evidenced greater norepinephrine and cortisol increases during the recovery period (Suarez et al., 1990). In addition, high Ho subjects, relative to low Ho subjects, showed higher levels of testosterone during baseline and greater testosterone changes to task, independent of condition.

Consistent with our observations, other researchers using a high conflict role-play task and unsolvable anagrams with misleading instructions have indicated a positive association between Ho scores and CV responses (Hardy & Smith, 1988; Smith & Allred, 1989; Weidner, Friend, Ficarotto, & Mendell, 1989). Also interesting to note is the fact that results from animal studies have indicated a similar "trait by situation" interaction in predicting severity of atherosclerosis. For example, studies have shown that dominant animals exhibited greater intimal damage and degree of atherosclerosis than subordinate animals, but only when exposed to a social stressor (Manuck et al., 1989).

Taken together, these studies suggest that exaggerated physiological reactivity to behavioral stressors is a plausible biological mechanism that could explain the increased risk of CHD associated with hostility. Equally as important, these data underscore the importance of situational factors in eliciting potentially pathogenic responses in high Ho persons. In our studies, Ho-related physiological effects could only be detected in the harassment condition, suggesting that the use of a social or interpersonal stressor is a necessary condition for demonstrating Ho differences in physiological reactivity.

INTERACTIVE MODULATORS OF REACTIVITY: TABP, HOSTILITY, AND AGE

Age is an important factor that has been overlooked in the research but is one that may have a moderating effect on the relationship between coronary-prone behaviors and reactivity. It is well known that aging is associated with a decrease in adrenergic system control of cardiac function (see Klausner & Schwartz, 1985; Roberts & Tumer, 1987, for references). A number of possibilities could account for this decline. One explanation is that the effectiveness of adrenergic stimulation on cardiac tissue is decreased as individuals age. Several investigators have suggested that the observed increase in circulating catecholamines with increasing age reflects a reduced sensitivity of adrenoceptors (Dochery & O'Malley, 1985; Ziegler, Lake, & Kopin, 1976). Given this scenario, it is possible that Type A or hostile persons, due to their propensity to exhibit excessive physiological responses to behavioral stimuli, hasten the effects of aging on adrenergic receptors. In other words, although a reduction in adrenergic sensitivity may be intrinsic to the aging process, hostile individuals may evidence reduced adrenergic receptor sensitivity at an earlier age. This further reduction of adrenoceptore sensitivity in middle-aged hostile persons may lead to an even higher level of circulating catecholamines during stress and nonstress periods.

That age and coronary-prone behaviors may act synergistically in altering physiological responses to behavioral stressors led us to investigate the potential effects of aging on the association between TABP, hostility, and stress-induced reactivity. The aim of the study (Williams, Suarez, Kuhn, Schanberg, & Zimmerman, 1991) was to compare the cardiovascular and neuroendocrine responses of middle-aged (aged 35–50) hostile Type A subjects and nonhostile Type B subjects to physiological responses of young (aged 18–24) Type A and B subjects during similar stressors. In that previous study of young males (Williams et al., 1982), comparisons between Type A and B subjects showed that Type A males, relative to Type Bs, showed greater increases in FBF, catecholamines (CA), and cortisol to MATH and greater testosterone increases to a vigilance task.

In contrast to the results of the young Type A/B men study (Williams et al., 1982), middle-aged Type A and B men did not differ in either cardiovascular or hormonal responses to either MATH or the word identification task (WIT). However, we did find remarkable and consistent significant differences in levels of plasma catecholamines and cortisol during pre-task, task, and recovery periods, such that Type As, relative to Type Bs, showed significantly higher elevations of neuroendocrines levels throughout the two laboratory sessions. These findings are remarkable given that the laboratory sessions were one week apart. Further substantiating the A/B differences in the level of plasma catecholamines, analysis of excretion rates of urinary catecholamines indicated that, Type Bs, Type As had significantly greater 24-hour excretion rates of catecholamines than did Type Bs.

In hostile Type A men, therefore, elevated levels of plasma norepinephrine (NE) and epinephrine (EPI) in conjunction with higher excretion rates of urine catecholamines suggests a potentially maladaptive process that can accelerate sympathetic function changes associated with aging. Thus, as the Type A male ages, the stress-induced SNS hyperresponsitivity often noted in young Type A males appears to manifest itself as a chronic elevation of plasma catecholamines. This chronic elevation of circulating catecholamines in high hostile Type As may be the result of a downregulation of adrenergic receptors due to repeated and/or prolonged exposure to circulating catecholamines (Lefkowitz, Stadel, Caron, 1983). A downregulation of beta-receptors could also explain the lack of A/B differences in baseline CV levels and task-related CV responses despite significant A/B differences in catecholamine levels during both tasks. Thus, by middle-age, hostile Type As may exhibit heightened levels of catecholamines that are characteristic of older individuals.

INTERACTIVE MODULATORS OF REACTIVITY: TABP, HOSTILITY, AND LIPIDS

The aim of most reactivity studies has been to demonstrate an association between coronary-prone behaviors and behaviorally induced reactivity.

However, recent studies have begun to examine the relationship between behaviorally induced physiological hyperreactivity and more traditional CHD risk factors such as lipid levels. For example, one study (Frederickson & Blumenthal, 1988) of post-myocardial infarction patients found that mental arithmetic evoked changes in EPI that were positively associated with the ratio of total serum cholesterol (TSC) to high density lipoprotein cholesterol (HDL). Results from another study (Frederickson, Lundber, Melin, & Frankenhaeuser, 1989) have suggested that, compared to persons with low TSC levels, persons with high TSC levels exhibit greater cardiovascular arousal to a number of laboratory challenges. Finally, Jorgensen, Nash, Lasses, Hymowotz, and Langer (1988) found that, relative to subjects with moderate stress-induced heart rate (HR) changes, individuals who responded to laboratory challenges with greater HR changes also exhibited higher levels of TSC and triglycerides. Taken together these preliminary findings suggest two hypotheses: (a) there is a significant positive relationship between stress-induced reactivity and TSC and, (b) individuals who exhibit both coronary-prone behaviors and elevated lipid levels may respond to stressors with the most extreme physiological changes, and thus be at greatest risk for CHD.

To investigate the hypothesis that coronary-prone behaviors and lipids produce a synergistic affect on cardiovascular and neurohormonal responsitivity to behavioral stressors, we re-analyzed data from our previous study of middle-aged Type A and B men (Williams et al., 1988). This re-analyses (Suarez et al., 1991) aimed at testing the hypothesis that physiological reactivity was potentiated by the presence of two factors such as lipid levels and hostility. The emphasis, therefore, was on the significance of the interaction between coronary-prone behaviors and lipid levels in predicting reactivity.

Results showed that the TABP by TSC interaction was significant for cortisol and catecholamine responses to MATH, such that for Type A subjects, TSC was positively and significantly associated with neurohormonal changes ($rs > .51$). In contrast (and somewhat to our surprise), in Type B subjects, TSC was negatively associated with cortisol ($r = -.65$) and unrelated to catecholamine responses. Substituting TCS with low-density lipoprotein (LDL) cholesterol in the analysis revealed similar results, such that LDL-cholesterol was positively associated with cortisol and NE responses to MATH in Type As ($rs > .48$) and was negatively associated with cortisol ($r = -.75$) in Type Bs.

Given the recent emphasis on hostility as a potential risk factor for CHD we also examined the interactive effects of hostility and lipids on reactivity. Results indicated that in subjects with Ho scores above 15, TSC was positively ($rs > .24$) associated with MATH-induced catecholamine and heart rate (HR) responses. In persons with low Ho scores (i.e., Ho < 15), however, TSC was unrelated with either MATH-induced HR or catecholamine changes ($.00 < rs < -.04$).

Hence, it appears that in hostile Type A middle-aged men, TSC and LDL-cholesterol are positively associated with heightened neurohormonal and HR responses to mental arithmetic. Surprisingly, in nonhostile Type B subjects, TSC and LDL-cholesterol were negatively associated or not related with neurohormonal responses. To date we know of only one other study (Schwertner, Troxler, Uhl, & Jackson, 1984) that has reported similar findings. Schwertner and colleagues found that in extreme Type A and coronary patients, cholesterol levels were negatively associated with cortisol levels during a glucose tolerance test. For Type Bs, however, the relationship between cortisol level and cholesterol was positive.

Plausible Mechanisms Accounting for the Divergence in the Relationships Between Lipids and Reactivity as a Function of Coronary-Prone Behaviors. The apparent hostility and A/B-related divergence in the associations between lipids and neurohormonal reactivity suggests potential differences in the effect of lipids on reactivity per se. The reasons for this divergence are not immediately obvious. However, two potential mechanisms that have opposite affect on adrenoreceptors may explain the A/B (and high/low hostility) differences: (a) the effect of TSC on beta-adrenergic receptor functions, and (b) the effect of circulating CA on adrenergic receptors.

Recent evidence has suggested a potential link between increased TSC and upregulation of beta-adrenergic receptors (Loh & Law, 1980). Several studies have indicated that elevated cholesterol is associated with both increased density (McMurchie, Patten, Charnock, & McLennan, 1987; McMurchie, Patten, McLennan, Charnock, & Nestel, 1988) and greater binding affinity (Kishi, Nishiyama, Numano, 1985; McMurchie & Patten, 1988) of beta-adrenergic receptors. Cholesterol-mediated upregulation of beta-adrenergic receptors can lead to enhancement of beta-receptor sensitivity to beta-agonists, as documented in one study (Rosendorf, Hoffman, Verrier, Rouleau, & Boerboom, 1981) that reported an augmentation of membrane responses to NE in hypercholesterolemic animals. It is possible, therefore, that our observations of reduced catecholamine responses in Type B middle-age men with elevated lipid levels are due to a TSC-related upregulation of adrenergic receptors.

If TSC-mediated upregulation of beta-receptors can account for our findings in low hostile Type Bs, what biological mechanism(s) could prevent or diminish the effects of TSC on beta-adrenergic receptor upregulation in hostile Type As, and thus explain the positive correlations TSC and catecholamine reactivity in them? One possible and well-documented mechanism that is known to cause downregulation of adrenergic receptors is prolonged exposure of receptors to beta-agonists, such as circulating catecholamines (Lefkowitz et al., 1983). Downregulation of adrenergic receptors would amount to a desensitization of beta-adrenergic receptors to agonist stimulation. Consistent with the hypothesis of downregulation of beta-adrenergic receptors by heightened levels of circulating catecholamines, we (Williams et al., 1991) found that Type As showed heightened levels of catecholamines throughout both laboratory sessions and during the 24-hour ambulatory monitoring period.

It is also interesting to note that circulating catecholamines affect LDL-receptor activity. Two recent studies (Krone, Naegele, Behnke, & Greten, 1988; Maziere, Maziere, Gardette, & Polonovski, 1985) have shown that increased levels of circulating EPI inhibit LDL-cholesterol binding and uptake by LDL-receptors and thus its degradation. LDL-receptors are responsible for incorporation of LDL-cholesterol into the cell membrane and represent one route of clearance of LDL-cholesterol from blood (Brown & Goldstein, 1986). Therefore, it is reasonable to assume that an increased EPI response to behavioral challenges could lead, via both increased lipolysis (Havel & Goldstein, 1959) and decreased LDL-receptor activity, to a higher TSC level. This explanation is compatible with our observation of a positive association between TSC and EPI reactivity in high hostile Type As.

Overall, these findings suggest an interactional model of behaviorally induced reactivity that includes both lipids and coronary-prone behaviors. As illustrated in Fig. 10.1, we hypothesized that physiological responses to behavioral stressors in hostile Type As and nonhostile Type Bs are linked to different underlying biological mechanisms regulating beta-adrenergic receptor functioning. Thus, in middle-aged low hostile Type Bs, reduced physiological response to MATH may be due to an upregulation of beta-adrenergic receptors by TSC, as indicated by the darkened arrow pointing from TSC to beta-adrenergic receptor (see Fig. 10.1). The potential upregulating effect of TSC on beta-adrenergic receptors is likely to contribute to smaller stress-induced CA responses without any discernable reduction in CV responses. For middle-aged high hostile Type As, on the other hand, prolonged exposure of beta-adrenergic receptors to high levels of circulating catecholamines appears to have diminished the effect of TSC on beta-adrenergic receptors by the process of desensitization. This effect is represented by the open arrow from circulating CA to beta-receptors downregulation.

Given the advent of receptor-binding techniques (Mills & Dimsdale, 1988) and the use of lymphocytes as a noninvasive model of beta-adrenergic receptors this model leads to certain testable hypotheses. Thus, we can directly test the interactive effect of TSC and coronary-prone behaviors on beta-adrenergic receptors on lymphocytes. In light of our previous findings, we expect that in middle-aged high hostile and Type A persons with significant and chronic elevations of basal catecholamine levels, higher lipid

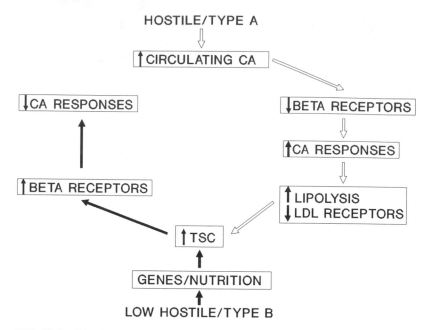

FIG. 10.1. Plausible pathways explaining the opposite associations between cholesterol (TSC) and stress-induced catecholamine (CA) responses as a function of hostility
and the Type A behavior pattern. In hostile Type As (opened arrows), excessive
elevations of circulating CA lead to downregulation of beta-adrenergic receptors.
Downregulation of beta-receptors has been linked with increased stress-induced CA
responses. Increased stress-induced CA responses can contribute to elevated TSC via
downregulation of LDL receptors and lypolysis. For low hostile Type Bs (closed
arrows), diet and genetics contribute to elevated TSC which may lead to an upregulation
of beta-adrenergic receptors. Upregulated receptors have been associated with smaller
CA responses to behavioral stressors.

levels will be associated with lower receptor density (Bmax), higher binding
affinity (Kd), and/or a decrease in the efficiency with which catecholamine
stimulate cyclic AMP, all indicative of downregulation of beta-adrenergic
receptors. Subsequently, correlations between TSC and/or Bmax and Kd
should be negative in hostile men. In contrast, we hypothesized that in
nonhostile and Type B persons, higher lipid levels will be associated with an
upregulation of beta-receptors, indicated by a high Bmax, low Kd, and/or
increased stimulation of cyclic AMP. Therefore, both Bmax and Kd should
be positively associated with TSC in nonhostile persons.

   In contrast to the hypotheses generated for middle-age men, young high
hostile men may not show a positive correlation between lipids and
neuroendocrine reactivity. We suspect that the chronic downregulation of
adrenergic receptors resulting from prolonged exposure to circulating
catecholamines has not occurred in young hostile males. It would be

unlikely, therefore, hostility-related differences in the association between lipid and reactivity would be observed.

PARASYMPATHETIC/SYMPATHETIC BALANCE

In addition to the potential pathogenic effects of the physiologic hyperreactivity to interpersonal conflicts and the potentiation of reactivity by elevated blood cholesterol levels in hostile persons, another line of research suggests that hostile Type A persons may also suffer from a deficient parasympathetic (vagal) antagonism of sympathetic effects on the heart.

The first indication that coronary-prone behaviors may be associated with altered autonomic balance came with our observation (Muranaka, Monou et al., 1988) of more prolonged EKG T-wave attenuation in response to isoproterenol infusions among young hostile Type A men as compared to low hostile Type B men. Because other beta receptor-mediated responses, including forearm blood flow, heart rate, and plasma cyclic-AMP, did not differ as a function of Type A or hostility, we hypothesized that the slower T-wave recovery among hostile Type A men relative to low hostile Type B men may be the result of a deficient, parasympathetic antagonism (for review see Vannoutte & Levy, 1980) of the isoproterenol effects on ventricular repolarization that are responsible for T-wave attenuation.

A second study (Muranaka, Lane et al., 1988) provided more direct evidence of diminished vagal responsivity in young Type A men. When the dive reflex was activated, via application of an ice-water pack to the upper face, both Type A and B men showed an identical heart rate slowing after 1 minute of application. After 2 minutes of application, however, the Type Bs showed further heart rate slowing, but the Type As show a return of heart rate to the baseline levels observed prior to application. This study shows that reflex activation of vagal outflow is attenuated more rapidly in young Type A men than in their Type B counterparts, thereby providing direct evidence for our hypothesis that parasympathetic function is diminished in persons displaying coronary-prone behaviors.

To provide still more direct evidence that the more prolonged T-wave attenuation to isoproterenol infusions in hostile Type As is due to their deficient vagal antagonism of the isoproterenol effects on the heart, we carried out a third study (Fukudo et al., 1989) in which atropine pretreatment was used to block any vagal effects on the T-wave responses to isoproterenol infusions. As in our first study, when placebo pretreatment was given, the hostile Type A subjects showed a more prolonged T-wave attenuation to the isoproterenol infusion. Atropine pretreatment had no effect on the T-wave response to isoproterenol infusion of the hostile Type

A subjects; among the low hostile Type Bs, however, following atropine pretreatment the T-wave attenuation to the isoproterenol infusion was significantly prolonged. This greater sensitivity to vagal blockade among the low hostile Type Bs enables us to infer (Eckberg, 1980) that their more rapid T-wave recovery on the placebo pretreatment day was due to stronger vagal antagonism of the isoproterenol effects on the heart that are responsible for the T-wave response.

Taken together, these findings suggest that coronary-prone behaviors, particularly high hostility and Type A behavior, are associated in young men with weaker vagal function than is present in low hostile, Type B men. Weaker vagal protection of the myocardium against the effects of sympathetic stimulation could provide yet another pathway (besides the increased reactivity to interpersonal conflicts described above) whereby hostility leads to increased disease risk.

There is already some evidence supporting a pathogenic role for weak vagal function among patients who already have clinical coronary disease present. Studies of post-MI patients have found evidence of weaker vagal function relative to controls whether heart rate variability during paced breathing (Airaksinen, Ikaheimo, Linnalouto, Niemela, & Takkunen, 1987) or heart rate slowing during cold water facial stimulation (Ryan, Hollenberg, Harvey, & Gwynn, 1976) was used to assess vagal function. More importantly, a prospective study (Kleiger, Miller, Bigger, & Moss, 1987) of 808 post-MI patients found decreased vagally mediated heart rate variability to be the strongest single predictor of mortality.

It appears that the decreased vagal function may not have been a response to myocardial damage, given that none of these clinical studies showed that the index of vagal function was related to extensive indices of cardiac function and disease severity. Rather, it may have been present all along and contributed to the development of coronary disease — a hypothesis that is consistent with our observations in three independent studies employing three different approaches to study vagal function that hostile Type As have diminished vagal functions.

IMPLICATIONS FOR FUTURE RESEARCH

Our findings suggest that models of reactivity should be interactional; hostile persons demonstrate excessive pathophysiological responses in the presence of certain classes of behavioral stimuli. Our laboratory evidence, in conjunction with results from other laboratories, clearly suggests the importance of social stressors in documenting exaggerated cardiovascular and neurohormonal responses in high Ho persons. Although an interactional model of trait-by-situation is congruent with our observations, this approach still lacks precision in predicting not only reactivity but also CHD risk. An additional area that could potentially contribute to a better understanding of these processes is the study of potential hostility-related differences in cognitive appraisal of behavioral stimuli. In our laboratory studies, the lack of significant hostility-related differences in the evaluations of the harassment procedure suggest that all participants interpreted the harassment as being antagonistic in nature. However, in daily living, situations may not be so clearly interpretable. Hostile individuals may appraise relatively nonhostile (and possibly benign) social situations as hostile encounters and thus respond more frequently with anger and irritation. Indeed, persons with high Ho scores report experiencing a greater number of daily anger-eliciting events (Smith & Frohm, 1985). Information on how hostile individuals perceive and interpret social situations would contribute to our understanding of the interactional processes leading to increased physiological hyperresponsiveness and CHD risk.

Equally as important, our data suggest a two-factor model of reactivity similar to that proposed by Manuck et al. (1989), with an interactive process between hostility on the one hand and affective responses to social stimuli on the other hand. Thus, we note, that only in high hostile persons did we observe a positive correlation between anger and irritation and physiological reactivity. This latter finding is particularly relevant given that, in a subsample of WCGS participants, anger and irritation significantly predict CHD incidence (Matthews, Glass, Rosenman, & Bortner, 1977).

In addition, our findings of interactive modulators of reactivity in middle-aged men suggest the importance of not only behaviors but also biological factors, such as lipids and age, in determining reactivity. Thus, we showed that the hyperreactivity noted in Type A and hostile persons may be more enhanced in those persons with elevated cholesterol levels. The presence of both increased reactivity and elevated cholesterol in hostile and Type A persons represents a synergistic union of two risk factors that could be highly pathogenic (see Fig. 10.2). In this case, cholesterol deposits would be highly probable, given the likelihood of greater endothelial damage attributed to enhanced physiological hyperreactivity. On the other hand, in nonhostile Type Bs, elevated cholesterol may not necessarily lead to increased risk of CHD in the absence of endothelial damage due to excessive physiological hyperresponsivity. Consistent with this notion is the fact that in the WCGS (Rosenman et al., 1975), Type B individuals, relative to Type As, (and we assume a similar relationship exits for hostile vs. nonhostile persons) were at lower risk for CHD at all levels of cholesterol.

Finally, our research points to a previously unappreciated mechanism whereby coronary-prone behaviors may be contributing to pathogenesis: deficient vagal antagonism of sympathetic effects on the heart. This work has focused on young male subjects selected on the basis of Type A

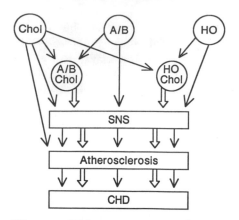

FIG. 10.2 Synergistic effects of lipids and coronary-prone behavior on reactivity and the development and progression of CHD. Elevated lipid levels, the Type A behavior pattern, and hostility have been independently linked to excessive stress-induced sympathetic nervous system (SNS) responses, increased severity of atherosclerosis, and CHD. The co-occurrance of these factors, however, may potentiate and hasten the atherogenic process. Thus, individuals who have elevated levels of both TSC and hostility may exhibit a more pronounced physiological response to stress (indicated by opened arrow) and possibly early onset of CHD.

behavior assessments. Yet it has been possible to document that hostility levels also correlate with the weakened vagal antagonism of sympathetic effects on the heart. Because vagal tone, as indexed by heart rate variability during paced breathing, has been found to decrease with age in normal men (Watkins & MacKay, 1980), our finding of diminished vagal function in young men who are Type A or score high on hostility suggests that such men may be displaying a form of premature aging with respect to autonomic balance.

It will be important, therefore, in future research to determine the effects of age on this difference in vagal function we have found between hostile Type A versus nonhostile Type B men. It could be the case, for example, that in middle-aged men the expected age-related decrease in vagal tone will be occurring to a far greater degree in hostile men, while vagal function in nonhostile men may be relatively intact. It will also be critical in future research on this phenomenon to evaluate the relationship between coronary-prone behaviors and vagal function in women of varying ages, as well as in other racial and ethnic groups.

With these observations at hand, what additional questions can be examined? First, future studies should aim at determining the generalizability of our laboratory findings with respect to both ambulatory cardiovascular and emotional activity in high and low hostile persons. Given our laboratory results, it would seem likely that hostile persons would show heightened levels of both ambulatory blood pressure and heart rate during emotionally stressful events, particularly during social interactions where anger and irritation may be provoked. Equally as important, behavioral ratings gathered throughout the day could shed light on hostility-related differences in the cognitive interpretations of social situations. We suspect that given an adequate sampling period and with a number of socially relevant situations being sampled, we could determine cognitive appraisal and emotional response differences between high and low hostile subjects. Already results from one study (Suarez & Blumenthal, 1991) suggest that among coronary patients with high Ho scores, higher SBP levels are significantly positively associated with self-reported ratings of emotional stress.

Second, our findings of a divergent relationship between lipids and reactivity in Type A and B persons as well as in hostile and nonhostile persons suggest a new avenue of research, that of biologically synergistic relationships between traditional CHD risk factors and hostility in determining reactivity. Thus, we can begin to ask the question: How do traditional risk factors alter the physiological responses patterns of high and low hostile subjects? Our preliminary data already suggest that lipids can moderate the response pattern associated with hostility, but other factors may also have a similar impact on hostility-related reactivity. For example, smoking has been associated with increased reactivity to stressful stimuli (MacDougall, Dembroski, Slaats, Herd, & Eliot, 1983). It would seem likely that hostile persons who smoke may be at greatest risk of CHD, and thus exhibit the greatest magnitude of reactivity to socially relevant stressors. Equally as important, nonhostile persons who smoke may obviate the "protective" quality afforded by being nonhostile, and thereby exhibit exaggerated physiological responses to behavioral stressors.

Third, it will be important to obtain measures of vagal tone in future studies of the generalizability of hostility effects and of the impact of lipids on reactivity. This will permit us to determine whether reactivity to interpersonal conflicts and the effects of lipids on this reactivity are mediated in any way by the weak parasympathetic function we are observing in coronary-prone person.

The aim of this chapter was to present new approaches that may prove useful in understanding the complexity of not only behaviorally induced reactivity but also the potential CHD risk associated with coronary-prone behaviors. At the very least we have made an attempt to develop new models that are based on empirical evidence while reflecting our conceptual and theoretical framework of the behavioral and biological links to CHD. What is clear from our approach is that future studies should aim at investigating the interactive effects of psychological, biological, and environmental factors on physiological reactivity and CHD risk.

REFERENCES

Airaksinen, K., Ikaheimo, M. J., Linnaluoto, M. K., Niemela, M., & Takkunen, J. T. (1987). Impaired vagal heart rate control in coronary artery disease. *British Heart Journal, 58,* 92–597.

Averill, J. R. (1982). *Anger and aggression: An essay on emotions.* New York: Springer-Verlag.

Barefoot, J. C., Dahlstrom, W. G., & Williams, R. B. (1983). Hostility, CHD incidence and total mortality: A 25-year follow-up study of 255 physicians. *Psychosomatic Medicine, 45,* 59–63.

Barefoot, J. C., Williams, R. B., Dahlstrom, W. G., & Dodge, K. A. (1987). Predicting mortality from scores on the Cook and Medley scale: A follow-up of 118 lawyers. *Psychosomatic Medicine, 49,* 210.

Brown, M., & Goldstein, J. (1986). A receptor-mediated pathway for cholesterol homeostasis. *Science, 232,* 34–47.

Buss, A. H., & Durkee, A. (1957). An inventory for assessing different kinds of hostility. *Journal of Consulting Psychology, 21,* 343–349.

Cook, W., & Medley, D. (1954). Proposed hostility and pharasaic-virtue scales for the MMPI. *Journal of Applied Psychology, 238,* 414–418.

Corse, C. D., Manuck, S. B., Cantwell, J. D., Giordani, B., & Matthews, K. A. (1982). Coronary-prone behavior pattern and cardiovascular response in persons with and without coronary heart disease. *Psychosomatic Medicine, 44,* 449–459.

Costa, P. T., & McCrae, R. R. (1985). *The NEO personality inventory manual.* Odessa FL: Psychological Assessment Resources.

Costa, P. T., McCrea, R. R., & Dembroski, T. M. (1989). Agreeableness versus antagonism: Explication of a potential risk factor for CHD. In A. W. Siegman & T. M. Dembroski (Eds.), *Search of coronary-prone behavior—Beyond Type A* (pp. 41–63). Hillsdale, NJ: Lawrence Erlbaum Associates.

Dembroski, T. M., MacDougall, J. M., Costa, P. T., & Crandits, G. A. (1989). Components of hostility as predictors of sudden death and myocardial infarction in the Multiple Risk Factor Intervention Trial. *Psychosomatic Medicine, 51,* 514–522.

Dembroski, T. M., MacDougall, J. M., & Lushene, R. (1979). Interpersonal interaction and cardiovascular response in Type A subjects and coronary patients. *Journal of Human Stress, 5,* 28–36.

Dembroski, T. M., MacDougall, J. M., Shields, J. L., Petitto, J., & Lushene, R. (1978). Components of the Type A coronary-prone behavior pattern and cardiovascular responses to psychomotor performance challenge. *Journal of Behavioral Medicine, 1,* 159–176.

Dochery, J. R., & O'Malley, K. (1985). Aging and alpha-adrenoceptors. *Clinical Science, 68*(Suppl 10), 133S–136S.

Eckberg, D. L. (1980). Parasympathetic cardiovascular control in human disease: A critical review of methods and results. *American Journal of Physiology, 239,* H581–H593.

Frederickson, M., & Blumenthal, J. A. (1988). Lipids, catecholamines and cardiovascular responses to stress in patients recovering from myocardial infarction. *Journal of Cardio-pulmonary Rehabilitation, 12,* 513–517.

Frederickson, M., Lundber, U., Tuomisto, M., Melin, B., & Frankenhaeuser, M. (1989). *Do serum cholesterol levels affect cardiovascular reactivity?* Manuscript submitted for publication.

Fukudo, S., Lane, J. D., Anderson, N. B., Kuhn, C. M., Schanberg, S. M., McCown, N. O., Muranaka, M., Suzuki, J., & Williams, R. B. (1989, March). *Vagal antagonism of cardiovascular and electrophysiologic responses to isoproterenol infusion is weaker in Type A than in Type B men.* Paper presented at annual meeting of American Psychosomatic Society, San Francisco, CA.

Glass, C. D., Lake, C. B., Contrada, R. J., Kehoe, K., & Erlanger, L. R. (1983). Stability of individual differences in physiological responses to stress. *Health Psychology, 2,* 317–341, 1983.

Harbin, T. J. (1989). The relationship between the Type A pattern and physiological responsivity: A quantitative review. *Psychophysiology, 26,* 110–119.

Hardy, J. H., & Smith, T. W. (1988). Cynical hostility and vulnerability to disease: Social support, life stress, and psychological response to conflict. *Health Psychology, 7,* 447–459.

Havel, R. J., & Goldstein, A. (1959). The role of sympathetic nervous system in the metabolism of free fatty acids. *Journal of Lipid Research, 1,* 102–108.

Hearn, M. D., Murray, D. M., & Luepker, R. V. (1989). Hostility, coronary heart disease, and total mortality: A 33-year follow-up study of university students. *Journal of Behavioral Medicine, 12,* 105–121.

Hecker, M. H. L., Chesney, M. A., Black, G. W., & Frautschi, N. (1989). Coronary-prone behavior in the Western Collaborative Group Study. *Psychosomatic Medicine, 50,* 153–164.

Henry, J. P. (1983). Coronary heart disease and arousal of the adrenal corticol axis. In T. M. Dembroski & T. Schmidt (Eds.), *Biobehavioral basis of coronary heart disease.* Basel, Switzerland: Karger.

Jorgensen, R. S., Nash, J. K., Lasses, N. L., Hymowotz, N., & Langer, A. W. (1988). Heart rate acceleration and its relationship to total serum cholesterol, triglycerides, and blood pressure reactivity in man with mild hypertension. *Psychophysiology, 25,* 39–44.

Keys, A., Taylor, H. L., Blackburn, J., Brozck, J., Anderson, J. T., & Somonson, E. (1971). Mortality and coronary heart disease among men studied for 23 years. *Archives of Internal Medicine, 128,* 201–214.

Kishi, Y., Nishiyama, K., & Numano, F. (1985). Cyclic AMP accumulation in rabbit aorta smooth muscle cells altered in the presence of hyperlipidemic serum. *Atherosclerosis, 6,* 213–222.

Klausner, S. C., & Schwartz, A. B. (1985). The aging heart, symposium on the aging process. *Clinics in Geriatric Medicine, 1,* 113–141.

Kleiger, R. E., Miller, J. P., Bigger, J. T., & Moss, A. J. (1987). Decreased heart rate variability and its association with increased mortality after acute myocardial infarction. *American Journal of Cardiology, 59,* 256–262.

Krantz, D. S., & Manuck, S. B. (1984). Acute psychophysiologic reactivity and risk of cardiovascular disease: A review and methodologic critique. *Psychological Bulletin, 96,* 435–464.

Krone, W., Naegele, H., Behnke, B., & Greten, H. (1988). Opposite effects of insulin and catecholamines on LDL-receptor activity in human mononuclear leukocytes. *Diabetes, 37,* 1386–1391.

Lefkowitz, R., Stadel, J., & Caron, M. (1983). Adenylate cyclase-coupled beta-adrenergic receptors: structures and mechanisms of activation and desensitization. *Analytic Review Biochemistry, 52,* 159–186.

Leon, G. R., Finn, S. E., Bailey, J. M., & Murray, D. (1988). Inability to predict cardiovascular disease from hostility scores or MMPI items related to Type A behavior. *Journal of Consulting and Clinical Psychology, 56,* 597–600.

Loh, H., & Law, P. Y. (1980). The role of membrane lipids in receptor mechanisms. *Analytic Review of Pharmacology and Taxicology, 20,* 201–234.

MacDougall, J. M., Dembroski, T. M., Slaats, S., Herd, J. A., Eliot, R. S. (1983). Cardiovascular effects of stress and cigarette smoking. *Journal of Human Stress, 9,* 13–21.

Manuck, S. B., Muldoon, M. F., Kaplan, J. R., Adams, M. R., & Polefrone, J. M. (1989). Coronary artery atherosclerosis and cardiac response to stress in cynomolgus monkeys. In A. W. Siegman & T. M. Dambroski (Eds.). *Search of coronary-prone behavior* (pp. 207–227). Hilldale, NJ: Lawrence Erlbaum Associates.

Matthews, K. A., Glass, D. C., Rosenman, R. H. H., & Bortner, R. W. (1977). Competitive drive, pattern A, and coronary heart disease: A further analysis of some data from the Western Collaborative Group Study. *Journal of Chronic Disease, 30,* 489–498.

Maziere, C., Maziere, J. C., Gardette, J., & Polonovski, J. (1985). Epinephrine decreases low density lipoprotein processing and lipid synthesis in cultured human fibroblast. *Biochemical and Biophysical Research Communications, 133,* 958–963.

McCranie, E. W., Watkins, L., Brandsma, J., & Sisson, B. (1986). Hostility, coronary heart disease incidence, and total mortality: Lack of association in a 25-year follow-up study of 478 physicians. *Journal of Behavioral Medicine, 29,* 119–125.

McMurchie, E., & Patten, G. (1988). Dietary cholesterol influences cardiac B-adrenergic receptor adenylate cyclase activity in the marmoset monkey by changes in membrane cholesterol status. *Biochimica et Biophysica Acta, 942,* 324–332.

McMurchie, E., Patten, G., Charnock, J., & McLennan, P. (1987). The interaction of dietary fatty acid and cholesterol on catecholamine-stimulated adenylate cyclase activity in the rat heart. *Biochimica et Biophysica Acta, 898,* 137–153.

McMurchie, E., Patten, G., McLennan, P., Charnock, J., & Nestel, P. (1988). The influence of dietary lipid supplementation on cardiac B-adrenergic receptors adenylate cyclase activity in marmoset monkeys. *Biochimica et Biophysica Acta, 937,* 347–358.

Mills, P. J., & Dimsdale, J. E. (1988). The promise of receptor studies in psychophysiologic research. *Psychosomatic Medicine, 50,* 555–566.

Muranaka, M., Lane, J. D., Suarez, E. C., Anderson, N. B., Suzuki, J., & Williams, R. B. (1988). Stimulus-specific patterns of cardiovascular reactivity in Type A and B subjects: Evidence for enhanced vagal reactivity in Type 3. *Psychophysiology, 2,* 330–338.

Muranaka, M., Monou, H., Suzuki, J., Lane, J. D., Anderson, N. B., Kuhn, C. M., Schanberg, S., McCown, N., & Williams, R. B. (1988). Physiological responses to catecholamine infusions in Type A and B men. *Health Psychology, 7*(Suppl.), 145–163.

Musante, L., MacDougall, J. M., Dembroski, T. M., & Costa, P. T. (1989). Potential for hostility and dimensions of anger. *Health Psychology, 8,* 343–354.

Ragland, D. R., & Brand, R. J. (1988). Type A behavior and mortality from coronary heart disease. *New England Journal of Medicine, 313,* 65–69.

Review Panel on Coronary-Prone Behavior and Coronary Heart Disease (1981). Coronary-prone behavior and coronary heart disease: A critical review. *Circulation, 63,* 1199.

Roberts, J., & Tumer, N. (1987). Age-related changes in autonomic function of catecholamines. In M. Rothstein (Ed.), *Review of biological research in aging* (Vol 3, pp. 257–298), New York: Alan R. Liss.

Rosendorf, C., Hoffman, J., Verrier, E., Rouleau, J., & Boerboom, L. (1981). Cholesterol potentiates the coronary artery response to norepinephrine in anesthesized and conscious dogs. *Circulation Research, 48,* 320–328.

Rosenman, R. H., Brand, R. J., Jenkins, C. D., Friedman, M., Straus, K., & Wurm, M. (1975). Coronary heart disease in the Western Collaborative Group study. Final follow-up experience of 8 1/2 years. *Journal of the American Medical Association, 233,* 872–877.

Ross, R., & Glomset, J. A. (1973). Atherosclerosis and the arterial smooth muscle cell. *Science, 180,* 1332–1339.

Ryan, C., Hollenberg, M., Harvey, D. B., & Gwynn, R. (1976). Impaired parasympathetic responses in patients after myocardial infarction. *American Journal of Cardiology, 37,* 1013–1018.

Sallis, M. A., Johnson, C. C., Treverron, T. R., Kaplan, R. M., & Hovell, M. F. (1987). The relationship between cynical hostility and blood pressure reactivity. *Journal of Psychosomatic Research, 31,* 111–126, 1987.

Schwertner, H. A., Troxler, R. G., Uhl, G. S., & Jackson, W. G. (1984). Relationship between cortisol and cholesterol in men with coronary heart disease and Type A behavior. *Arteriosclerosis, 4,* 59–64.

Shekelle, R. B., Gale, M., Ostfeld, A. M., & Paul, O. (1983). Hostility, risk of coronary disease and mortality. *Psychosomatic Medicine, 45,* 109–114.

Siegman, A. W., Dembroski, T. M., & Ringel, N. (1987). Components of hostility and the severity of coronary artery disease. *Psychosomatic Medicine, 49,* 127–135.

Smith, T. W., & Allred, K. D. (1989). Blood pressure responses during social interaction in high and low cynically hostile males. *Journal of Behavioral Medicine, 12,* 135–143.

Smith, T. W., & Frohm, K. (1985). What's so bad about hostility? Construct validity and psychosocial correlates of the Cook and Medley Hostility Scale. *Health Psychology, 4,* 503–520.

Smith, M. A., & Houston, B. K. (1987). Hostility, anger expression, cardiovascular responsivity, and social support. *Biological Psychology, 24,* 39–48, 1987.

Sparrow, D., Tifft, C. P., Rosner, B., & Weiss, S. T. (1984). Postural changes in diastolic blood pressure and the risk of myocardial infarction: The normative aging study. *Circulation, 4,* 533–537.

Spieberger, C. D., Johnson, E. H., Russell, S. F., Crane, R. J., Jacobs, G. A., & Worden, T. J. (1985). Experience and expression of anger: Construction and validation of an anger expression scale. In M. A. Chesney & R. H. Rosenman (Eds.), *Anger and hostility in cardiovascular and behavioral disorders* (pp. 5–30). Washington DC: Hemisphere.

Suarez, E. C., & Blumenthal, J. A. (1991). Cardiovascular levels during environmental challenges in high and low hostile patients with a recent myocardial infarction. *Journal Cardiopulmonary Rehabilitation, 11,* 169–175.

Suarez, E. C., & Williams, R. B. (1989). Situational determinants of cardiovascular and emotional responses in high and low hostile men. *Psychosomatic Medicine, 51,* 404–418.

Suarez, E. C., & Williams, R. B. (1990). The relationships between dimensions of hostility and cardiovascular reactivity as a function of task characteristics. *Psychosomatic Medicine, 2,* 8–70.

Suarez, E. C., Williams, R. B., Harlan, E. S., & Peoples, M. K. (1990). *The relationship of hostility and harassment to cardiovascular responses in high and low hostile women.* Paper presented at the 11th annual meeting of the Society of Behavioral Medicine, Chicago.

Suarez, E. C., Williams, R. B., Harlan, E. S., Peoples, M. C., Kuhn, C. M., & Schanberg, S. M. (1990). *Cook-Medley Ho scores predict neuroendocrine, testosterone, and cardiovascular responses to harassment.* Paper presented at the 11th annual meeting of the Society of Behavioral Medicine, Chicago.

Suarez, E. C., Williams, R. B., Kuhn, C. M., Schanberg, S. M., Zimmerman, E. (1991). Biobehavioral basis of coronary-prone behavior in middle-aged men. Part II: Serum Cholesterol, the Type A behavior pattern, and hostility as interactive modulators of physiological reactivity. *Psychosomatic Medicine, 53,* 528–537.

Vanhoutte, P. M., & Levy, M. N. (1980). Prejunctional cholinergic modulation of adrenergic neurotransmission in the cardiovascular system. *American Journal of Physiology, 238,* H275-H281.

Watkins, R. J., & MacKay, J. D. (1980). Cardiac denervation in diabetic neuropathy. *Annals of Internal Medicine, 92,* 304–307.

Weidner, G., Friend, R., Ficarotto, T. J., & Mendell, N. R. (1989). Hostility and cardiovascular reactivity to stress in women and men. *Psychosomatic Medicine, 51,* 36–45.

Williams, R. B. (1987a). Psychological factors in coronary artery disease. Epidemiologic evidence. *Circulation, 76,* 117–123.

Williams, R. B. (1987b). Refining the Type A hypothesis: Emergence of the hostility complex. *American Journal of Cardiology, 60,* 27–32.

Williams, R. B., Haney, T. L., Lee, K. L., Kong, Y., Blumenthal, J., & Whalen, R. (1980). Type A behavior, hostility, and coronary atherosclerosis. *Psychosomatic Medicine, 42,* 539–549.

Williams, R. B., Lane, J. D., Kuhn, C. M., Melosh, W., White, A. D., & Schanberg, S. M. (1982). Type A behavior and elevated physiological and neuroendocrine responses to cognitive tasks. *Science, 218,* 483–485.

Williams, R. B., Suarez, E. C., Kuhn, C. M., Schanberg, S. M., & Zimmerman, E. (1991). Biobehavioral basis of coronary-prone behavior in middle-aged men. Part I. Evidence for chronic sympathetic nervous system activation in Type As. *Psychosomatic Medicine, 53,* 517–527.

Ziegler, M. G., Lake, C. B., & Kopin, I. J. (1976). Plasma noradrenaline increases with age. *Nature (London), 261,* 333–33.

11 Insulin Sensitivity and Blood Pressure

Jay S. Skyler
Jennifer B. Marks
Novelette E. Thompson
Michael D. Fili
Neil Schneiderman
University of Miami

Hypertension, glucose intolerance, obesity, and hyperlipidemia are extremely prevalent problems in Western society, and each confers increased risk for coronary heart disease (CHD; Donahue, Skyler, Schneiderman, & Prineas, 1990). This cluster of disorders is so commonly associated as to suggest common pathogenetic mechanisms. Hyperinsulinemia and insulin resistance have been proposed to be the underlying link between these disorders (Christlieb, Krolewski, Warram, & Soeldner, 1985; Donahue et al., 1990; Ferrari & Weidmann, 1990; Krieger & Landsberg, 1988; Reaven & Hoffman, 1987; Sims, 1982; Swislocki, 1990), which collectively have been dubbed the GOH (glucose intolerance–obesity–hypertension) syndrome by Modan et al. (1985), "Syndrome X" by Reaven (1988), the "deadly quartet" by Kaplan (1989), the "chronic disease risk factor syndrome" by Zimmet (1989), and the "insulin resistance syndrome" by DeFronzo and Ferrannini (1990).

It is well established that hyperinsulinemia and insulin resistance are characteristic features both of obesity and of glucose intolerance (both impaired glucose tolerance [IGT] and Type II diabetes mellitus; DeFronzo, 1988; Olefsky, 1981; Reaven, 1988). More recently, evidence has been developed relating hyperinsulinemia and decreased insulin sensitivity (i.e., insulin resistance) to elevated blood pressure. Before reviewing the evidence, it is helpful to review the methodology that has been used.

MEASUREMENT OF INSULIN SENSITIVITY/INSULIN RESISTANCE

A variety of methods have been developed to quantify tissue sensitivity to insulin. Insensitivity to insulin, or insulin resistance, may be defined as being present whenever normal concentrations of insulin elicit a less than normal biological response (Kahn, 1978). Typically, the measured biological responses relate to the glucoregulatory properties of insulin because these are the most readily appreciated responses and because plasma glucose concentration is the most important signal regulating insulin secretion. In nondiabetic individuals, insulin resistance may be recognized by the presence of hyperinsulinemia in the absence of hypoglycemia. In any subject, insulin resistance can be demonstrated by a subnormal response to either endogenous or exogenous insulin. Although there may be circulating factors responsible for insulin resistance (such as high titers of anti-insulin antibodies in rare patients with immunologic insulin resistance, or antibodies directed against the insulin receptor), most insulin resistance is a consequence of impaired insulin sensitivity at the level of target cells.

Because insulin resistance is defined as being present whenever normal concentrations of insulin elicit a subnormal biological response, insulin resistance may be inferred by finding either basal (fasting) hyperinsulinemia or a greater than normal insulin response to a provocative challenge (e.g., an oral glucose tolerance test [OGTT] or an intravenous glucose tolerance test [IVGTT]). Clearly, differences between groups will be magnified by the provocative challenge of glucose. The insulin response to such challenge often is expressed as the "insulin/glucose ratio" (I/G), often calculated as the area under the curve.

Insulin sensitivity may be quantified by measuring the biological response to exogenous insulin under controlled conditions. A number of protocols have been devised to standardize the conditions for insulin administration (the challenges) and to provide uniformity of measurement of the response variables (Reaven, 1983).

In the insulin tolerance test (ITT), a fixed dose of insulin (e.g., 0.1 units/kg) is given as an intravenous bolus, with the response variable being the rate of decline of plasma glucose (the K_I value) obtained from serial samples over a short period (i.e. 30–60 minutes; Lebovitz & Feinglos, 1980; Lebovitz, Feinglos, Bucholtz, & Lebovitz, 1977). The ITT, however, is of relatively limited utility due to K_I being measured at a time coinciding with glucose mixing, the nonsteady state plasma insulin levels, variable counter-regulatory hormone response, and the notion that the rate of change of plasma glucose may be influenced by the basal plasma glucose level.

The insulin suppression test is based on the premise that infusion of fixed amounts of glucose and insulin will result in steady state plasma glucose (SSPG) concentrations that reflect overall responsiveness to exogenous steady state plasma insulin (SSPI), assuming that endogenous insulin is suppressed (Harano et al., 1977; Nagulesparan, Savage, Unger, & Bennett, 1979; Ratzmann, Besch, Witt, & Schulz, 1981; Reaven & Miller, 1979;

Shen, Reaven, & Farquhar, 1970). Several protocols have been developed to suppress endogenous insulin, with infusions either of epinephrine plus propranolol or of somatostatin. In such protocols, the higher the level of SSPG, the greater the degree of insulin resistance.

The insulin clamp technique has been widely used and has become the gold standard for quantitation of insulin sensitivity (Andres, Swerdloff, Pozefsky, & Coleman, 1966; DeFronzo, Tobin, & Andres, 1979; Del Prato, Ferrannini, & DeFronzo, 1986). The method involves infusion of insulin at a fixed rate designed to achieve a steady state plasma insulin concentration. Plasma glucose level is maintained constant (clamped) at a predetermined level (usually either euglycemia or the basal plasma glucose level, depending on the protocol) by virtue of continuous infusion of a variable amount of glucose, the amount determined by every 1- to 5-minute sampling of plasma glucose, with computer guided adjustment of the glucose infusion (Andres et al., 1966; DeFronzo et al., 1979), or by use of an artificial pancreas (Clemens, Hough, & Dorazio, 1982; Ponchner et al., 1984). Once a steady state glucose infusion rate is achieved, this is considered a parameter of insulin action because the steady state glucose infusion rate (SSGIR) would equal the rate of glucose metabolism (M), less any urinary glucose losses. If the clamp is performed at basal glucose concentration, glucose clearance (glucose infusion rate divided by plasma glucose) may serve as a parameter of insulin action. Greater precision of measurement can be achieved by simultaneously determining glucose fluxes using isotopic glucose. This permits calculation of hepatic glucose production and peripheral glucose utilization (DeFronzo, Simonson, & Ferrannini, 1982; Finegood, Bergman, & Vranic, 1987; Kolterman, Insel, Saekow, & Olefsky, 1980; Kolterman et al., 1981).

The clamp technique has some limitations and some advantages. Theoretical limitations are a consequence of the fixed hyperinsulinemia induced by the procedure. This precludes assessment of the effects of glucose on glucose utilization rate, and mandates additional clamp experiments to ascertain insulin sensitivity at more than one level of insulinemia. The procedure is technically tedious and generally requires the presence of two investigators throughout. For accurate results, it is necessary to sample arterialized venous blood obtained by creating an arterial venous shunt through warming of the hand in a hot box or heating pad (Forster, Dempsey, Thomson, Vidruk, & DoPico, 1972; McGuire, Helderman, Tobin, Andres, & Berman, 1976). Advantages of the clamp technique include the potential for simultaneously determining glucose flux rates; for coupling the clamp technique to simultaneous indirect calorimetry, thus identifying how the glucose is being metabolized (DeFronzo et al., 1981); and for studying the effects of insulin on parameters other than glucose, for example, effects on water and mineral metabolism (DeFronzo, Cooke, Andres, Faloona, & Davis, 1975), or effects on the sympathetic nervous system (Rowe et al., 1981).

The minimal model approach, developed by Bergman and colleagues, assesses insulin sensitivity during a frequently sampled intravenous glucose tolerance test (FSIGT; Bergman, 1989; Bergman, Finegood, & Ader, 1985). The model describes glucose restoration rate based on two factors: (a) the effect of glucose independent of any increase in insulin, glucose effectiveness or S_G, and (b) the effect of glucose that is enhanced by insulin, expressed as insulin sensitivity or S_I. The minimal model computer program assesses estimates of S_I and S_G from the dynamic relationship between plasma insulin and the glucose time course. S_I reflects the total effect of insulin on glucose economy (i.e., the increment in glucose utilization plus the decrement in endogenous [hepatic] glucose production). The original technique for performance of the FSIGT was modified to include addition of an injection of tolbutamide 20 minutes after the glucose injection, in order to provoke additional endogenous insulin secretion beyond that of glucose alone, thus enhancing the ability of the computer to estimate the model parameters (Beard, Bergman, Ward, & Porte, 1986; Yang, Youn, & Bergman, 1987). This has been labeled the *modified minimal model* (MMM). S_I, obtained from the FSIGT, have been compared to insulin sensitivity estimates obtained by the clamp technique in both dogs and human beings (Beard et al., 1986; Bergman, Prager, Volund, & Olefsky, 1987; Donner et al., 1985; Finegood, Pacini, & Bergman, 1984). In two separate human studies, using the MMM protocol, the correlation between S_I and clamp values was found to be $r = 0.84$ by the Seattle group (Beard et al., 1986), and $r = 0.89$ by the San Diego group (Bergman et al., 1987). Most recently, the experimental procedure has been simplified such that a reduced schedule of blood samples can be used for the modeling calculations (Bergman, 1989; Cutfield, Bergman, Menon, & Sperling, 1990; Steil, Volund, & Bergman, 1991).

The minimal model approach has some limitations and some advantages. Specifically, extreme insulin resistance cannot be easily measured because the calculation of insulin sensitivity is dependent on secreted insulin having a measurable influence on plasma glucose level. Conversely, insulin sensitivity cannot be easily measured when there is marked impairment in endogenous insulin secretion because the calculations depend on insulin dynamics, although it may be possible to circumvent this difficulty by administering exogenous insulin in lieu of tolbutamide in the MMM (Finegood, Hramiak, & Dupre, 1990). With the exception of these extremes, the model has been widely used to estimate insulin sensitivity in studies of a variety of groups of subjects. An advantage of using the FSIGT for measuring insulin sensitivity is that one can also derive indices of glucose tolerance (K_G) and prehepatic beta cell secretion simultaneously (Watanabe, Volund, Roy, & Bergman, 1989). Another advantage is that it is not necessary to use arterialized venous blood, as comparable values are obtained with and without use of a "hot box" to arterialize venous blood (Bergman, Beard, & Chen, 1986).

INSULIN SENSITIVITY AND BLOOD PRESSURE

Insulinemia and Blood Pressure in Different Populations

The first report of hyperinsulinemia in hypertensive patients, both treated and untreated, was by Welborn, Breckenbridge, Rubinstein, Dollery, and Fraser (1966), who found higher plasma insulin concentrations both fasting and after an oral glucose challenge in a group of 19 hypertensive men with normal glucose tolerance. Berglund et al. (1976) reported that 106 hypertensive men had higher plasma insulin concentrations than 41 normotensive men, and that although there was also a greater frequency of obesity and impaired glucose tolerance in the men with hypertension, the differences were sustained after matching for body fat.

A number of studies have found correlations between plasma insulin concentration and blood pressure in different populations. Modan et al. (1985) studied 2,475 Israelis participating in a health survey, and found that hypertensives had higher fasting and post glucose insulin levels, especially if they were not taking antihypertensive medications. However, 83.4% of their hypertensive subjects were either obese or had glucose intolerance, thus confounding the interpretation of the relationship between insulin and blood pressure. Nevertheless, the finding persisted after ranking for obesity and for frank diabetes. Pyrola, Savolainen, Kaukola, and Haapakoski (1985), reporting data from the Helsinki Policemen Study ($n = 982$), found correlations between plasma insulin levels and both systolic and diastolic blood pressure, but again the relationship could be partly explained by obesity. Lucas, Estigarribia, Darga, and Reaven (1985) found plasma insulin levels and blood pressure to be correlated in 33 obese women. Lowenthal, Pim, Hillson, Dhar, and Hockaday (1985) found that among 215 newly diagnosed diabetic subjects, fasting insulin correlated with blood pressure. Christlieb et al. (1985) found that among 195 individuals with impaired glucose tolerance, plasma insulin levels were higher in those with diastolic hypertension (who also were more obese) than those who had only systolic hypertension or who were normotensive.

In a study of 248 hospital workers (111 men and 137 women) having routine health examinations, only 4% of whom were hypertensive, Fournier

Gadia, Kubrusly, Skyler, and Sosenko (1986) found that fasting plasma insulin concentrations correlated with both systolic and diastolic blood pressure in both men and women. Our sample was mostly White (88% of men, 68% of women) relatively young (mean age 41.9 for men, 44.2 for women), and were nondiabetic. In the Beaver County study, among 170 young adults (age 20–24), fasting insulin was correlated with diastolic blood pressure in men, and with systolic blood pressure in both sexes (Donahue, Orchard, Becker, Kuller, & Drash, 1987). Nagasaki et al. (1986) studied 2,927 Japanese living in Hiroshima, Los Angeles, or Hawaii, and found that those who had the highest quintile of fasting plasma insulin, had a higher frequency of hypertension, but also were more obese and had a higher rate of diabetes. Rose, Yalow, Schwertzer, and Schwartz (1986) found that post glucose insulin levels correlated strongly with blood pressure in a group of young amputees. Modan et al. (1987) in 1,211 Israeli subjects found insulinemia to be related to obesity, impaired glucose tolerance, hypertension, hyperuricemia, abnormal lipid profiles, and altered cation balance. In Finland, Uusitupia, Niskanen, Siitonen, and Pyorala (1987) studied 133 newly diagnosed diabetic subjects, in comparison to 144 controls. They found that fasting and post glucose insulin levels correlated with blood pressure in control men (but not women) and in diabetic men and women, and that the relationship persisted even after adjustment for obesity.

In a series of reports from Parma, Italy, a number of interesting statistical relationships have been found. In one report of 367 subjects, including normotensive and untreated mildly hypertensive individuals, overall there was no independent relationship between insulinemia and blood pressure, but after controlling for age and weight, insulinemia was correlated with diastolic blood pressure, and amongst their nonobese subjects ($n = 247$), insulinemia correlated with both systolic and diastolic blood pressure (Bonora et al., 1987). In a subsequent report (Zavaroni et al., 1989), these workers confined their analyses to 247 nonobese normotensive nondiabetic subjects. They found 32 individuals who had plasma insulin greater than 2 SD above the mean and matched these for age, gender, and body mass index with 32 individuals who had plasma insulin within 1 SD of the mean. The hyperinsulinemia group had higher systolic and diastolic blood pressures, higher triglyceride and cholesterol levels, and lower HDL-cholesterol levels.

Among 489 White premenopausal women, Wing, Bunker, Kuller, and Matthews (1989) found fasting insulin and body mass index to be correlated both with blood pressure and lipid levels. In the CARDIA study, which examined 4,576 young adults (ages 18–30), fasting insulin correlated directly with both systolic and diastolic blood pressures, higher triglyceride and total and LDL-cholesterol levels, and inversely with HDL-cholesterol levels (Manolio et al., 1990). In the CARDIA study, multivariate analysis that controlled for weight indices suggested that insulinemia was only partly explanatory for the relationships with cardiovascular risk factors (Folsom et al., 1989). In a recent Italian study, Marigliano et al., (1990) examined 36 essential hypertensives and 12 subjects with renovascular hypertension, all newly diagnosed and untreated, in comparison to 69 normotensives. Fasting insulin was increased in the essential hypertensives, but not in those with renovascular hypertension. Also, blood pressure correlated with fasting insulin in the essential hypertensives.

Not all studies, however, find insulinemia to be related to blood pressure. In the Bogalusa Heart Study, which examined 3,313 children age 7–15, although fasting insulin was directly related to systolic and diastolic blood pressure, this became nonsignificant after adjustment for age and weight (Burke et al., 1986). In their study of 204 obese individuals, Weinsier et al. (1986) failed to find a correlation between insulinemia and blood pressure when they corrected for weight, body fat, fat mass, body build, and upper body fat pattern. Likewise, Cambien et al. (1987), in their study of 2,144 middle-aged normotensive nondiabetic French men, failed to find a relationship between insulinemia and blood pressure when they corrected for plasma glucose and body mass index. They did note that a simultaneous increase of BMI, plasma glucose, and insulin is strongly correlated with blood pressure. Interestingly, in an earlier study from the same group, among 7,246 middle-aged nondiabetic French men, there was a relationship between insulinemia and overall cardiovascular disease risk (Ducimetiere et al., 1980). Mbanya, Thomas, Wilkinson, Alberti, and Taylor (1988) studied four groups of subjects, normotensives and hypertensives with and without diabetes, matched for age, gender, body mass index, renal function, and in the diabetics glycemic control and duration of disease. They found hyperinsulinemia to be a feature of hypertension only within the diabetic group. Their data, in which C-peptide was not concomitantly elevated, suggested that decreased hepatic extraction may contribute to the hyperinsulinemia. Alberti et al. (1989) studied 5,036 adults among four ethnic groups living in Maritius. Although they found a relationship between fasting insulin and blood pressure, this accounted for less than 1% of the variance in blood pressure.

Insulin Resistance (or Inference Thereof)

Several studies have inferred that insulin resistance is present in hypertension by virtue of the finding of a greater insulin response during an oral glucose tolerance test (OGTT) in hypertensive subjects than in normotensive nondiabetic controls. Singer, Godicke, Voigt, Hajdu, and Weiss (1985) from East Germany reported increased insulin responses both during

OGTTs and diurnal profiles in 8 hypertensive men versus 22 normotensive men. Manicardi, Camellini, Bellodi, Coscelli, and Ferrannini (1986) reported higher insulin levels at 1 hour of an OGTT in 18 moderately obese hypertensive subjects versus 17 normotensive subjects. Fuh, Shieh, Wu, Chen, and Reaven (1987) studied 40 middle-aged Taiwanese men, 20 with untreated hypertension, and 20 normotensive controls. The insulin response to OGTT was higher in the hypertensive men, and was directly correlated with both systolic and diastolic blood pressure. Resnick, Gupta, Gruenspan, Alderman, and Laragh (1990) found that the integrated insulinemic response during an OGTT was greater in 20 hypertensives than in 20 normotensives.

In the Bogalusa Heart Study, Voors, Radhakrishramurthy, Srinivasan, Webber, and Berenson (1981) examined the relationship between blood pressure and a peripheral insulin resistance index (PRI), defined as the product of the 1-hour glucose and 1-hour insulin values. Examining 272 youth (ages 7–15) who represented a stratified sample of 3,524 participants, they compared the upper and lower blood pressure quintiles and found a higher PRI in the high blood pressure strata for White males. The relationship was not seen for Blacks, but the latter were more insulin resistant as a group and a relationship may have been obscured due to restriction of range.

Two studies have used the insulin suppression test to compare insulin sensitivity in hypertensives versus normotensives. Shen et al. (1988) studied three groups of age- and weight-matched Taiwanese men, 8 with normal blood pressure, 8 with untreated hypertension, and 8 with hypertension treated with thiazide diuretics and beta-blockers. They found that SSPG was higher in both hypertensive groups, signifying insulin resistance. It should be noted that both hypertensive groups also had higher levels of both glucose and insulin during an OGTT. Swislocki, Hoffman, and Reaven (1989) studied lean White men of similar age and weight, divided in four groups: 16 normotensives, 14 untreated hypertensives, 9 hypertensives treated with diuretics, and 8 hypertensives treated with diuretics and beta-blockers. They, too, found higher SSPG levels in the hypertensive groups, with treated subjects showing higher values than untreated subjects. Again, OGTTs revealed higher levels of both glucose and insulin in hypertensives.

Several studies have used the euglycemic insulin clamp technique to compare insulin sensitivity in hypertensives versus normotensives. Ferrannini et al. (1987) studied 13 young Italian untreated hypertensives of normal body weight and with normal glucose tolerance, in comparison to 11 normotensive controls. They found markedly reduced insulin sensitivity (M) in the hypertensive subjects, and that M was inversely correlated with both systolic and mean arterial blood pressure. Moreover, they demonstrated that the decreased insulin sensitivity was a consequence of a reduction in nonoxidative glucose metabolism (glycogen synthesis and glycolysis), with glucose oxidation remaining normal. OGTTs revealed higher levels of both glucose and insulin in the hypertensives. Verza et al. (1988) studied 12 elderly Italian hypertensives of normal body weight, in comparison to 12 normotensives of similar age, gender, and weight. They too found reduced insulin sensitivity (M) in the hypertensive subjects, and again reported higher levels of both glucose and insulin in the hypertensives during OGTTs, and higher insulin levels during IVGTTs. Pollare, Lithell, and Berne (1990) performed clamp studies in 51 normotensive, 58 nonobese hypertensive, and 85 obese hypertensive subjects participating in a health survey in Sweden. The hypertensives included 90 men and 53 women. They found reduced insulin sensitivity (M) in both hypertensive groups, with obese hypertensives showing the most insulin resistance. The changes persisted after adjustment for gender, age, body mass index, and waist/hip ratio. Most recently, in healthy, normotensive volunteers, we have found that insulin sensitivity (M) correlated inversely with both systolic and diastolic blood pressure, indicating that subjects who were more insulin resistant had higher blood pressure (Thompson et al., in press).

Parallel Changes in Insulin and Blood Pressure

Support for the relationship between insulin and blood pressure can be gained by examining the relationship of these parameters and their change in response to various interventions. It has long been established that weight reduction is associated with reduction of blood pressure (Berchtold, Jorgens, Kemmer, & Berger, 1982; Kannel, Brand, Skinner, Dawber, & McNamara, 1967; Kempner, Newborg, Peschel, & Skyler, 1975; Schotte & Stunkard, 1990) and with reduction of insulinemia and insulin resistance (Olefsky, Reaven, & Farquhar, 1974).

Physical training lowers blood pressure and increases insulin sensitivity. Krotkiewski et al. (1979) found that a 6-month physical training program in obese women resulted in reductions in both plasma insulin and blood pressure, and that the reductions were correlated. Rocchini, Katch, Schork, and Kelch (1987) found that weight loss in obese adolescents resulted in a decrease of plasma insulin and of blood pressure, and that the change in blood pressure was directly correlated both with change in weight and change in plasma insulin, and that these changes were particularly related to the exercise these adolescents had.

Other maneuvers have also shown parallel reductions in blood pressure and insulinemia. Sims (1982) reported a strong correlation between decrements in blood pressure and decrements in insulin in a group of 12 obese hypertensive subjects participating in a 12-week weight reduction program with or without a concomitant exercise prescription. Carretta et al. (1989) found that in response to a somatostatin infusion, which markedly lowered plasma insulin, there was a reduction in mean arterial blood pressure in obese hypertensive subjects (but not in nonobese normotensive subjects). Tedde, Sechi, Marigliano, Papa, and Seano (1989) found that with a reduction of insulin dosage in diabetic subjects, there was a concomitant increase in urine volume and in sodium excretion, and a decrease in both weight and blood pressure. On the other hand, Hall, Coleman, and Mizelle (1989) found that a 7- to 28-day insulin infusion into healthy dogs had no effect on blood pressure or on angiotensin-II induced blood pressure response.

Effects of Antihypertensive Therapy on Insulin Sensitivity

In a series of studies from Uppsala University (reviewed by Lithell, Pollare, & Berne, 1990), the effects of various antihypertensive agents on insulin sensitivity have been examined using serial euglycemic insulin clamp measurements before and after treatment periods of 12, 16, or 24 weeks in one or another study. These investigators found that there was a decrease of insulin sensitivity in subjects treated with the selective beta 1-adrenoceptor blockers atenolol and metoprolol (Pollare, Lithell, Morlin et al., 1989; Pollare, Lithell, Selinus, & Berne, 1989) and the diuretic hydrochlorothiazide (Pollare, Lithell, & Berne 1989). They found no change in insulin sensitivity with the calcium channel blocker diltiazem (Pollare, Lithell, Morlin et al., 1989). In contrast, they reported improvement in insulin sensitivity both with the alpha 1-adrenoceptor blocker prazosin (Pollare et al 1988) and with the angiotensin converting enzyme inhibitor captopril (Pollare, Lithell, & Berne, 1989). Jauch et al. (1987) also found that captopril increased insulin sensitivity, when given as a single oral dose during an insulin clamp procedure.

Sheu, Swislocki, Hoftman, Chen, and Reaven (1991) used the insulin suppression test to assess insulin sensitivity in hypertensive subjects treated with the beta 1-adrenoceptor blocker atenolol or the calcium channel blocker nifedipine. They found a slight, but statistically significant, decrease in insulin sensitivity with atenolol; and very slight, but nonetheless statistically significant, improvement in insulin sensitivity with nifedipine.

There are a number of ongoing studies examining the effects of various antihypertensive agents on insulin sensitivity. It is likely that effects on insulin sensitivity will become an important characteristic for consideration when selecting pharmacologic agents for the management of hypertension, particularly in patients with either Type II diabetes or impaired glucose tolerance, and perhaps in the hypertensive population at large.

ETHNICITY IN RELATION TO INSULIN AND BLOOD PRESSURE

As noted earlier, in the Bogalusa Heart Study, Voors et al. (1981) found no relationship between blood pressure and an insulin resistance index in Black children, although they did in Whites. In the CARDIA study, the correlation of fasting insulin with blood pressure was very weak in Blacks, particularly after adjustment for body mass index (Manolio et al., 1990).

Saad et al. (1990) studied 2,873 Pima Indians. Although hypertension could be related to fasting insulin concentration, this relationship was not found in the subjects who were not taking antihypertensive medications. It should be noted, however, that as a group Pimas have extraordinarily high plasma insulin levels, profound insulin resistance, a high frequency of diabetes, and an extremely high prevalence of obesity. It is possible that this may have obscured other relationships. In a second study, Saad et al. (1991) examined the relationship between blood pressure and both plasma insulin and insulin sensitivity (using the clamp technique) in normotensive nondiabetic subjects in three ethnic groups — Pima Indians ($n = 116$), Caucasians ($n = 53$), and Blacks ($n = 42$). They found mean arterial blood pressure to be directly related to plasma insulin, and inversely related to insulin sensitivity in Whites, but not in Pimas or Blacks.

In the San Antonio Heart Study, Mexican Americans have been found to have a high frequency of diabetes (Haffner, Stern, Hazuda, Pugh, & Patterson, 1986), and it has been shown that diminished insulin sensitivity, measured by the minimal model, and a hyperinsulinemic response to OGTT, are present in young nonobese normoglycemic individuals (Haffner, Stern, Dunn et al., 1990). This suggests that insulin resistance precedes development of obesity and diabetes in Mexican Americans. It is interesting to note that in this group, the prevalence of hypertension is decreased in comparison to Whites (Haffner, Stern, Hazuda, Mitchell, & Patterson, 1990), and is almost always associated with concomitant obesity and diabetes. In spite of the decreased prevalence of hypertension, there is a direct relationship between plasma insulin level and blood pressure in high risk individuals prior to onset of diabetes (Haffner, Mitchell, Stern, Hazuda, & Patterson, 1990c).

These data suggest that it may be beneficial to examine the relationships among insulinemia and insulin resistance, blood pressure, adiposity and fat distribution, and glucose tolerance in different ethnic groups that vary in their relative frequency of hypertension, obesity, and glucose intolerance.

In the United States, Blacks are twice as likely as non-Hispanic Whites to be hypertensive (Hypertension Detection and Follow-up Program, 1977). Blacks are also more likely than non-Hispanic Whites to develop diabetes mellitus and impaired glucose tolerance (Harris, 1990). The race disparity is most apparent for both conditions when the prevalence rates for women are compared. In 1976–1980, 39.8% of Black women had hypertension, compared to 20% of White women; 24.6% of Black women had glucose intolerance, compared to 18.3% of White women (Harris, 1990; Hypertension Detection and Follow-up Program, 1977). The prevalence rates of both diseases increase progressively with age. In Blacks, both diseases are associated with increased morbidity and mortality, compared to Whites. Less data are available for Cubans. However, age-adjusted prevalence of hypertension is lowest amongst Cubans (compared to Blacks and non-Hispanic Whites) in spite of the fact that obesity is more prevalent in Cubans than non-Hispanic Whites (Dept. of Health, Education, and Welfare, 1989). For women, the age-adjusted prevalence rates for overweight are: Blacks 44.4%, Whites 23.9%, Cubans 31.6%. In contrast, the age-adjusted prevalence rates for hypertension in women are: Blacks 43.8%, Whites 25.1%, Cubans 14.4%. The prevalence of diabetes parallels that of overweight, with Cubans intermediate between Blacks and Whites. Thus, despite the higher prevalence of overweight and diabetes in Cubans, their proportion of hypertension is markedly lower. These findings suggest that there may be measurable differences among interacting risk factors among these ethnic groups.

Risk of Hypertension and Hyperinsulinemia in Relatives of Glucose Intolerant Individuals

Berntorp and Lindgarde (1986) noted that among nonobese men with normal glucose tolerance, those who had a family history of diabetes ($n = 22$) had higher blood pressure than those without a family history ($n = 51$), and that there was a direct relationship between blood pressure and postglucose insulinemia. Haffner et al. (1989) have reported that nondiabetic subjects with a positive parenteral history of Type II diabetes mellitus (and insulin resistance) have higher systolic and diastolic blood pressure than individuals with a negative parental history of diabetes. Zavaroni et al. (1990) have reported that offspring of subjects with impaired glucose tolerance had hyperinsulinemia, higher systolic and diastolic blood pressures, and higher triglyceride levels than controls. These data suggest that the changes in blood pressure and plasma insulin may antedate clinical disease.

INSULIN AND SODIUM EXCRETION

The antinatriuretic effect of insulin is well established (DeFronzo, 1981). As early as the 1930s, Atchley, Loeb, Richards, Benedict, and Driscoll (1933) suggested that insulin therapy of diabetes resulted in a marked reduction of renal sodium excretion. Miller and Bogdonoff (1954) were the first to perform controlled studies that showed that insulin administration in normal subjects reduced urinary sodium excretion. Meticulous studies by DeFronzo et al. (1975), using the euglycemic clamp technique, demonstrated that hyperinsulinemia in normal subjects resulted in a reductions of urinary sodium excretion, $U_{Na} \cdot V$; sodium clearance, C_{Na}; and fractional excretion of sodium, FE_{Na}. These changes were shown in the absence of changes in glomerular filtration rate, renal plasma flow, filtered load of glucose, or plasma aldosterone concentration. Additional studies by DeFronzo, Goldberg, and Agus (1976) in dogs combined euglycemic clamp studies with renal micropuncture, and suggested that insulin's antinatriuretic effect is at the level of the distal tubule. Hall et al. (1989) found that although a 7- to 28-day insulin infusion into healthy dogs had no effect on blood pressure, it did result in sodium retention.

Skott et al. (1989) performed two insulin dose clamp studies in normal human subjects, and demonstrated a dose response relationship for insulin's effect on reducing sodium clearance and fractional excretion of sodium, and also provided data suggesting that the insulin effect is in the distal tubule. On the other hand, Baum (1987), using isolated rabbit proximal tubules, found that insulin stimulated volume absorption, including active sodium chloride transport. Human studies by Trevisan et al. (1990) also suggested that hyperinsulinemia increases proximal tubule sodium reabsorption. Their study also demonstrated differences between normotensives and hypertensives in sodium excretion in response to a saline challenge. Although their data also demonstrated that induced hyperinsulinemia reduced sodium excretion, their clamp studies were only carried out in normotensive subjects, thus precluding any conclusions about potential differences between normotensives and hypertensives in sodium excretion in response to insulin. O'Hare et al. (1989) compared responses to hyperinsulinemia in obese men and lean men, and surprisingly found that whereas lean men showed the anticipated reduction in sodium excretion, the obese men had an increase in sodium excretion in response to hyperinsulinemia. No explanation was offered for this finding. It indicates the need for more careful studies that assess renal sodium response to insulin in relationship to body composition, insulin sensitivity, and ethnicity.

INSULIN, SYMPATHETIC NERVOUS SYSTEM (SNS), AND CARDIOVASCULAR FUNCTION

Young and Landsberg (1982) suggested that insulin may be the major link between changes in dietary intake and changes in sympathetic outflow, and that these changes may be responsible for the hypertension of obesity. The parallel reductions in blood pressure, insulinemia, and SNS activity following caloric restriction, weight loss, and exercise in obese subjects, has been taken as support for this linkage (Krieger & Landsberg, 1988).

Early studies of insulin effects on SNS activity and cardiovascular function were complicated by the induction of hypoglycemia and the subsequent counterregulatory response of catecholamines and/or by the presence of diabetes with varying degree of glycemia (Christensen, 1979; Hilsted et al., 1984; Mogensen, Christensen, & Gundersen, 1980). Pereda, Eckstein, and Abboud (1962) did attempt to examine cardiovascular responses to insulin in the absence of hypoglycemia in dogs, but their design was complicated by the presence of hyperglycemia and the administration of glucagon together with the insulin. Nevertheless, they found that insulin increased arterial blood pressure, cardiac output, and right atrial pressure, and that these responses appeared to be centrally mediated. Later, Liang et al. (1982) performed studies in dogs, in which they infused glucose to reverse or prevent hypoglycemia, and demonstrated that acute insulin infusion resulted in increments of plasma norepinephrine (and epinephrine when hypoglycemia occurred), along with increases in heart rate, mean arterial blood pressure, cardiac output, and left ventricular contractility indices. These investigators also examined the effects of insulin infusion on blood flow to various organs.

The direct effects of insulin, independent of hypoglycemia, can be studied by maintenance of euglycemia with the clamp technique. Using this approach, Rowe et al. (1981) demonstrated that in young, healthy, nonobese volunteers, the induction of acute pharmacologic hyperinsulinemia, in a dose response manner, results in increased plasma levels of norepinephrine, and increases in heart rate (HR), pulse pressure (SBP-DBP), mean arterial blood pressure (MAP) and double product (HR*SBP), a noninvasive measure of myocardial oxygen consumption. It should be noted that the insulin doses used raised mean plasma insulin to pharmacologic levels of 154 mcU/ml (low dose infusion) and 601 mcU/ml (high dose infusion). In the elderly, using an identical protocol with the clamp technique, in response to acute pharmacologic hyperinsulinemia, both the norepinephrine response and the changes in cardiovascular indices were markedly blunted (Minaker et al., 1982). On the other hand, when comparing young lean men and young obese men, in response to acute pharmacologic hyperinsulinemia with the clamp technique (lower dose infusion only), there were no differences in norepinephrine response, heart rate increment, or MAP (although both basal heart rate and MAP were higher in the obese), despite the fact that the obese subjects were insulin resistant (O'Hare et al., 1989). Surprisingly, the obese men did not statistically differ from the lean men in insulin sensitivity (M), although they had higher fasting plasma insulin levels.

In healthy medical students, the effects of moderate physiologic acute hyperinsulinemia (raising mean plasma insulin levels to 92 mcU/ml) studied with the clamp technique during continuous heart rate monitoring and intermittent echocardiography, did not result in any change in plasma catecholamines, heart rate, blood pressure, left ventricular end-diastolic diameter, or ejection phase indices (Airaksinen, Lahetla, Ikaheimo, Sotaniemi, & Takkunen, 1985). Likewise, Natali et al. (1990) found that local intraarterial moderate physiologic hyperinsulinemia (raising mean plasma insulin levels to 125 mcU/ml) had no acute hemodynamic effects on forearm blood flow, forearm vascular resistance, heart rate, or blood pressure. Trovati et al. (1988; Trovati et al., 1989) also failed to demonstrate a catecholamine response to hyperinsulinemia, in spite of having raised mean plasma insulin levels to 160 mcU/ml, perhaps because the duration of the hyperinsulinemia was but 30 minutes, much shorter than the time course of effects in other studies. In healthy volunteers, we have found that moderate physiologic hyperinsulinemia (raising the mean plasma insulin to 100 mcU/ml with the euglycemic clamp technique) results in a small increase in blood pressure and in increased cardiac sympathetic tone, as measured by three indices (QT/QX, PEP/LVET, and Heather Index) calculated from simultaneous continuous electrocardiography, phonocardiography, and impedance cardiography (Marks et al., 1991). Interestingly, we found that subjects who were more insulin sensitive (in terms of glucoregulatory effects) also had greater increases of blood pressure in response to hyperinsulinemia, suggesting that the acute effects of insulin blood pressure regulation become dampened by chronic insulin resistance (Thompson et al., 1991).

Collectively, these findings suggest that the changes in cardiovascular function observed by Rowe et al. (1981) may have been mediated via the SNS, through changes in norepinephrine, or that any direct effects of insulin are only seen at higher more sustained plasma levels. It should also be noted that the presence of hyperglycemia and of insulin resistance may influence the vascular response to hyperinsulinemia. The San Diego group reported that in the face of moderate physiologic hyperinsulinemia (mean plasma insulin levels of 72 mcU/ml), progressive hyperglycemia (to a level of 380 mg/dl) resulted in a doubling of leg blood flow in healthy nonobese subjects (Edelman et al., 1990), but not in obese men (Laakso et al., 1990).

In vitro, insulin has been shown to directly elicit a positive inotropic effect on cardiac muscle (Lee & Downing, 1976). On the other hand, insulin has an inhibitory effect on the inotropic action of norepinephrine (Lee & Downing, 1976), and the vasoconstrictive responses to both norepinephrine and angiotensin II (Alexander & Oake, 1977; Yagi et al., 1988). On the other hand, pharmacological hyperinsulinemia (with the clamp technique) in normal man did not modify the pressor response to angiotensin II (Vierhapper, Waldhausl, & Nowotny, 1983). In response to acute hyperinsulinemia (mean plasma insulin levels of 160 mcU/ml with the clamp), there are elevations of both plasma renin activity and angiotensin II, with decrease of aldosterone, all of which are obviated by concomitant potassium infusion (Trovati et al., 1989).

Increased SNS activity is a feature of essential hypertension, especially early in the course of the disease and in borderline hypertensives (Folkow, 1989; Goldstein, 1983; Julius, 1990). It is clear from the studies reviewed here that the interactions between insulin and SNS activity are complex. Insulin appears both to increase SNS activity and to modulate the pressor effects of norepinephrine (at least in vitro). Further studies are needed to clarify the nature of the interactions among insulin, insulin sensitivity, catecholamine secretion, and cardiovascular response.

PREGNANCY, INSULIN RESISTANCE, GLUCOSE TOLERANCE, AND BLOOD PRESSURE

Two of the most common complicating problems seen during pregnancy are the appearance of gestational diabetes (Freinkel, 1980, 1985) and of hypertension (National High Blood Pressure Education Program, 1990). Both of these conditions are more likely to occur during late pregnancy and both usually abate in the postpartum period. Both herald an increased risk for future development of disease. Their course is such that both may be attributed to arising as a consequence of the progressive insulin resistance characteristic of pregnancy that abates postpartum, but may have unmasked an underlying predisposition to subsequent disease development.

O'Sullivan (1984) followed 943 women for a quarter century postpartum. Of the 615 who had developed gestational diabetes, life table analysis projected a 74% prevalence of diabetes after a follow-up of 24 years, in contrast to a prevalence of 11.2% in women with normal glucose tolerance during pregnancy. Stowers, Sutherland, & Kerridge (1985) reported a prevalence of impaired glucose tolerance of 35% after a mean follow-up of approximately 13 years of 112 women who had gestational diabetes. Thus, gestational diabetes presages future glucose intolerance. Moreover, O'Sullivan (1984) found that among former gestational diabetic women, after a follow-up of 20 years, there were higher levels of plasma cholesterol and triglyceride, higher systolic blood pressure, and higher frequencies of hypertension and of EKG abnormalities. Therefore, it appears that gestational diabetes portends the chronic disease risk factor insulin resistance syndrome.

Pregnancy is a screening test for risk of ultimate hypertension. Women who are normotensive during pregnancy, especially after the age of 25, have a low risk of future hypertension (Fisher, Luger, Spargo, Lindheimer, 1981). Gestational hypertension, labeled *transient hypertension* by the newest recommendations (National High Blood Pressure Education Program, 1990), distinct from preeclampsia, foretells future risk of hypertension (Chesley, 1980). The literature on this subject is confusing, because clear distinction has not been made in most studies between gestational hypertension and preeclampsia. The evidence is that preeclampsia does not appear to constitute a risk factor for future hypertension (Chesley, 1980). If one requires that women with a true diagnosis of preeclampsia have significant proteinuria (i.e., at least 300 mg/l in a 24-hour collection or 1 g/l in a random collection) and if one assumes that true preeclampsia occurs in primagravida, then one can infer a diagnosis of gestational hypertension either if proteinuria is absent or in the absence of data on proteinuria if the pregnancy is in a multiparous woman. The data have been analyzed this way by Chesley (1980; Chesley, Annitto, & Cosgrove, 1976) for a number of studies, and they find that the future prevalence of hypertension in women who have had gestational hypertension is 40%–74%. In two subsequent series, the prevalence was 36% and 42% (Lindeberg, Ayelsson, Jorner, Maluberg, & Sandstrom, 1988; Svensson, Aldersch, & Hansson, 1983). The prevalence of diabetes developing many years after gestational hypertension is four times the expected rate (Chesley et al., 1976), again signifying the overlap between ultimate risk of hypertension and of diabetes.

During the course of gestation, there is a progressive increase in maternal insulin response to glucose (Bleicher, O'Sullivan, & Freinkel, 1964; Spellacy & Goetz, 1963), thus inferring insulin resistance. We demonstrated this directly by performing euglycemic clamp studies in the third trimester of pregnancy (Ryan, Enns, O'Sullivan, & Skyler, 1988; Ryan, O'Sullivan, & Skyler, 1985). Insulin resistance was found to be characteristic of pregnancy per se, and abated to a large degree postpartum. Moreover, there was a greater degree of insulin resistance in women with either gestational diabetes or impaired glucose tolerance. Using the minimal model technique, Cousins, Rea, and Crawford (1988) found a progressive increase in insulin resistance from the first through the third trimester, returning to normal postpartum. In women with previous gestational diabetes,. despite appearing clinically normal, decreased insulin sensitivity has been demonstrated in comparison to carefully matched controls, both by the clamp technique (Catalano et al., 1986) and by the minimal model technique (Ward et al., 1985). Decreased insulin sensitivity has also been unmasked in such women by oral contraceptive administration (Skouby, Andersen, Saurbrey, Kuhl, 1987).

Women with hypertension during the third trimester of pregnancy have been shown to have hyperinsulinemia in response to an oral glucose tolerance test, in comparison to normotensive control women (Bauman, Maimen, & Lauger, 1988). Both groups of women had similar normal glucose tolerance curves, and had equivalent circulating levels of placental lactogen, thought to be one factor conferring the insulin resistance of pregnancy. Thus, gestational hypertension, like gestational diabetes, appears to be associated with an even greater degree of insulin resistance than that normally seen in pregnancy.

CONCLUSIONS

The evidence relating elevated blood pressure to reduced insulin sensitivity has been reviewed. It is important to note that when there is reduced sensitivity to the glucoregulatory effects of insulin, hyperinsulinemia ensues. In contrast to the reduced sensitivity to the glucoregulatory effects of insulin, there may be preservation of sensitivity to other effects of insulin. Thus, hyperinsulinemia may result in increased stimulation of pathways that contribute to maintenance of blood pressure, and consequently raise such pressure. The pathways involved in regulation of blood pressure are complex and multifactorial. Thus, much further investigation is required to provide further insights and definition to the mechanisms involved in insulin's effects on blood pressure. Concomitantly, such studies may also better explain the nature of the "chronic high risk factor syndrome," one of the most important public health problems in the world today.

ACKNOWLEDGMENT

This chapter was supported by grant #P01-HL-36588 from the National Institutes of Health, U.S. Public Health Service.

REFERENCES

Airaksinen, J., Lahtela, J. T., Ikaheimo, M. J., Sotaniemi, E. A., & Takkunen, J. T. (1985). Intravenous insulin has no effect on myocardial contractility or heart rate in healthy subjects. *Diabetologia, 28,* 649–652.

Alberti, K. G. M. M., Dowse, G., Finch, C., Zimmet, P., Gareeboo, H., Brigham, L., Mauritius, N. C. D. Study Group. (1989). Is blood pressure related to peripheral insulin levels? – A community study in mauritius. *Diabetes, 38*(Suppl 2), 92A.

Alexander, W. D., & Oake, & R. J. (1977). The effect of insulin on vascular reactivity to norepinephrine. *Diabetes, 26,* 611–614.

Andres, R., Swerdloff, R., Pozefsky, T., & Coleman, D. (1966). Manual feedback technique for the control of blood glucose concentration. In L. T. Skeggs (Ed.), *Automation in analytical chemistry* (pp. 486–491). New York: Mediad.

Atchley, D. W., Loeb, R. F., Richards, D. W., Benedict, E. M., & Driscoll, M. E. (1933). On Diabetic Acidosis. *Journal of Clinical Investigation, 12,* 297–326.

Baum, M. (1987). Insulin stimulates volume absorption in the rabbit proximal convoluted tubule. *Journal of Clinical Investigation, 79,* 1104–1109.

Bauman, W. A., Maimen, M., & Langer, O. (1988). An association between hyperinsulinemia and hypertension during the third trimester of pregnancy. *American Journal of Obstetrics and Gynecology, 159,* 446–450.

Beard, J. C., Bergman, R. N., Ward, W. K., & Porte, D. (1986). The insulin sensitivity index in nondiabetic man: Correlation between clamp-derived and IVGTT-derived values. *Diabetes, 35,* 362–369.

Berchtold, P., Jorgens, V., Kemmer, F. W., & Berger, M. (1982). Obesity and hypertension: Cardiovascular response to weight reduction. *Hypertension, 4* (Suppl III), I11SO-11155.

Berglund, G., Larsson, B., Anderson, O., Larsson, O., Svardsudd, K., Bjorntorp, P., & Wilhelmsen, L. (1976). Body composition and glucose metabolism in hypertensive middle-aged males. *Acta Medica Scandinavica, 200,* 163–169.

Bergman, R. N. (1989). Toward physiological understanding of glucose tolerance: Minimal model approach. *Diabetes, 38,* 1512–1527.

Bergman, R. N., Beard, J. C., & Chen, M. (1986). The minimal model method. Assessment of insulin sensitivity and beta cell function in vivo. In W. L. Clarke, J. Larner, & S. L. Pohl (Eds.), *Methods in diabetes research, Vol. II clinical methods* (pp. 15–34). New York: J Wiley.

Bergman, R. N., Finegood, D. T., & Ader, M. (1985). Assessment of insulin sensitivity in vivo. *Endocrine Review, 6,* 45–86.

Bergman, R. N., Prager, R., Volund, A., Olefsky, J. M. (1987). Equivalence of the insulin sensitivity index in man derived by the minimal model method and the euglycemic glucose clamp. *Journal of Clinical Investigation, 79,* 790–800.

Berntorp, K., & Lindgarde, F. (1986). Familial aggregation of Type II diabetes mellitus as an etiological factor in hypertension. *Diabetes Research in Clinical Practices, 1,* 307–313.

Bleicher, S. J., O'Sullivan, J. B., & Freinkel, N. (1964). Carbohydrate metabolism in pregnancy. *New England Journal of Medicine, 271,* 866–872.

Bonora, E., Zavaroni, I. Alpi, O., Pezzarossa, A., Bruschi, F., Dall'Aglio, E., Guerra, L., Coscelli, C., & Butturini, U. (1987). Relationship between blood pressure and plasma insulin in non-obese and obese non-diabetic subjects. *Diabetologia, 30,* 719–723.

Burke, G. L., Webber, L. S., Srinivasan, S. R., Radhakrishnamurthy, B., Freedman, D. S., & Berenson, G. S. (1986). Fasting plasma glucose and insulin levels and their relationship to cardiovascular risk factors in children: Bogalusa Heart Study. *Metabolism, 35,* 441–446.

Cambien, F., Warnet, J.-M., Eschwegel, E., Jacqueson, A., Richard, J. L., & Rosselin, G. (1987). Body mass, mlood pressure, glucose, and lipids. Does plasma insulin explain their relationship? *Arteriosclerosis, 7,* 197–202.

Carretta, R., Fabris, B., Fischetti, F., Costantini, M., DeBiasi, F., Muiesan, S., Bardelli, M., Vran, F., & Companacci, L. (1989). Reduction of blood pressure in obese hyperinsuli-naemic hypertensive patients during somatostatin infusion. *Journal of Hypertension, 7*(Suppl 6), S196–S197.

Catalano, P. M., Bernstein, I. M., Wolfe, R. R., Srikanta, S., Tyzbir, E., Sims, E. A. H. (1986). Subclinical abnormalities of glucose metabolism in subjects with previous gestational diabetes. *American Journal of Obstetrics and Gynecology, 155,* 1255–1262.

Chesley, L. C. (1980). Hypertension in pregnancy: Definitions, familial factor, and remote prognosis. *Kidney International, 18,* 234–240.

Chesley, L. C., Annitto, J. E., & Cosgrove, R. A. (1976). The remote prognosis of eclamptic women. Sixth periodic report. *American Journal of Obstetrics and Gynecology, 124,* 446–459.

Christensen, N. J. (1979). Catecholamines and diabetes mellitus. *Diabetologia, 16,* 211–224.

Christlieb, A. R., Krolewski, A. S., Warram, J. H., & Soeldner, J. S. (1985). Is insulin the link between hypertension and obesity? *Hypertension, 7*(Suppl II), 1154–1157.

Clemons, A. H., Hough, D. L., & DOrazio, P. A. (1982). Development of the biostator glucose clamping algorithm. *Clinical Chemistry, 28,* 1899–1904.

Cousins, L., Rea, C., & Crawford, M. (1988). Longitudinal characterization of insulin sensitivity and body fat quantitation in normal and gestational diabetic pregnancies. *Diabetes, 37*(Suppl 1), 251A.

Cutfield, W. S., Bergman, R. N., Menon, A. K., & Sperling, M. A. (1990). The modified minimal model: Application to measurement of insulin sensitivity in children. *Journal of Clinical Endocrinology and Metabolism, 70,* 1664–1650.

DeFronzo, R. A. (1981). The effect of insulin on renal sodium metabolism. *Diabetologia, 21,* 165–171.

DeFronzo, R. A. (1988). The triumvirate: B-cell, muscle, liver. A collusion responsible for NIDDM. *Diabetes, 37,* 667–687.

DeFronzo, R. A., Ferrannini, E. (1990). Insulin resistance: A multi-faceted syndrome. *Diabetes Care, 13.*

DeFronzo, R. A., Cooke, C. R., Andres, R., Faloona, G. R., & Davis, P. J. (1975). The effect of insulin on renal handling of sodium, potassium, calcium, and phosphate in man. *Journal of Clinical Investigation, 55,* 845–855.

DeFronzo, R. A., Goldberg, M., & Agus, Z. S. (1976). The effects of glucose and insulin on renal electrolyte transport. *Journal of Clinical Investigation, 58,* 83–90.

DeFronzo, R. A., Jacot, E., Jequier, E., Maeder, E., Wahren, J., & Felber, J. P. (1981). The effect of insulin on the disposal of intravenous glucose: Results from indirect calorimetry and hepatic and femoral venous catheterization. *Diabetes, 30,* 1000–1007.

DeFronzo, R. A., Simonson, D., & Ferrannini, E. (1982). Hepatic and peripheral insulin resistance: A common feature of Type II (non-insulin-dependent) and Type I (insulin-dependent) diabetes mellitus. *Diabetologia, 23,* 313–319.

DeFronzo, R. A., Tobin, J. D., & Andres, R. (1979). Glucose clamp technique: A method for quantifying insulin secretion and resistance. *American Journal of Physiology, 237,* E214–223.

Del Prato, S., Ferrannini, E., & DeFronzo, R, A, (1986). Evaluation of insulin Sensitivity in man. In W. L. Clarke, J. Larner, & S. L. Pohl (Eds.), *Methods in diabetes research, Vol. II, clinical methods* (pp. 35–76). New York: J Wiley.

Department of Health, Education, and Welfare. (1989). *Nutrition monitoring in the United States* (DHH5 Publication #89-1255). Washington, DC.

Donahue, R. P., Orchard, T. J., Becker, D. J., Kuller, L. H., & Drash, A. L. (1987). Sex differences in the coronary heart disease risk profile: A possible role for insulin. *American Journal of Epidemiology, 125,* 650–657.

Donahue, R. P., Skyler, J. S., Schneiderman, N., & Prineas, R. J. (1990). Hyperinsulinemia and elevated blood pressure: Cause, confounder, or coincidence? *American Journal of Epidemiology, 132,* 827–836.

Donner, C. C., Fraze, E., Chen, Y. D. I., Hollenbeck, C., Foley, J. E., & Reaven, G. M. (1985). Presentation of a new method for specific measurement of in vivo insulin stimulated glucose disposal in humans: Comparison of this approach with the insulin clamp and minimal model techniques. *Journal of Clinical Endocrinology and Metabolism, 60,* 723–726.

Ducimetiere, P., Eschwege, E., Papoz, L., Richard, J. L., Claude, J. R., & Rosselin, G. (1980). Relationship of plasma insulin levels to the incidence of myocardial infarction and coronary heart disease mortality in a middle-aged population. *Diabetologia, 19,* 205–210.

Edelman, S. V., Laakso, M., Wallace, P., Brechtel, G., Olefsky, J. M., & Baron, A. D. (1990). Kinetics of insulin-mediated and non-insulin-mediated glucose uptake in humans. *Diabetes, 39,* 995–964.

Ferrannini, E., Buzzigoli, G., Bonadonna, R., Giorico, M. A., Oleggini, M., Graziadei, L., Pedrinelli, R., Brandi, L., & Bevilacqua, S. (1987). Insulin resistance in essential hypertension. *New England Journal of Medicine, 31,* 350–357.

Ferrari, P., & Weidmann, P. (1990). Insulin, insulin sensitivity and hypertension. *Journal of Hypertension, 8,* 491–500.

Finegood, D. T., Bergman, R. N., & Vranic, M. (1987). Estimation of endogenous glucose production during hyperinsulinemic-euglycemic glucose clamps. *Diabetes, 36,* 914–924.

Finegood, D. T., Hramiak, I. M., & Dupre, J. (1990). A modified protocol for estimation of insulin sensitivity with the minimal model of glucose kinetics in patients with insulin dependent diabetes mellitus. *Journal of Clinical Endocrinology and Metabolism, 71,* 1538–1589.

Finegood, D. T., Pacini, G., & Bergman, R. N. (1984). The insulin sensitivity index. Correlation in dogs between values determined from the intravenous glucose tolerance test and the euglycemic glucose clamp. *Diabetes, 33,* 362–368.

Fisher, H. A., Luger, A., Spargo, B. H., Lindheimer, M. D. (1981). Hypertension in pregnancy: Clinical-pathological correlations and remote prognosis. *Medicine, 60,* 267–276.

Folkow, B, (1989). Sympathetic nervous control of blood pressure. Role in primary hypertension. *American Journal of Hypertension, 2,* 103S-111S.

Folsom, A. R., Burke, G. L., Ballew, C., Jacobs, D. R., Jr., Haskell, W. L., Donahue, R. P., Liu, K., & Hilner, J. E. (1989). Relation of body fatness and its distribution to cardiovascular risk factors in young blacks and whites. *American Journal of Epidemiology, 130,* 911–924.

Forster, H. V., Dempsey, J. A., Thomson, J., Vidruk, E., & DoPico, G. A. (1972). Estimation of arterial pO_2, pCO_2, pH, and lactate from arterialised venous blood. *Journal of Applied Physiology, 32,* 134–137.

Fournier, A. M., Gadia, M. T., Kubrusly, D. B., Skyler, J. S., & Sosenko, J. M. (1986). Blood pressure, insulin, and glycemia in nondiabetic subjects. *American Journal of Medicine, 80,* 861–864.

Freinkel, N. (1980). Of pregnancy and progeny. *Diabetes, 29,* 1023–1035.

Freinkel, N. (Ed.). (1985). Proceedings of the second international workshop-conference on gestational diabetes mellitus. *Diabetes, 34*(Suppl 2), 1–126.

Fuh, M. M.-T., Shieh, S.-M., Wu, D.-A., Chen, Y.-D. I., & Reaven, G. M. (1987). Abnormalities of carbohydrate and lipid metabolism in patients with hypertension. *Archives of Internal Medicine, 147,* 1035–1038.

Goldstein, D. S. (1983). Plasma catecholamines and essential hypertension. An analytical review. *Hypertension, 5,* 86–252.

Haffner, S. M., Mitchell, B. D., Stern, M. P., Hazuda, H. P., & Patterson, J. K. (1990). Decreased prevalence of hypertension in Mexican Americans. *Hypertension, 16,* 225–232.

Haffner, S. M., Stern, M. P., Dunn, J., Mobley, M., Blackwell, J., & Bergman, R. N. (1990). Diminished insulin sensitivity and increased insulin response in nonobese nondiabetic Mexican Americans. *Metabolism, 39,* 842–847.

Haffner, S. M., Stern, M. P., Hazuda, H. P., Mitchell, B. D., Patterson, J. K., & Ferrannini, E. (1989). Parental history of diabetes is associated with increased cardiovascular risk factors. *Arteriosclerosis, 9,* 929–933.

Haffner, S. M., Stern, M. P., Hazuda, H. P., Mitchell, B. D., & Patterson, J. K. (1990). Cardiovascular risk factors in confirmed prediabetic individuals. *JAMA, 263,* 2893–2898.

Haffner, S. M., Stern, M. P., Hazuda, H. P., Pugh, J. A., & Patterson, J. K. (1986). Hyperinsulinemia in a population at high risk for non-insulin-dependent diabetes mellitus. *New England Journal of Medicine, 315,* 220–224.

Hall, J. E., Coleman, T. G., & Mizelle, H. L. (1989). Does chronic hyperinsulinemia cause hypertension? *American Journal of Hypertension, 2,* 171–173.

Harano, Y., Ohgaku, S., Hidake, H., Haneda, K., Kikkawa, R., Shigeta, Y., & Abe, H. (1977). Glucose, insulin and somatostatin infusion for the determination of insulin sensitivity. *Journal of Clinical Endocrinology and Metabolism, 45,* 1124–1127.

Harris, M. I. (1990). Noninsulin-dependent diabetes mellitus in Black and White Americans. *Diabetes/Metabolism Review, 6,* 71–90.

Hilsted, J., Bonde-Peterson, F., Norgaard, M.-B., Greninman, M., Christensen, N. J., Parving, H.-H., & Suzuki, M. (1984). Haemodynamic changes in insulin-induced hypoglycaemia in normal man. *Diabetologia, 26,* 328–332.

Hypertension Detection and Follow-up Program. (1977). Race, education and prevalence of hypertension. *American Journal of Epidemiology, 106,* 351–361.

Jauch, K. W., Hartl, W., Guenther, B., Wicklmayr, M., Rett, K., & Dietze, G. (1987). Captopril enhances insulin responsiveness of forearm muscle tissue in non-insulin-dependent diabetes mellitus. *European Journal of Clinical Investigation, 17,* 448–454.

Julius, S. (1990). Hemodynamic and neurohumoral evidence of multifaceted pathophysiology in human hypertension. *Journal of Cardiovascular Pharmacology, 15*(Suppl 5), 553–558.

Kahn, C. R. (1978). Insulin resistance, insulin insensitivity, and insulin unresponsiveness: A necessary distinction. *Metabolism, 27,* 1893–1902.

Kannel, W. B., Brand, N., Skinner, J. J., Dawber, T. R., & McNamara, P. M. (1967). The relation of adiposity of blood pressure and development of hypertension. The Framingham Study. *Annals of Internal Medicine, 67,* 48–60.

Kaplan, N. M. (1989). The deadly quartet. Upper-body obesity, glucose intolerance, hypertriglyceridemia, and hypertension. *Archives of Internal Medicine, 149,* 1514–1519.

Kempner, W., Newborg, B. C., Peschel, R. L., & Skyler, J. S. (1975). Treatment of massive obesity with Rice/Reduction Diet Program. *Archives of Internal Medicine, 135,* 1575–1584.

Kolterman, O. G., Gray, R. S., Griffin, J., Burstein, P., Insel, J., Scarlett, J. A., & Olefsky, J. M. (1981). Receptor and post-receptor defects contribute to insulin resistance in non-insulin dependent diabetes mellitus. *Journal of Clinical Investigation, 68,* 957–969.

Kolterman, O. G., Insel, J., Saekow, M., & Olefsky, J. M. (1980). Mechanisms of insulin resistance in human obesity—evidence for receptor and postreceptor defects. *Journal of Clinical Investigation, 65,* 1273–1284.

Krieger, D. R., & Landsberg, L. (1988). Mechanisms in obesity-related hypertension: Role of insulin and catecholamines. *American Journal of Hypertension, 1,* 84–90.

Krotkiewski, M., Mandroukas, K., Sjostrom, L., Sullivan, L., Wetterqvist, H., & Bjorntorp, P. (1979). Effects of long-term physical training on body fat, metabolism, and blood pressure in obesity. *Metabolism, 28,* 650–658.

Laakso, M., Edelman, S. V., Olefsky, J. M., Brechtel, G., Wallace, P., & Baron, A. D. (1990). Kinetics of in vitro muscle insulin-mediated glucose uptake in human obesity. *Diabetes, 39,* 965–974.

Lebovitz, H. E., & Feinglos, M. N. (1980). Therapy of insulin independent diabetes mellitus. General considerations. *Metabolism, 29,* 474–481.

Lebovitz, H. E., Feinglos, M. N., Bucholtz, H. K., Lebovitz, F. L. (1977). Potentiation of insulin action: A probable mechanism for the anti-diabetic action of sulfonylurea drugs. *Journal of Clinical Endocrinology and Metabolism, 45,* 601–604.

Lee, J. C., & Downing, S. E. (1976). Effects of insulin on cardiac muscle contraction and responsiveness to norepinephrine. *American Journal of Physiology, 230,* 1360–1365.

Liang, C.-S., Doherty, J. U., Faillace, R., Maekawa, K., Arnold, S., Gavras, H., & Hood, W. B. (1982). Insulin infusion in conscious dogs. Effects on systemic and coronary hemodynamics, regional blood flows, and plasma catecholamines. *Journal of Clinical Investigation, 69,* 1321–1336.

Lindeberg, S., Axelsson, O., Jorner, U., Malmberg, L., & Sandstrom, B. (1988). A prospective controlled five-year follow-up study of primiparas with gestational hypertension. *Acta Obstetrics Gynecologie Scandinavica, 67,* 605–609.

Litheil, H. O., Pollare, T., & Berne, C. (1990). Insulin sensitivity in newly detected hypertensive patients: Influence of Captopril and other antihypertensive agents on insulin sensitivity and related biological parameters. *Journal of Cardiovascular Pharmacology, 15*(Suppl 5), 546–552.

Lowenthal, L. M., Pim, B., Hillson, R. M., Dhar, H., & Hockaday, T. D. R. (1985). Blood pressure at diagnosis of Type II diabetes correlates with plasma insulin concentration but not during the next 5 years. *Diabetes Research, 2,* 65–69.

Lucas, C. P., Estigarribia, J. A., Darga, L. L., & Reaven, G. M. (1985). Insulin and blood pressure in obesity. *Hypertension, 7,* 702–706.

Manicardi, V., Camellini, L., Bellodi, G., Coscelli, C., & Ferrannini, E. (1986). Evidence for an association of high blood pressure and hyperinsulinemia in obese man. *Journal of Clinical Endocrinology and Metabolism, 62,* 1302–1304.

Manolio, T. A., Savage, P. J., Burke, G. L., Liu, K., Wagenknecht, L. E., Sidney, S., Jacobs, D. R., Jr., Roseman, J. M., Donahue, R. P., & Oberman, A. (1990). Association of fasting insulin with blood pressure and lipids in young adults. A CARDIA study. *Arteriosclerosis, 10,* 430–436.

Marigliano, A., Tedde, R., Sechi, L. A., Pala, A., Pisanu, G., & Pacifico, A. (1990). Insulinemia and blood pressure. Relationships in patients with primary and secondary hypertension, and with or without glucose metabolism impairment. *American Journal of Hypertension, 3,* 521–526.

Marks, J. B., Hurwitz, B. E., Ansley, J., Quillian, R. E., Thompson, N. E., Olsson-Istel, G. M., Spitzer, S., Schneiderman, N., & Skyler, J. S. (1991). Effects of induced hyperinsulinemia on blood pressure & sympathetic tone in healthy volunteers. *Diabetes, 40*(Suppl 1), 367A.

Mbanya, J.-C. N., Thomas, T. H., Wilkinson, R., Alberti, K. G. M. M., & Taylor, R. (1988). Hypertension and hyperinsulinaemia: A relation in diabetes but not essential hypertension. *Lancet, 1,* 733–734.

McGuire, E. A. H., Helderman, J. H., Tobin, J. D., Andres, R., & Berman, M. (1976). Effects of arterial versus venous sampling on analysis of glucose kinetics in man. *Journal of Applied Physiology, 41,* 565–573.

Miller, J. H., & Bogdonoff, M. D. (1954). Antidiuresis associated with administration of insulin. *Journal of Applied Physiology, 6,* 509–512.

Minaker, K. L., Rowe, J. W., Young, J. B., Sparrow, D., Pallotta, J. A., & Landsberg, L. (1982). Effect of age on insulin stimulation of sympathetic nervous system activity in man. *Metabolism, 31,* 1181–1184.

Modan, M., Halkin, H., Almog, S., Lusky, A., Eshkol, A., Shefi, M., Shitrit, A., & Fuchs, Z. (1985). Hyperinsulinemia. A link between hypertension, obesity and glucose intolerance. *Journal of Clinical Investigation, 75,* 809–817.

Modan, M., Halkin, H., Fuchs, Z., Lusky, A., Chetrit, A., Segal, P., Eshkol, A., Almog, S., & Shefi, M. (1987). Hyperinsulinemia—A link between glucose intolerance, obesity, hypertension, dyslipoproteinemia, elevated serum uric acid and internal cation imbalance. *Diabetes Metabolism, 13,* 375–380.

Mogensen, C. E., Christensen, N. J., & Gundersen, H. J. G. (1980). The acute effect of insulin on heart rate, blood pressure, plasma noradrenaline and urinary albumin excretion. *Diabetologia, 18,* 453–457.

Nagasaki, K., Hara, H., Ogawa, J., Egusa, G., et al. (1986). Relationship between hyperinsulinemia and risk factors of atherosclerosis. *Japanese Journal of Medicine, 3,* 270–277.

Nagulesparan, M., Savage, P. J., Unger, R. H., & Bennett, P. H. (1979). A simplified method using somatostatin to assess in vivo insulin resistance over a range of obesity. *Diabetes, 28,* 980–983.

Natali, A., Buzzigoli, G., Taddei, S., Santoro, D., Cerri, M., Pedrinelli, R., & Ferrannini, E. (1990). Effects of insulin on hemodynamics and metabolism in human forearm. *Diabetes, 39,* 490–500.

National High Blood Pressure Education Program. (1990). Working group report on high blood pressure in pregnancy. *American Journal of Obstetrics and Gynecology* and *DHHS Publication #90–3029,* 1–38.

O'Hare, J. A., Minaker, K. L., Meneilly, G. S., Rowe, J. W., Pallotta, J. A., & Young, J. B. (1989). Effect of insulin on plasma norepinephrine and 3, 4-dihydroxyphenylalanine in obese men. *Metabolism, 38,* 322–329.

Olefsky, J. (1981). Insulin resistance and insulin action: An in vitro and in vivo perspective. *Diabetes, 30,* 148–162.

Olefsky, J., Reaven, G. M., & Farquhar, J. W. (1974). Effects of weight reduction on obesity. Studies of lipid and carbohydrate metabolism in normal and hyperlipoproteinemic subjects. *Journal of Clinical Investigation, 53,* 64–76.

O'Sullivan, J. B. (1984). Subsequent morbidity among gestational diabetic women. In H. W. Sutherland & J. M. Stowers (Eds.), *Carbohydrate metabolism in pregnancy and the newborn* (pp. 174–180). Edinburgh: Churchill Livingstone.

Pereda, S. A., Eckstein, J. W., & Abboud, F. M. (1962). Cardiovascular responses to insulin in the absence of hypoglycemia. *American Journal of Physiology, 202,* 249–252.

Pollare, T., Lithell, H., & Berne, C. (1989). A comparison of the effects of hydrochlorothiazide and captopril on glucose and lipid metabolism in patients with hypertension. *New England Journal of Medicine, 321,* 868–873.

Pollare, T., Lithell, H., & Berne, C. (1990). Insulin resistance is a characteristic feature of primary hypertension independent of obesity. *Metabolism, 39,* 169–174.

Pollare, T., Lithell, H., Morlin, C., Prantare, H., Hvarfner, A., & Ljunghall, S. (1989). Metabolic effects of diltiazem and atenolol: Results from a randomized, double blind study with parallel groups. *Journal of Hypertension, 7,* 551–559.

Pollare, T., Lithell, H., Selinus, I., & Berne, C. (1988). Application of prazosin is associated with an increase of insulin sensitivity in obese patients with hypertension. *Diabetologia, 31,* 415–420.

Pollare, T., Lithell, H., Selinus, I., & Berne, C. (1989). Sensitivity to insulin during treatment with atenolol and metoprolol: A randomized, double blind study of effects on carbohydrate and lipoprotein metabolism in hypertensive patients. *British Medical Journal, 298,* 1152–1157.

Poncher, M., Heine, R. J., Pernet, A., Hanning, I., Francis, A. J., Cook, D., Orskov, H., & Alberti, K. G. M. M. (1984). A comparison of the artificial pancreas (glucose controlled insulin infusion system) and a manual technique for assessing insulin sensitivity during euglycaemic clamping. *Diabetologia, 26,* 420–425.

Pyorala, K., Savolainen, E., Kaukola, S., & Haapakoski, J. (1985). Plasma insulin as coronary heart disease risk factor: Relationship to other risk factors and predictive value during 9-½ year follow-up of the Helsinki policemen study population. *Acta Medica Scandinavica, 701,*(Suppl), 38–52.

Ratzmann, K. P., Besch, W., Witt, S., & Schulz, B. (1981). Evaluation of insulin resistance during inhibition of endogenous insulin and glucagon secretion by somatostatin in non-obese subjects with impaired glucose tolerance. *Diabetologia, 21,* 192–197.

Reaven, G. M. (1983). Insulin resistance in non-insulin dependent diabetes mellitus. Does it exist and can it be measured? *American Journal of Medicine, 74,* 1A:3–17.

Reaven, G. M. (1988). Role of insulin resistance in human disease. *Diabetes, 37,* 1595–1607.

Reaven, G. M., & Hoffman, B. B. (1987). A role for insulin in the aetiology and course of hypertension? *Lancet, 2,* 435–437.

Reaven, G. M., & Miller, R. G. (1979). An attempt to define the nature of chemical diabetes using a multidimensional analysis. *Diabetologia, 16,* 17–24.

Resnick, L. M., Gupta, R. K., Gruenspan, H., Alderman, M. H., & Laragh, J. H. (1990). Hypertension and peripheral insulin resistance. Possible mediating role of intracellular free magnesium. *American Journal of Hypertension, 3,* 373–379.

Rocchini, A. P., Katch, V., Schork, A., & Kelch, R. P. (1987). Insulin and blood pressure during weight loss in obese adolescents. *Hypertension, 10,* 267–273.

Rose, H. G., Yalow, R. S., Schweitzer, P., & Schwartz, E. (1986). Insulin as a potential factor influencing blood pressure in amputees. *Hypertension, 8,* 793–800.

Rowe, J. W., Young, J. B., Minaker, K. L., Stevens, A. L., Pallotta, J., & Landsberg, L. (1981). Effect of insulin and glucose infusions on sympathetic nervous system activity in normal man. *Diabetes, 30,* 219–225.

Ryan, E. A., Enns, L., O'Sullivan, M. J., & Skyler, J. S. (1988). Insulin action in pregnancy. In H. J. Goren (Eds.), *Insulin action and diabetes* (pp. 191–201). New York: Raven Press.

Ryan, E. A., O'Sullivan, M. J., & Skyler, J. S. (1985). Insulin action during pregnancy. Studies with the euglycemic clamp technique. *Diabetes, 34,* 380–389.

Saad, M. F., Knowler, W. C., Pettitt, D. J., Nelson, R. G., Mott, D. M., Bennett, P. H. (1990). Insulin and hypertension: Relationships to obesity and glucose intolerance in Pima Indians. *Diabetes, 39,* 1430–1435.

Saad, M. F., Lillioja, S., Nyomba, B. L., Castillo, C., Ferrano, R., DeGregorio, M., Ravussin, E., Knowler, W. C., Bennett, P. H., Howard, B. V., & Bogardus, C. (1991). Racial differences in the relation between blood pressure and insulin resistance. *New England Journal of Medicine, 324,* 733–739.

Schotte, D. E., & Stunkard, A. J. (1990). The effects of weight reduction on blood pressure in 301 obese patients. *Archives of Internal Medicine, 150,* 1701–1704.

Shen, D.-C., Shieh, S.-M., Fuh, M. M.-T., Wu, D.-A., Chen, Y.-D. I., & Reaven, G. M. (1988). Resistance to insulin-stimulated-glucose uptake in patients with hypertension. *Journal of Clinical Endocrinology and Metabolism, 66,* 580–583.

Shen, S. W., Reaven, G. M., & Farquhar, J. (1970). Comparison of impedance to insulin-mediated glucose uptake in normal subjects and in subjects with latent diabetes. *Journal of Clinical Investigation, 49,* 2151–2160.

Sheu, W. H. H., Swislocki, A. L. M., Hoffman, B., Chen, Y. D. I., & Reaven, G. M. (in press). Comparison of the effects of atenolol and nifedipiine on glucose, insulin, and lipid metabolism in patients with hypertension. *American Journal of Hypertension, 4.*

Sims, E. A. M. (1982). Mechanisms of hypertension in the overweight. *Hypertension, 4*(Suppl III), III43–III49.

Singer, P., Godicke, W., Voigt, S., Hajdu, I., & Weiss, M. (1985). Postprandial hyperinsulinemia in patients with mild essential hypertension. *Hypertension, 7,* 182–186.

Skott, P., Hother-Nielsen, O., Bruun, N. E., Giese, J., Nielsen, M. D., Beck-Nielsen, H. B., & Parving, H. H. (1989). Effects of insulin on kidney function and sodium excretion in healthy subjects. *Diabetologia, 32,* 694–699.

Skouby, S. O., Andersen, O., Saurbrey, N., & Kuhl, C. (1987). Oral contraception and insulin sensitivity: In vivo assessment in normal women and women with previous gestational diabetes. *Journal of Clinical Endocrinology and Metabolism, 64,* 519–523.

Spellacy, W. N., & Goetz, F. C. (1963). Plasma insulin in normal late pregnancy. *New England Journal of Medicine, 268,* 988–991.

Steil, G. M., Volund, A., & Bergman, R. N. (1991). *Reduced sampling schedule to calculate Insulin sensitivity and glucose effectiveness from the minimal model.* Manuscript submitted for review.

Stowers, J. M., Sutherland, H. W., & Kerridge, D. F. (1985). Long-range implications for the mother. *Diabetes, 34*(Suppl 2), 106–110.

Svensson, A., Ahdersch, B., & Hansson, L. (1983). Prediction of later hypertension following a hypertensive pregnancy. *Journal of Hypertension, 1*(Suppl 1), 94–96.

Swislocki, A. (1990). Insulin resistance and hypertension. *American Journal of Medical Science, 300,* 104–115.

Swislocki, A. L. M., Hoffman, B. B., & Reaven, G. M. (1989). Insulin resistance, glucose intolerance and hyperinsulinemia in patients with hypertension. *American Journal of Hypertension, 2,* 419–423.

Tedde, R., Sechi, L. A., Marigliano, A., Papa, A., & Scano, L. (1989). Antihypertensive effect of insulin reduction in diabetic-hypertensive patients. *American Journal of Hypertension, 2,* 163–170.

Thompson, N. E., Marks, J. B., Hurwitz, B. E., Quillian, R. E., Ansley, J., Spitzer, S., Schneiderman, N., & Skyler, J. S. (1991). Insulin resistance dampens the acute effects of insulin on blood pressure regulation. *Diabetes, 40*(Suppl 1): 366A.

Trevisan, R., Fioretto, P., Semplicini, A., Opocher, G., Mantero, F., Rocco, S., Remuzzi, G., Morocutti, A., Zanette, G., Donadon, V., Perico, N., Giorato, C., & Nosadini, R. (1990). Role of insulin and atrial natriuretic peptide in sodium retention in insulin-treated IDDM patients during isotonic volume expansion. *Diabetes, 39,* 289–298.

Trovati, M., Anfossi, G., Cavalot, F., Massucco, P., Mularoni, E., & Emanuelli, G. (1988). Insulin directly reduces platelet sensitivity to aggregating agents. Studies in vitro and in vivo. *Diabetes, 37,* 780–786.

Trovati, M., Massucco, P., Anfossi, G., Cavalot, F., Mularoni, E., Mattiello, L., Rocca, G., & Emanuelli, G. (1989). Insulin influences the renin-angiotension-aldosterone system in humans. *Metabolism, 38,* 501–503.

Uusitupa, M., Niskanen, L., Siitonen, O., & Pyorala, K. (1987). Hyperinsulinemia and hypertension in patients with newly diagnosed non-insulin-dependent diabetes. *Diabetes Metabolism, 13,* 639–374.

Verza, M., D-Avino, M., Cacciapuoti, F., Aceto, E., D'Errico, S., Varricchio, M., & Giugliano, D. (1988). Hypertension in the elderly is associated with impaired glucose metabolism independently of obesity and glucose intolerance. *Journal of Hypertension, 6*(Suppl 1), S45–S48.

Vierhapper, H., Waldhausl, W., & Nowotny, P. (1983). The effect of insulin on the rise in blood pressure and plasma aldosterone after angiotensin II in normal man. *Clinical Science, 64,* 383–386.

Voors, A. W., Radhakrishnamurthy, B., Srinivasan, S. R., Webber, L. S., & Berenson, G. S. (1981). Plasma glucose level related to blood pressure in 272 children, ages 7–15 years, sampled from a total biracial population. *American Journal of Epidemiology, 113,* 347–356.

Ward, W. K., Johnston, C. L. W., Beard, J. C., Benedetti, T. J., Halter, J. B., Porte, D. (1985). Insulin resistance and impaired insulin secretion in subjects with histories of gestational diabetes mellitus. *Diabetes, 34,* 861–869.

Watanabe, R. M., Volund, A., Roy, S., & Bergman, R. N. (1989). Prehepatic beta cell secretion during the intravenous glucose tolerance test in humans: Application of a combined model of insulin and C-peptide kinetics. *Journal of Clinical Endocrinology and Metabolism, 69,* 790–797.

Welborn, T. A., Breckenridge, A., Rubinstein, A. H., Dollery, C. T., & Fraser, T. R. (1966). Serum-insulin in essential hypertension and in peripheral vascular disease. *Lancet, 1,* 1336–1337.

Weinsier, R. L., Norris, D. J., Birch, R., Bernstein, R. S., Pi-Sunyer, F. X., Yang, M. U., Wang, J., Pierson, R. N., Jr., & Vanltallie, T. B. (1986). Serum insulin and blood pressure in an obese population. *International Journal of Obesity, 10,* 11–17.

Wing, R. R., Bunker, C. H., Kuller, L. H., & Matthews, H. A. (1989). Insulin, body mass index, and cardiovascular risk factors in premenopausal women. *Arteriosclerosis, 9,* 479–484.

Yagi, S., Takata, S., Kiyokawa, H., Yamamoto, M., Noto, Y., Ikeda, T., & Hattori, N.

(1988). Effects of insulin on vasoconstrictive responses to norepinephrine and angiotensin II in rabbit femoral artery and vein. *Diabetes, 37,* 1064–1067.

Yang, Y. J., Youn, J. H., & Bergman, R. N. (1987). Modified protocols improve insulin sensitivity estimation using the minimal model. *American Journal of Physiology, 253,* E596–E602.

Young, J. B., & Landsberg, L. (1982). Diet-induced changes in sympathetic nervous system activity: Possible implications for obesity and hypertension. *Journal of Chronic Diseases, 35,* 879–886.

Zavaroni, I., Bonora, E., Pagliara, M., Dall'Aglio, E., Luchetti, L., Buonanno, G., Bonati, P. A., Bergonzani, M., Gnudi, L., Passeri, M., & Reaven, G. (1989). Risk factors for coronary artery disease in healthy persons with hyperinsulinemia and normal glucose tolerance. *New England Journal of Medicine, 320,* 702–706.

Zavaroni, I., Mazza, S., Luchetti, L., Buonanno, G., Bonati, P. A., Bergonzani, M., Passeri, M., & Reaven, G. M. (1990). High plasma insulin and triglyceride concentrations and blood pressure in offspring of people with impaired glucose tolerance. *Diabetes Medicine, 7,* 494–498.

Zimmet, P. (1989). Non-insulin-dependent (Type II) diabetes mellitus: Does it really exist? *Diabetes Medicine, 6,* 728–735.

12 Insulin Resistance as a Determinant of Cardiovascular Reactivity

Bonita Falkner
Sonia Hulman
Harvey Kushner
Hahnemann University

Essential hypertension (EH) is a health problem of major magnitude. Dysregulatory mechanisms evolving into hypertensive states have their onset in the young (Londe, Bourgoigne, Robson, & Goldring, 1971; Task Force on Blood Pressure Control in Children, 1977; Zinner, Levy, & Kass, 1971). Investigations in the young have characterized level of blood pressure, identified related parameters (Cornoni-Huntley, Harlan, & Leaverton, 1979; Harlan, Cornoni-Huntley, & Leaverton, 1979; Prineas, Gillum, Horibe, & Hannan, 1980), and provided evidence of hemodynamic changes in the young at risk for EH (Falkner, Lowenthal, Affreme, & Hamstra, 1982; Schieken, Clark, & Lauer, 1981; Zahka, Neill, Kidd, Cutilleta, & Cutilleta, 1983).

One line of investigation has concerned the sympathetic nervous system (Folkow, 1982). There is a correlation of stress-induced enhanced sympathetic nervous system activity in EH (Baumann et al., 1973; Nestle, 1969) and in the young with a family history of EH (Falkner, Onesti, Angelakos, Fernandez, & Langman, 1979; Manuck, & Proietti, 1982). Based on the experimental design of these studies, it has been assumed that the neurogenic hyperresponsivity has been related to greater beta-adrenergic activity. However, many of the clinical studies on neurogenic-cardiovascular interaction have used racially mixed populations. Fredrickson (1986) compared racial differences in cardiovascular reactivity to mental stress in EH. He observed that although the Black sample was small, compared to Whites, Blacks had lesser cardiac sympathomimetic responses but had greater vascular responses to mental stress. Light and Obrist (1980) have investigated the racial differences in the cardiovascular response to active coping stressors in college-age males. Young Blacks were compared to Whites in both normotensive and marginally hypertensive groups. Hypertensives demonstrated a greater response than normotensives. The blood pressure response was greatest in the Black hypertensives but without an attendant increase in heart rate (Light & Obrist 1980). The investigators proposed that this response reflects a greater peripheral resistance in the marginally hypertensive young Blacks. This observation varies from the more classic description of borderline hypertension. Based on extensive hemodynamic studies, Julius (1977) characterized borderline hypertension as a condition of high blood pressure, high cardiac output, and normal peripheral resistance. The theoretic basis for this model of borderline hypertension is that neurogenic stimulation provokes an enhanced beta-adrenergic response that in turn effects an increased cardiac output (Folkow, 1982). However, Light and colleagues have provided preliminary evidence that in young adult Blacks, stress-mediated neurogenic stimulation may have a greater effect on peripheral vascular resistance.

CARDIOVASCULAR REACTIVITY TO CENTRAL STRESS

We have conducted a series of investigations in the young on dysregulatory blood pressure mechanisms that contribute to the development of EH. The initial line of investigation concerned the family history of EH, the sympathetic nervous system, and the relationship of cardiovascular response to adrenergic stimulation. We demonstrated that adolescent offspring of parents with EH exhibited a significantly greater heart rate and blood pressure response to the central stress of difficult mental arithmetic than did offspring of normotensive parents (Falkner, 1979). The relationship of family history of EH to stress-induced cardiovascular reactivity has been confirmed by other investigators (Light & Obrist, 1980; Manuck & Proietti, 1982). With the known association of environmental stress with EH, the correlation of mental stress-induced cardiovascular reactivity in adolescents with parental EH may provide a model of gene-environmental interaction. In a 5-year longitudinal study on the predictability of stress-induced reactivity, we characterized adolescents who progressed from borderline or variable blood pressure to persistent hypertension. The characteristics of high EH risk in adolescents included: parental EH, high resting heart rate, high stress-induced cardiovascular reactivity, and in females, excessive body weight (Falkner, Kushner, Onesti, & Angelakos, 1981). These characteristics were consistent with a neurogenic pattern in the early phase of EH.

The data on cardiovascular reactivity was analyzed further with Fourier analysis and mathematical modeling (Kushner & Falkner, 1981). Figures

12.1 and 12.2 depict the systolic and diastolic blood pressure response during stress, as percent change from baseline, for normotensive and early hypertensive adolescents. In the initial minutes of mental stress, the systolic and diastolic blood pressure response is quite similar for the two groups. With continued stress, the normotensives appear to recover or counterregulate the blood pressure toward baseline. However, the hypertensives display persistence of the blood pressure elevation with limited ability to counterregulate the pressure toward baseline. The statistically significant difference in the stress reactivity between the two groups is most marked in the later phase of the stress protocol. These data suggested that processes other than the initial neurogenic-mediated response alone may be operative in the response differences of the hypertensive versus normotensive.

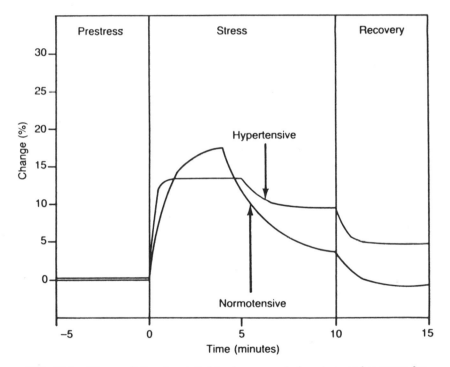

FIG. 12.1. The reactivity of systolic blood pressure during stress and recovery for hypertensives and normotensives expressed as percent change from baseline or prestress period. Note that the early response of the normotensive group peaks higher than the early response of the hypertensive group (although the hypertensives' rate of increase is greater). A "control factor" changes the direction of the response. This factor occurs earlier in the normotensives and is more effective in allowing recovery of normal systolic blood pressure after the cessation of stress. The hypertensive group remained elevated after the 5-minute recovery period. The control factor is blunted in the hypertensives.

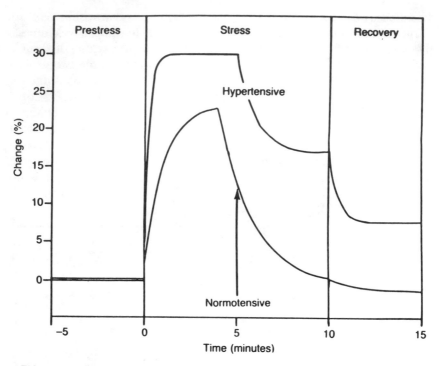

FIG. 12.2. The reactivity of diastolic pressure during stress and recovery for normotensives and hypertensives expressed as percentage of change from baseline or prestress period. When diastolic blood pressure is plotted against time, the hypertensive group showed a greater and more rapid rise than the normotensives. A "control factor" reduces the stress response by about the 5-minute point. The normotensive group was able to approach baseline blood pressure before the end of stress, whereas the hypertensive group did not. The diastolic pressure of the hypertensive group remained elevated after the 5-minute recovery period.

BLOOD PRESSURE SENSITIVITY TO SODIUM

We hypothesized that the differences in neurogenic-mediated cardiovascular response patterns may be related to altered vascular tone relative to sodium and volume balance. A study on young adults 18 to 23 years of age was conducted to investigate the interaction of sodium sensitivity with stress-induced cardiovascular reactivity. Young adult Blacks were compared to Whites in their blood pressure response to chronic oral sodium loading. The cardiovascular reactivity to stress was studied before and after sodium loading. In this study, we again replicated our earlier finding that the stress-induced reactivity was greater in offspring of hypertensives than offspring of normotensive. However, we also found that Whites exhibited great central stress reactivity than Blacks (Falkner & Kushner, 1989).

Prevalence of sodium sensitivity was greater in young Blacks than in young Whites. In sodium sensitive subjects, the sodium load raised baseline blood pressure and sodium excretion was blunted compared to sodium insensitive subjects (both normotensive and borderline hypertensive). However, the stress-induced cardiovascular reactivity was not altered by the sodium load (Falkner & Kushner, 1990). Subsequently, we used the same design to study the effect of potassium loading on central stress-induced reactivity in Blacks. Following chronic potassium load, potassium-sensitive subjects had a reduction in baseline blood pressure. However, the mental stress-induced cardiovascular reactivity was not altered by the potassium load. Data from these investigations indicate that shifts in sodium/potassium balance do not interact with the beta-adrenergic mediated cardiovascular reactivity. In Blacks, the baseline blood pressure change induced by the shifts in sodium/potassium balance appear to be related to functional changes in peripheral vascular resistance. Light et al. (1987), and Dimsdale, Grahm, Ziegler, Zusman, and Berry (1987) reported data that are consistent with this concept. Several studies have now reported greater beta-mediated cardiac responsivity in Whites and greater alpha-mediated adrenergic activity in Blacks (Anderson, Lane, Muranka, Williams, & Houseworth, 1988; Fredrickson, 1986). These reports are also consistent with our findings on racial differences in reactivity (Falkner & Kushner, 1989).

With our extensive studies on cardiovascular reactivity, we have demonstrated that the cardiovascular reactivity response to a central neurogenic-stimulus is reproducible within individuals over time and is consistently greater in borderline hypertensives and in offspring of hypertensive parents. Therefore, centrally induced reactivity appears to be useful as a predictor of hypertension. However, this model alone is limited within clinical investigations to explain the mechanism of developing EH.

INSULIN RESISTANCE

Data were indicating that functional and possibly structural changes were occurring in the peripheral vasculature that were mediating the hypertensive process. Because of its trophic effect on vascular smooth muscle, insulin may contribute to the pathogenesis of EH (Kaiser, Tur-Sinai, Hasin, & Cerasi, 1985; King, Goodman, Buzney, Moses, & Kuhn, 1985). Variation in insulin action, or insulin resistance, was also a hypothetical mechanism that could account for the variations in adrenergic activity, sodium sensitivity, and cation transport, which we have described in a young population. It was hypothesized that the anabolic effects of insulin could affect growth; both somatic growth and growth of the peripheral vasculature.

We performed a pilot study on a subgroup of young adult Black males who had been subjects in our previous investigations. The purpose of this study was to determine if insulin resistance could be detected at an early phase of EH. The confounding effects of obesity and carbohydrate intolerance were excluded by enrolling lean males (body mass index [BMI] < 27 kg/m^2) who had a normal oral glucose tolerance test. Subjects were classified as normotensive (systolic < 135, diastolic < 85 mmHg) or marginal hypertensive (systolic ≥ 135 and/or diastolic ≥ 85 mmHg). Hypertensives (diastolic > 95 mmHg) were excluded. Insulin-stimulated glucose uptake was studied using the euglycemic hyperinsulinemic clamp technique ("clamp"). The two groups were matched for age, BMI, and triceps skinfold thickness. Blood pressures were significantly greater in the marginal hypertensives. The clamp method establishes hyperinsulinemia with a steady-state insulin infusion. The primed insulin infusion was calculated to raise the fasting insulin to 100 uU/ml above fasting. Euglycemia was maintained during hyperinsulinemia by a simultaneous glucose infusion. The rate of glucose infusion (GIR) then becomes an index of sensitivity (or resistance) to the action of insulin.

In this pilot study, we found that fasting glucose was the same in both groups. The clamped glucose was also the same in both groups and indicated the euglycemia was maintained in both groups. Fasting insulin, although within normal clinical range, was significantly greater in the hypertensives ($p < .05$), despite the small sample size. Insulin-directed exogenous glucose metabolism as determined by the GIR during steady-state hyperinsulinemia was significantly lower in the marginal hypertensives ($p < .02$) indicating that they were insulin resistant compared to normotensive controls. We analyzed the relationship of blood pressure with GIR for the entire population and found a significant negative correlation between GIR and systolic blood pressure ($p < .01$). Additionally, previous data from each subject on their cardiovascular response to stress was related to the index of insulin-stimulated glucose metabolism. Despite a small sample size, significant correlations again emerged. There was a significant negative correlation of GIR with stress systolic pressure ($r = -.685$, $p < 0.01$) and stress diastolic pressure ($r = -.613$, $p < 0.01$). Therefore, these data suggest a functional relationship of adrenergic activity and insulin resistance.

DISCUSSION

Epidemiologic and clinical studies have recently addressed the overlap of EH with non-insulin dependent diabetes mellitus (NIDDM) and obesity. NIDDM and obesity are characterized by hyperinsulinemia, which in itself is regarded as a cardiovascular disease risk factor. Data are also emerging that indicate that hyperinsulinemia or insulin resistance correlates with EH, independent of NIDDM or obesity. Fuh, Shieh, Wu, Chen, and Reaven

(1987) demonstrated an augmented insulin response to oral glucose, as well as fasting hyperlipidemia, in hypertensives. Shen et al. (1988) studied lean Chinese males with the insulin suppression test, and found blunted glucose disposal in hypertensives. In a rigorous experimental study, Ferrannini et al. (1987) utilized a euglycemic hyperinsulinemic clamp technique to study insulin resistance in lean, hypertensive adults with normal glucose tolerance. Compared to age- and weight-matched normotensive controls, the hypertensives exhibited marked impairment of glucose uptake in response to the insulin infusion. Their data provide substantial evidence that EH is associated with insulin resistance independent of obesity or carbohydrate intolerance in middle-aged adults. Zavaroni et al. (1989) demonstrated, in a population of 247 lean subjects with normal glucose tolerance, that fasting insulin concentration greater than 2 *SD* above the mean predicted hypertriglyceridemia as well as elevated blood pressure. They also found that augmented insulin response during oral glucose tolerance testing in this group was correlated with elevated blood pressure. They concluded that hyperinsulinemia in the absence of impaired glucose tolerance predicts elevated blood pressure. The sum of evidence from these studies is that insulin resistance is a determinant of blood pressure in adults and may also be engaged in the pathogenesis of EH.

An alteration in sympathetic nervous system activity may also be involved in insulin resistance. Chronic insulin release has been shown to be stimulated by beta-mediated sympathetic activity (which is regarded to be higher in EH). It had been suggested that the peripheral uptake of glucose would decrease with increasing beta-receptor mediated sympathetic activity, resulting in decreased insulin sensitivity (Berglund et al., 1976). However, more recently Rowe et al. (1981) utilized the hyperinsulinemic euglycemic clamp technique to demonstrate a significant increase in plasma norepinephrine levels in response to euglycemic hyperinsulinemia. Cardiovascular measurements demonstrated a concurrent increase in blood pressure. This study indicates that elevated levels of plasma insulin may increase sympathetic nervous system activity in the absence of changes in blood glucose.

Fasting suppresses sympathetic nervous system activity and refeeding stimulates sympathetic nervous system activity (O'Hare, 1988). The interrelationship of carbohydrate intake, insulin resistance, and sympathetic nervous system activity remains to be clarified. However, there is presently evidence that supports a role of this adrenergic-metabolic interaction at an early phase in the pathogenesis of hypertension and cardiovascular disease.

REFERENCES

Anderson, N. B., Lane, J. D., Muranka, M., Williams, R. B., & Houseworth, S. J. (1988). Racial differences in blood pressure and forearm vascular responses to the cold face stimulus. *Psychosomatic Medicine, 50,* 57–63.

Baumann, R., Ziprian, H., Godicke, W., Hartrodt, W., Naumann, E., & Lauter, J. (1973). The influence of acute psychi stress situations and vegetative parameters of essential hypertensives at the early stage of the disease. *Psychotheraphy and Psychosomatics, 22,* 131.

Berglund, G., Larsson, B., Anderson, O. W. E., Larsson, O., Svardsudd, K., Bjorntorp, P., & Wilhelmsen, L. (1976). Body composition and glucose metabolism in hypertensive middle-aged males. *Acta Medica Scandinavica, 200,* 163–169.

Cornoni-Huntley, J., Harlan, W. R., & Leaverton, P. E. (1979). Blood pressure in adolescence. United States Health Examination Survey. *Hypertension, 1,* 566.

Dimsdale, J. E., Grahm, R., Ziegler, M. G., Zusman, R., Berry, C. C. (1987). Age, race, diagnosis, and sodium effects on the pressor response to infused norepinephrine. *Hypertension, 10,* 564–569.

Falkner, B., & Kushner, H. (1989). Racial differences in stress induced reactivity in young adults. *Health Psychology, 8,* 613–617.

Falkner, B., & Kushner, H. (1990). The effect of chronic oral sodium loading on the cardiovascular response to stress in young blacks and whites. *Hypertension, 15,* 36–43.

Falkner, B., Kushner, H., Onesti, G., & Angelakos, E. T. (1981). Cardiovascular characteristics in adolescents who develop essential hypertension. *Hypertension, 3,* 251.

Falkner, B., Lowenthal, D. T., Affrime, M. B., & Hamstra, B. (1982). R wave amplitude change in hypertensive children. *American Journal of Cardiology, 50,* 152–156.

Falkner, B., Onesti, G., Angelakos, E. T., Fernandez, M., & Langman, C. (1979). Cardiovascular response to mental stress in normal adolescents with hypertensive parents. *Hypertension, 1,* 23.

Folkow, B. (1982). Physiological aspects of primary hypertension. *Physiological Reviews, 62,* 347–504.

Fredrickson, M. (1986). Racial differences in cardiovascular reactivity to mental stress in essential hypertension. *Journal of Hypertension, 4,* 325–331.

Ferrannini, E., Buzzigoli, G., Bonadonna, R., Giorico, M. A., Oleggini, M., Gradizdei, L., Pedrinelli, R., Brandi, L., & Bevilacgua, S. (1987). Insulin resistance in essential hypertension. *New England Journal of Medicine, 317,* 350–357.

Fuh, M., Shieh, S. M., Wu, D. A., Chen, Y. D., & Reaven, G. M. (1987). Abnormalities of carbohydrate and lipid metabolism in patients with hypertension. *Archives of Internal Medicine, 147,* 1035–1038.

Harlan, W. R., Cornoni-Huntley, J., & Leaverton, P. E. (1979). Blood pressure in childhood. National Health Examination Survey. *Hypertension, 1,* 566.

Julius, S. (1977). Borderline hypertension: An overview. *Medical Clinics of North America, 61,* 595.

Light, K. C., Obrist, P. A., Shervood, A., James, S. A., & Strogats, P. S. (1987). Effects of race and marginally elevated blood pressure on responses to stress. *Hypertension, 10,* 555–563.

Kaiser, N., Tur-Sinai, A., Hasin, M., & Cerasi, E. (1985). Binding, degradation and biological activity of insulin in vascular smooth muscle cells. *American Journal of Physiology, 429,* E292–E298.

King, G. L., Goodman, D., Buzney, S., Moses, A., & Kahn, C. R. (1985). Receptors and growth-promoting effects of insulin and insulin-like growth factors on cells from bovine retinal capillaries and aorta. *Journal of Clinical Investigation, 75,* 1028–1036.

Kushner, H., & Falkner, B. (1981). A harmonic analysis of cardiac response of normotensive and hypertensive adolescents during stress. *Journal of Human Stress, 7,* 21–27.

Light, K. C., & Obrist, P. A. (1980). Cardiovascular reactivity to behavioral stress in young males with and without marginally elevated casual systolic pressures: Comparison of clinic, home, and laboratory measures. *Hypertension, 2,* 802.

Londe, S., Bourgoignie, J. J., Robson, A. M., & Goldring, D. (1971). Hypertension in apparently normal children. *Journal of Pediatrics, 78,* 569.

Manuck, S. B., & Proietti, J. M. (1982). Parental hypertension and cardiovascular response to cognitive and isometric challenge. *Psychophysiology, 19,* 481–489.

Nestle, R. J. (1969). Blood pressure and catecholamine excretion after mental stress in labile hypertension. *Hypertension, 1,* 692.

O'Hare, J. A. (1988). The enigma of insulin resistance and hypertension. *American Journal of Medicine, 84,* 505–510.

Prineas, R. J., Gillum, P. F., Horibe, H., & Hannan, P. J. (1980). Minneapolis Children's blood pressure study. Part 2: Multiple determinants of blood pressure. *Hypertension, 2*(Suppl), I-24.

Report of the Task Force on Blood Pressure Control in Children. (1977). *Pediatrics, 58*(Suppl) 797.

Rowe, J. W., Young, J. B., Minaker, K. L., Stevens, A. L., Pallotta, J., & Landsberg, L. (1981). Effect of glucose and insulin infusions on sympathetic nervous system activity in normal men. *Diabetes, 30,* 219–225.

Schieken, P. M., Clark, W. R., & Lauer, P. M. (1981). Left ventricular hypertrophy in children in the upper guintile of blood pressure distribution. The Muscatine Study. *Hypertension, 3,* 699.

Shen, D. C., Shieh, S. M., Fuh, M. M., Wu, D. A., Chen, Y. D., & Reaven, G. M. (1988). Resistance to insulin-stimulated glucose uptake in patient with hypertension. *Journal of Clinical Endocrinology and Metabolism, 66,* 580–583.

Zahka, K. G., Neill, C. A., Kidd, L., Cutilleta, M. A., & Cutilleta, A. F. (1983). Cardiac involvement in adolescent hypertension. *Hypertension, 3,* 664–668.

Zavaroni, I., Bonora, E., Pagliara, M., Dall'Aglio, E., Luchetti, L., Buonanno, G., Bonati, P. A., Bergonzani, M., Gnudi, L., & Passeri, M. (1989). Risk factors for coronary artery disease in healthy persons with hyperinsulinemia and normal glucose tolerance. *New England Journal of Medicine,* 702–706.

Zinner, S. A., Levy, P. S., & Kass, E. H. (1971). Family aggregation of blood pressure in childhood. *New England Journal of Medicine, 283,* 461.

13 Glycemic Responsivity To Adrenergic Stimulation and Genetic Predisposition to Type II Diabetes

Richard S. Surwit
Duke University Medical Center

Since the 1980s, great strides have been made in the understanding of pathophysiology at the molecular level. Reverse genetic methods have been used to identify the mechanisms by which genetic defects cause a cascade of biochemical events leading to the development of disease. The promise of the molecular genetics has overshadowed much of the importance of conventional physiology and has shifted the focus of many scientists from the whole organism to microparticles. However, it is important to realize that ultimate potential of the molecular approach depends on a thorough understanding of how the organism functions in its environment. The reverse genetic methodology of molecular biology utilizes conventional genetics to map, localize, and clone genes related to disease. This approach is limited by our ability to identify individuals who show the phenotype of a particular disease. Diseases with "variable penetrance" are difficult to study genetically because the phenotype may not always be present in individuals who carry the genotype. One important lesson to come from behavioral medicine research is that many disease phenotypes result from the interaction of environmental stress and genetic predisposition. Acting through neuroendocrine pathways, stress disturbs the function of vulnerable end organ systems in predisposed individuals. This disturbance, if chronic, can lead to a permanent breakdown in function.

Behavioral research may, therefore, be useful in identifying individuals who carry the genotype for susceptibility to the deleterious effects of stress. For instance, recent studies on cardiovascular reactivity have suggested that individuals with family histories of cardiovascular disease will show greater reactivity of cardiovascular responses during acute laboratory stressors (see

Matthews et al., 1986, for review). In theory, these laboratory tests may be useful as markers to identify individuals who are at risk for cardiovascular disease. Once individuals carrying genetic predisposition to disease are properly identified, underlying neurobiologic defects, which make them reactive to the effects of stress, can be studied, even if the disease itself has not developed. In addition to helping to identify individuals who show the disease phenotype, these neurobiologic defects may, in turn, suggest novel candidate genes not directly related to diseased organ systems. For instance, if predisposition to the development of hypertension is related to a neurochemical defect, then genes regulating neurochemical expression may be appropriate candidate genes for genetic analysis. In this fashion, behavioral medicine promises to offer the molecular biologist new insights into pathophysiology that may help in the search for the genes that predispose individuals to disease.

TYPE II DIABETES: BEHAVIORAL AND GENETIC ANALYSIS

An example of how behavioral research can lead to new genetic hypotheses can be seen in our recent work on Type II diabetes. Type II diabetes is thought to be a highly heritable condition. Some investigators have shown concordance for the disease in 95% of identical twins (Barnett, Eff, Leslie, & Pyke, 1979) and abnormal glucose tolerance in as many as 30% of relatives of patients with Type II diabetes (Kobberling, 1971). Nevertheless, little is known about the specific inherited defects that predispose individuals to the disease. In certain populations, a form of Type II diabetes appears to be inherited in a complex fashion, with insulin resistance and impaired pancreatic activity segregating separately (Lillioja et al., 1988; O'Rahilly, Turner, & Matthews, 1988). Defects in both the insulin gene and insulin receptor gene have been postulated factors in the etiology of this disease (Lillioja et al., 1988; O'Rahilly, Turner, & Matthews, 1988; O'Rahilly, Wainscoat, & Turner, 1988). However, there has been no clear relationship between restriction–fragment–length polymorphism at these loci and the presence of Type II diabetes (O'Rahilly, Wainscoat, & Turner, 1988).

Part of the difficulty in studying the genetics of Type II diabetes stems from the fact that the expression of the phenotype often depends on numerous environmental factors. It is widely believed that proper diet and exercise habits can prevent the expression of diabetes in individuals with the genetic predisposition to develop the disease (O'Rahilly, Wainscoat, & Turner, 1988). For example, although diabetes was almost completely unknown in Pima Indian Native Americans two generations ago, it now affects almost 60% of the adult population. Therefore, the disease can have variable penetrance and not be present at all unless favorable environmental conditions bring it on.

An additional problem is the late onset of Type II diabetes. Type II diabetes often does not occur until the fifth or sixth decade at which time the parents of the proband are usually no longer living. Finally, Type II diabetes is probably a heterogeneous condition, with different genetic factors involved in the various forms of the disease. One phenotype does not exist in all diabetic patients. Banerji and Lebovitz (1989) have described two forms of Type II diabetes, one in which insulin sensitivity is normal and a significant pancreatic defect exists, and another in which there is a mild impairment of glucose-stimulated insulin secretion accompanied by significant insulin resistance. Still another form of Type II diabetes, Maturity Onset Diabetes of Youth (MODY), is different from other forms in that it is apparently transmitted in an autosomal dominant fashion (Fajans, 1982). For these reasons, analysis of the human disease has been considered a particularly difficult genetic problem (O'Rahilly et al., 1988).

Animal models of Type II diabetes offer simpler systems that are often more amenable to genetic analysis. Inbred mouse strains have been of particular interest in that several forms of Type II diabetes can be found in mice (Coleman, 1978). Furthermore, mice breed rapidly and inbred strains provide large numbers of genetically identical individuals that are homozygous at each genetic locus. Finally, the mouse genome has been extensively mapped and much of it has been shown to be conserved in humans (Hedrich, 1981; Searle et al., 1987).

ANIMAL MODELS OF TYPE II DIABETES

Syndromes resembling Type II diabetes have been identified in several animal species, but many of these models have other problems that make them less than an ideal model of this disease. For instance, the obese mouse (C57BL/6J *ob/ob*) develops insulin resistance and hyperglycemia in conjunction with massive obesity and has multiple associated endocrine abnormalities. In contrast, two species of desert rodents display diabetes after diet-induced obesity (Dunlin, Gerristen, & Chang, 1983). However, because these animals are not inbred strains, they are not well suited to genetic analysis.

In an early series of experiments (Kuhn, Cochrane, Feinglos, & Surwit, 1987; Surwit, Feinglos, Livingston, Kuhn, & McCubbin, 1984), we investigated the role of stress and adrenergic responsivity in the hyperglycemia of the obese mouse. We found that this animal was only mildly hyperglycemic when left undisturbed, but would show a substantial hyperglycemic response to stress (Fig. 13.1) or adrenergic stimulation (Fig. 13.2) when compared to the lean C57BL/6J (BL/6) mouse. In another study, we demonstrated that even the lean BL/6 mouse showed exaggerated glycemic reactivity to adrenergic stimulation when compared to other strains (Surwit, Feinglos, Cochrane, & Kuhn, 1986). Furthermore, like the obese mouse, the BL/6 mouse shows an abnormal metabolic response to opiodergic stimulation, also implying differences in autonomic control of glucose metabolism in this strain (Surwit, McCubbin, Kuhn, Cochrane, & Feinglos, 1989).

These findings suggest the presence of abnormalities in autonomic control of glucose metabolism in the BL/6 strain. If these abnormalities are related to the pathophysiology of Type II diabetes, the BL/6 background strain should carry the genotype for diabetes. This hypothesis is supported by the fact that the BL/6 mouse is the background strain for the obese mouse as well as other diabetic mutations (Coleman, 1978). To test this hypothesis, we studied the effects of diet-induced obesity on glucose metabolism in BL/6 and A/J mice (Surwit, Kuhn, Cochrane, McCubbin, &

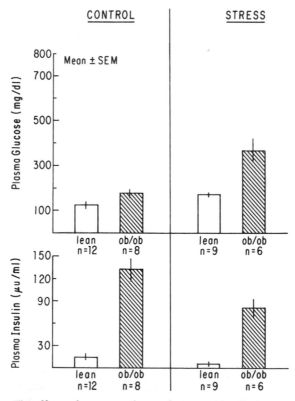

FIG. 13.1.   The effects of stress on plasma glucose and insulin in C57BL/6J *ob/ob* mice and their lean littermates (mean ± SEM).

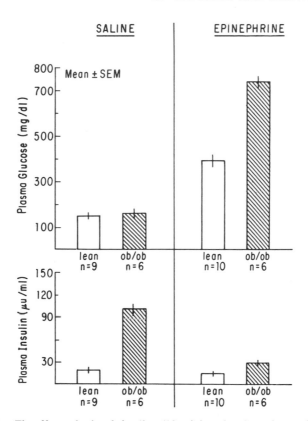

FIG. 13.2.   The effects of epinephrine (3 ug/10 g, injected s.c.) on plasma glucose and inslin in C57BL/6J *ob/ob* mice and their lean litermates (mean ± SEM).

Feinglos, 1988). Diet-induced obesity is associated with the onset of Type II diabetes in humans. We showed that the BL/6 inbred mouse will develop an analogue of Type II diabetes if weaned onto a high fat, high carbohydrate diet and allowed to become obese. Although animals raised on ordinary laboratory chow remain lean and euglycemic, animals on the experimental diet developed obesity, hyperinsulinemia, and hyperglycemia, with fasting blood glucose levels above 230 mg/d. When obese, fasting blood glucose levels of BL/6 and A/J animals are at least 3 *SD* apart. Furthermore, the elevation in fasting blood glucose produced by obesity in the BL/6 animals is at least 2 *SD* from that in lean animals (Fig. 13.3).

This finding is consistent with a report (Kaku, Fiedorek, Province, & Permutt, 1988) in which investigators compared glucose tolerance in a number of lean inbred mouse strains. They concluded that, of those studied, the BL/6 mouse was the most glucose intolerant of all of the strains studied and appears to show a defect in first-phase insulin release that has been linked to the development of Type II diabetes. Furthermore, they

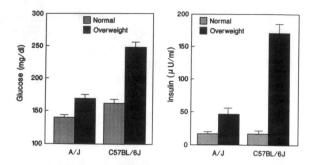

FIG. 13.3.   The effect of diet-induced obesity on fasting serum glucosed and inslin in fasting normal (hatched bars) and overweight (solid bars) C57BL/6J and A/J mice. All values are mean ± SEM.

showed that when the BL/6 mouse is crossed with the C3H/HeJ mouse and the F_1 hybrid is backcrossed to the BL/6 parent strain, the distribution of glucose tolerance in the backcrosses is consistent with a polygenic mode of inheritance.

GENETICS OF DIABETES IN THE BL/6 MOUSE

In a recent series of studies (Surwit, Seldin, Kuhn, Cochrane, & Feinglos, 1991), we continued to explore the genetics of Type II diabetes in the BL/6 mouse. We studied the effects of diet-induced obesity on glucose metabolism in BL/6 mice, A/J mice, F_1 crosses (BXA) and backcrosses on the BL/6 parent strain [(BL/6 × A/J female)F_1 X BL/6] as well as backcrosses on the A/J strain [(BL/6 × A/J female)F_1 X A/J] (see Fig. 13.4). The

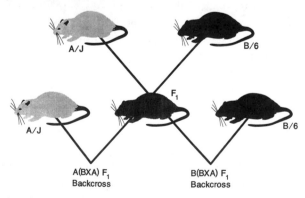

FIG. 13.4.   Method of producing F_1 and backcross strains from C57BL/6J and A/J parentals.

values for glucose, insulin, weight, and insulin sensitivity are depicted in Fig. 13.4. BL/6 mice fed the control diet had slightly higher glucose values than the A/J or F_1 mice given this diet, but insulin levels, insulin sensitivity, and body weight were the same as that of A/J and F_1 animals. The experimental diet raised glucose, insulin levels, and body weight of all animals, but this effect was much more pronounced for the diabetes prone BL/6 mice.

The F_1 mice on the diabetogenic diet showed glucose and insulin levels as well as body weights that were intermediate between the parental strains; these values were significantly lower than BL/6 mice, but not significantly different from those of A/J mice (Fig. 13.5), suggesting a recessive mode of inheritance. The diabetogenic diet greatly reduced the insulin sensitivity of BL/6 mice, but did not affect insulin sensitivity of A/J mice. In contrast, the insulin sensitivity values for F_1 animals on the experimental diet were less than those of A/J mice, but not significantly greater than those of BL/6 mice suggesting a dominant mode of inheritance.

Data from backcross animals suggested that hyperglycemia and insulin resistance were controlled by different genetic factors. There was no correlation between glucose and insulin sensitivity in either backcross. Furthermore, there was no correlation between insulin and body weight in the [(BL/6 × A/J) F_1 × BL/6] backcross mice despite a strong correlation in the diabetic BL/6 mice and a lower but significant correlation in [(BL/6 × A/J) F_1 × A/J] backcross mice. This finding implies that, although environmental factors that control weight and/or insulin result in parallel changes in the genetically identical diabetic BL/6 mice, the genetic factors influencing these abnormalities may be largely independent.

In order to further investigate the inheritance of genes predisposing to the diabetic phenotype, nine BXA recombinant inbred (RI) strains were examined. RI strains are derived from crosses between two inbred progenitor strains in which the mice from the F_2 generation and each subsequent generation are mated in accordance with a strict inbreeding program. After 20 generations, each of the resultant RI strains has a unique contribution from each original progenitor where the alleles from either progenitor strain have become fixed at each locus. Thus, observations may be made on different individuals each of which has an identical genotype. Mice from each of these strains are homozygous at each locus but each strain contains a unique contribution of the two progenitor strains. As shown in Fig. 13.6, there is no relationship between serum glucose values and insulin sensitivities. These data support the conclusion that insulin resistance and hyperglycemia are determined by different genetic factors in this murine model.

Is there a relationship between altered adrenergic sensitivity seen in lean BL/6 mice and their predisposition to develop Type II diabetes? Preliminary data suggests that like hyperglycemia, glycemic hyperresponsivity to

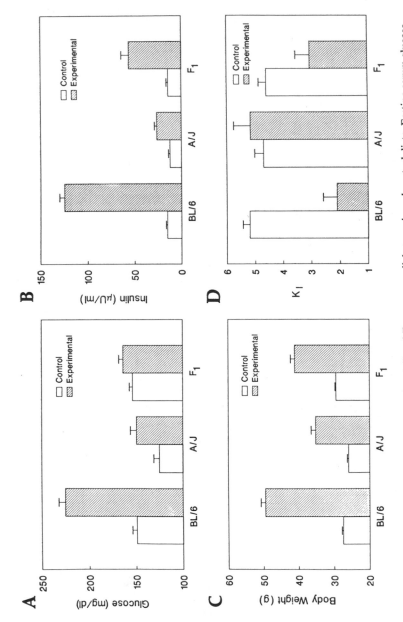

FIG. 13.5. Metabolic parameters of C57BL/6J, A/J and F₁ crosses on diabetogenic and control diets. Fasting serum glucose, insulin, and body weight after 5 months and insulin sensitivity (K₁) after 4.5 months on control (open bars) or diabetogenic diet (hatched bars). All values are mean ± SEM.

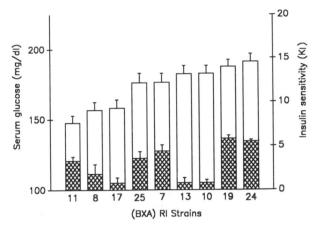

FIG. 13.6. Serum glucose and insulin sensitivity (K_I) of recombinant inbred (RI) strains on the diabetogenic diet (Mean ± SEM).

adrenergic stimulation is a recessive trait. When (AXB) F_1 mice are given epinephrine, their glycemic response is similar to that of A/J mice and not to BL/6 (Fig. 13.7). Thus, glycemic response to adrenergic stimulation, even in the lean state, like the tendency to develop Type II diabetes on the high fat, high-simple carbohydrate diet, is inherited in a recessive fashion. Whether these phenomena are controlled by the same genetic factors, remains to be determined.

IMPLICATIONS FOR THE UNDERSTANDING OF HUMAN DIABETES

These data allow us to draw several conclusions about the inheritance of Type II diabetes in the BL/6 mouse. Of primary importance is that insulin

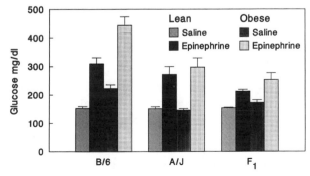

FIG. 13.7. Serum glucose values in response to saline or epinephrine (3 ug/10 g, injected s.c.) for C57BL/6J, A/J or F_1 mice. All values are mean ± SEM.

resistance and hyperglycemia are controlled by different genetic factors. Three lines of evidence allow us to reach this conclusion. First, in both backcross groups, fasting glucose and insulin sensitivity do not correlate together, indicating that insulin resistance and hyperglycemia segregate independently. Furthermore, insulin sensitivity did not correlate with fasting insulin levels in the [(BL/6 × A/J) F × BL/6] group of backcross animals, suggesting that separate genetic factors determine insulin resistance and pancreatic secretory ability in the mouse strains studied. Second, the differential dominance of blood glucose levels and insulin sensitivity in the F_1 crosses show that although insulin resistance is inherited in a dominant fashion, hyperglycemia appears to be a recessive trait. Third, and most conclusively, hyperglycemia and insulin sensitivity segregated independently in RI strains. Thus, two distinct genetic factors appear necessary for the appearance of Type II diabetes characteristic of the BL/6 mouse.

Although one cannot immediately generalize these findings to the phenomenon of human diabetes, they may be of great relevance to our understanding of human Type II diabetes. The question of whether impaired pancreatic secretory ability or insulin resistance is the primary defect in Type II diabetes has been debated for many years. One school of thought holds that diabetes develops when severe insulin resistance finally exhausts pancreatic secretory ability (Gerich, 1988). Another point of view is that a defect in pancreatic secretory ability is primary and that insulin resistance is a secondary phenomenon (Kahn & Porte, 1988). Our data support several recent studies that have suggested that insulin sensitivity and impaired pancreatic activity may be separate phenomena that do not have to occur together (Banerji & Lebovitz, 1989; Erikkson et al., 1989; Reaven, 1988) in human Type II diabetes. Lillioja et al. (1988) found that impaired glucose tolerance in Pima Indians was due to insulin resistance, whereas the development of frank hyperglycemia was associated with a defect in pancreatic function. More recently, studying a Scandinavian population, Eriksson et al. (1989) showed that even insulin sensitivity alone could not explain impaired glucose tolerance; that a defect in first-phase insulin release had to be present as well. Finally, as noted earlier, Banerji and Lebovitz (1989) have described two forms of Type II diabetes, one in which insulin sensitivity is normal and a significant pancreatic defect exists and another in which there is a mild impairment of glucose-stimulated insulin secretion accompanied by significant insulin resistance. Reaven (1988) has suggested that insulin resistance is a very common problem, and therefore cannot be, by itself, the cause of Type II diabetes. Our data support the conclusion that impaired insulin sensitivity does not cause hyperglycemia in the BL/6 mouse and that the development of diabetes in this animal model is primarily dependent on some other genetic factor.

Several other conclusions can be reached from our data. Hyperinsulinemia in BL/6 mice is not simply a function of body weight. Although body weight correlated significantly with insulin levels in the diabetic BL/6 mice, there was no correlation in the nondiabetic A/J mice. Because the variance of weights was similar in the two strains, the results suggest that the effect of weight on fasting insulin levels is dependent on genetic background. That insulin is correlated more strongly with body weight in BL/6 and F_1 suggests that this is a property of insulin-resistant animals. Thus, insulin resistance may be inherited independent of obesity.

Studies in several human populations have suggested similar conclusions. Lillioja et al. (1987) reported that the familial component of insulin action and hyperinsulinemia occurs in addition to the effects of obesity in Pima Native Americans, and Haffner, Stern, Hazuda, Mitchell, and Patterson (1988) found a similar independence of genetic and environmental effects in Mexican Americans. Furthermore, in the Pima population, insulin resistance appears to be trimodally distributed among nondiabetic individuals, suggesting that this trait is determined by one codominant gene (Bogardus et al., 1989). An additional recessive gene(s) is thought to be responsible for the development of overt diabetes. Therefore, similar modes of inheritance may be operative in the genetics of diabetes in BL/6 mice and in some human populations.

Exaggerated glycemic reactivity to behavioral stress also appears to be characteristic of at least some people who are predisposed to developing Type II diabetes. Pima Indian Native Americans are at high risk for developing Type II diabetes. Approximately 60% of Pima Indian Native Americans eventually develop Type II diabetes in adulthood, compared to 5% of the Caucasian population. In a recent study (Surwit, McCubbin, Feinglos, Esposito-Del Puente, & Lillioja, 1990), we observed that young, euglycemic Pima Indians show a disturbed glycemic response to behavioral stress compared to Caucasians. We gave a group of Pima Indians and Caucasians a mixed meal that was followed 2 hours later by a 10-minute mental arithmetic stressor. Although all subjects showed normal glucose tolerance in response to the meal, 10 of 13 Pima Indians show a hyperglycemic response to a mental arithmetic stressor, whereas 7 of 8 Caucasian controls did not. In that both groups showed similar cardiovascular and neuroendocrine responses to the stress, it appears as though the diabetes-prone Pimas have a specific glucoregulatory defect that becomes apparent during such stimulation. As a marker for the development of Type II diabetes, the direction of glycemic response to this stressor has a sensitivity of 76% and a specificity of 87%. In that only approximately 60% of our Pima sample will develop diabetes, the sensitivity of the test may be much higher!

How might altered glycemic responses to adrenergic stimulation be related to the pathophysiology of Type II diabetes? In that no defect in the insulin receptor or insulin gene have been identified as a reliable marker of diabetic populations, some other genetic loci must be involved in this disease. Furthermore, our research shows that insulin resistance and hyperglycemia are controlled by different genetic factors, implying that some physiologic mechanism other than insulin resistance is responsible for the hyperglycemia in obese BL/6 mice. One possible contributor to glucose intolerance in BL/6 mice is impaired first-phase insulin release. Although overall insulin response to glucose is normal or exaggerated in BL/6 mice, like human Type II diabetics, these mice show a blunted immediate response to the introduction of a glucose load (Kaku et al., 1988). Insulin release is, in large part, directly controlled by blood glucose level. However, first-phase insulin release may depend on appropriate vagal activity (Havel & Taborsky, 1989). In that we have shown that pancreatic secretory function is abnormally sensitive to inhibition by adrenergic stimulation in BL/6 mice (Surwit et al., 1986; Surwit et al., 1988), it is possible that this defect in first-phase insulin release is caused by altered adrenergic sensitivity. Furthermore, altered adrenergic sensitivity in the liver and in adipose tissue could enhance the effects of adrenergic stimulation upon hepatic glucose output and lypolyis leading to further metabolic disregulation as well.

These observations may have relevance for the understanding of Type II diabetes at the molecular level. Attempts to identify genetic defects in the insulin gene or in the insulin-receptor gene in individuals with Type II diabetes have been unfruitful to date (Lillioja et al., 1988). Although more work needs to be done to delineate the specific autonomic defects that may contribute to Type II diabetes, the notion that an autonomic mechanism may contribute to hyperglycemia in Type II diabetes offers an alternative hypothesis to the notion that something is wrong with the beta-cell or the insulin receptor per se. This hypothesis would suggest that the genetic defect may be found in those genes involved in the expression of adrenergic sensitivity in the pancreas and liver. Once the autonomic defect is better specified, genes that are known to control these functions can be looked at as candidate genes for study in diabetic mice or selected human diabetic populations. Finally, observations that altered adrenergic control of glucose metabolism precede the development of Type II diabetes may be helpful in conducting standard genetic analysis. Because of the variable expression of Type II diabetes, family pedigree studies cannot be meaningfully performed. Utilizing abnormalities in autonomic control of glucose metabolism as a phenotype may improve our understanding of the inheritance of this disorder and facilitate genetic analysis. In this manner, observations resulting from behavioral medicine research may prove to be relevant in the understanding of the pathophysiology of diabetes.

REFERENCES

Banerji, M. A., & Lebovitz, H. E. (1989). Insulin-sensitive and insulin resistant variants in NIDDM. *Diabetes, 38,* 784–792.

Barnett, A. K., Eff, C., Leslie, R. D. G., & Pyke, D. A. (1979). Diabetes in identical twins: A study of 200 pairs. *Diabetoloaia, 17,* 333–343.

Bogardus, C., Lillioja, S., Nyomba, B. L., Swinburn, B., Espositodel Puente, A., Knowler, W. C., Ravussin, E., Mott, D. M., & Bennett, P. (1989). Distribution of in vivo insulin action in Pima Indians as mixture of three normal distributions. *Diabetes, 38,* 1423–1432.

Coleman, D. L. (1978). Obese and diabetes: Two mutant genes causing diabetes-obesity syndromes in mice. *Diabetoloqia, 14,* 141–148.

Dunlin, W. E., Gerristen, G. C., & Chang, A. Y. (1983). Experimental and spontaneous diabetes in animals. In M. Ellenberg & H. Rifkin (Eds.), *Diabetes mellitus, theory and practice* (3rd ed., pp. 361–408). New Hyde Park, NY: Medical Examination Publishing.

Erikkson, J., Franssila-Killunki, A., Estrand, A., Saloranta, C., Widen, S., Schalin, C., & Groop, L. (1989). Early metabolic defects in persons at increasing risk for non-insulin-dependent diabetes mellitus. *New England Journal of Medicine, 321,* 339–343.

Fajans, S. S. (1982). Heterogeneity between families with non-insulin dependent diabetes of the MODY type. In J. Kobberling & R. Tattersall (Eds.), *The genetics of diabetes mellitus* (pp. 221–286). New York: Academic Press.

Gerich, J. E. (1988). Role of insulin resistance in the pathogenesis of type II (non-insulin-dependent) diabetes mellitus. *Bailliere's Clinical Endocrinology and Metabolism, 2,* 307–326.

Haffner, S. M., Stern, M. P., Hazuda, H. P., Mitchell, B. D., & Patterson, J. K. (1988). Increased insulin concentrations in nondiabetic offspring of diabetic parents. *New England Journal of Medicine, 319,* 1297–1301.

Havel, F. J., & Taborsky, G. J. (1989). The contributions of the autonomic nervous system to changes in glucagon and insulin secretion during hypoglycemic stress. *Endocrine Reviews, 10,* 332–350.

Hedrich, H. J. (1981). Genetic monitoring. In H. L. Foster, J. D. Small, & J. G. Fox (Eds.), *The mouse in biomedical research* (Vol. 1; pp. 159–176). New York: Academic Press.

Kahn, S. E., Porte, D., Jr. (1988). Islet dysfunction in non-insulin-dependent diabetes mellitus. *American Journal of Medicine, 85*(Suppl. 5A), 4–8.

Kaku, K., Fiedorek, F. T., Province, M., & Permutt, M. A. (1988). Genetic analysis of glucose tolerance in inbred mouse strains: Evidence of polygenic control. *Diabetes, 37,* 707–713.

Kobberling, J. (1971). Studies on the genetic heterogeneity of diabetes mellitus. *Diabetologia, 7,* 46–49.

Kuhn, C. M., Cochrane, C., Feinglos, M. N., & Surwit, R. S. (1987). Exaggerated peripheral responsivity to catecholamines contributes to stress-induced hyperglycemia in the ob/ob mouse. *Physiological Biochemistry and Behavior, 26,* 491–495.

Lillioja, S., Mott, D. M., Howard, V., Bennett, P. H., Hannele, Y. J., Freymond, D., Nyomba, B. L., Zurlo, F., Swinburn, B., & Bogardus, C. (1988). Impaired glucose tolerance as a disorder of insulin action: Longitudinal and cross-sectional studies in Pima Indians. *New England Journal of Medicine, 318,* 1217–1224.

Lillioja, S., Mott, D. M., Zawadski, K., Young, A. A., Abbott, W. G., Knowler, W. C., Bennett, P. H., Moll, P., & Bogardus, C. (1987). In vivo insulin action is familial characteristic in Nondiabetic Pima Indians. *Diabetes, 36,* 1329–1335.

Matthews, H. A., Weiss, S. M., Detre, T., Dembroski, T. M., Falkner, B., Manuck, S. B., & Williams, R. B. (Eds.). (1986). *Handbook of stress, reactivity, & cardiovascular disease.* New York: Wiley.

O'Rahilly, S., Turner, R. C., & Matthews, D. R. (1988). Impaired pulsatile secretion of insulin in relatives of patients with noninsulin-dependent diabetes. *New England Journal of Medicine, 318,* 1225–1230.

O'Rahilly, S., Wainscoat, J. S., & Turner, R. C. (1988). Type II (non-insulindependent) diabetes mellitus: New genetics for old nightmares. *Diabetologia, 31,* 407–414.

Reaven, G. M. (1988). Role of insulin resistance in human disease. *Diabetes, 37,* 1595–1607.

Searle, A. G., Peters, J., Lyon, M. F., Evans, E. P., Edwards, J. H., & Buckle, W. (1987). Chromosome maps of man and mouse, III. *Genomics, 1,* 3–18.

Surwit, R. S., Feinglos, M. N., Cochrane, C., & Kuhn, C. M. (1986). Altered alpha-adrenergic responsivity in C57BL/6J mice. *Diabetes, 35*(Supp 1), 19A (Abstract).

Surwit, R. S., Feinglos, M. N., Livingston, E. G., Kuhn, C. M., & McCubbin, J. A. (1984). Behavioral manipulation of the diabetic phenotype in ob/ob mice. *Diabetes, 33,* 616–618.

Surwit, R. S., Kuhn, C. M., Cochrane, C., McCubbin, J. A., & Feinglos, M. N. (1988). Diet-induced type II diabetes in C57BL/6J mice. *Diabetes, 37,* 1163–1167.

Surwit, R. S., McCubbin, J. A., Feinglos, M. N., Esposito-Del Peunte, A., & Lillioja, S. (1990). Glycemic reactivity to stress: A biologic marker development of type II diabetes. *Diabetes, 39*(Suppl 1), 8A.

Surwit, R. S., McCubbin, J. A., Kuhn, C. M., Cochrane, C., & Feinglos, M. N. (1989). Differential glycemic effects of morphine in diabetic and normal mice. *Metabolism, 38,* 282–85.

Surwit, R. S., Seldin, M. F., Kuhn, C. M., Cochrane, C., & Feinglos, M. N. (1991). Control of expression of insulin resistance and hyperglycemia in diabetic C57BL/6J mice by difference genetic factors. *Diabetes, 40,* 82–87.

14 Psychosocial Aspects of Childhood Diabetes: A Multivariate Framework

Annette M. La Greca
Dante S. Spetter
University of Miami

Insulin-dependent diabetes mellitus (IDDM), previously known as juvenile-onset diabetes and also referred to as Type I diabetes, is the most common metabolic disorder of childhood. Estimates indicate that approximately 120,000 youngsters in the United States are affected by this disease. For these individuals, survival depends on exogenous insulin administration and a very demanding and complex treatment regimen to balance insulin levels with food intake and energy expenditure, in an effort to approximate normal glucose metabolism.

Among individuals with IDDM, persistently high levels of plasma glucose (hyperglycemia) have been implicated in the development of diabetes-related health complications (Klein, Klein, & Moss, 1985; Krolewski et al., 1986; Skyler, 1987). Chronic complications associated with the disease include retinopathy, neuropathy, and renal disease (Keen & Jarrett, 1982). Diabetic retinopathy, for instance, is the leading cause of adult blindness in the United States (Klein, 1988). Moreover, virtually all youngsters with IDDM eventually develop at least background diabetic retinopathy, and this typically emerges during early adulthood (Klein, 1988).

In order to prevent or forestall associated disease complications, medical management of IDDM emphasizes the maintenance of adequate or, if possible, near normal levels of glycemia. This is a very difficult and challenging task for most youngsters with diabetes and their families. Daily management of IDDM requires a complicated, multicomponent treatment regimen that includes: daily insulin administration (typically two shots or more), multiple daily glucose tests, dietary regulation, careful timing of meals and snacks, and monitoring of exercise and activity level (Davidson, 1986a; Schiffrin, 1987).

Although achieving a balance among diet, insulin, and exercise has long been an important consideration for the management of diabetes, it is only recently that health-care professionals have begun to recognize the contributions of behavioral and psychological factors to diabetes care (Hamburg, Lipsett, Inoff, & Drash, 1979). This growing awareness has spurred a wealth of research into psychosocial factors related to treatment adherence and glycemic control among youngsters with diabetes and their families.

The purpose of this chapter is to describe current research on psychological aspects of childhood diabetes, and to present a multivariate model for conceptualizing this research. This chapter draws upon material presented at the Academy of Behavioral Medicine Research (La Greca, 1989), and from other recent sources (La Greca, 1988; La Greca & Skyler, 1991). In the context of the discussion, several cautions and caveats for future research are also considered.

EARLY RESEARCH ON PSYCHOLOGICAL ASPECTS OF CHILDHOOD DIABETES

Initial psychosocial research on childhood diabetes attempted to identify psychological sequelae specific to this chronic disorder. Youngsters with diabetes were compared with healthy children across a variety of personality and psychological adaptation parameters, such as behavior problems, self-esteem, and symptoms of psychiatric dysfunction. However, few consistent findings emerged from this literature. In their review of studies from 1940 to 1979, Dunn and Turtle (1981) concluded that little support could be found for differences between youngsters with diabetes and healthy controls. Similarly, Hauser and Pollets (1979) noted that the few studies that indicated higher rates of psychopathology among children with diabetes relied heavily on psychiatric interviews and categorical clinical judgments, whereas studies employing large sample sizes and less subjective clinical assessments typically did not find those with diabetes to differ from controls. These and other reviews (Dunn & Turtle, 1981; Fisher, Delamater, Bertelson, & Kirkley, 1982; Hauser & Pollets, 1979; Johnson, 1980) seriously questioned existing studies on a number of methodological grounds, including the use of inappropriate control groups, the absence of standardized methods for assessing psychological functioning, and bias in subject selection methods.

Even with the advent of more sophisticated psychological measures and multivariate statistical procedures, more recent work reveals remarkably few, if any, consistent differences between youngsters with diabetes and controls (e.g., Gross, Delcher, Snitzer, Bianchi, & Epstein, 1985; Jacobson et al., 1986; Kovacs, Brent, Steinberg, Paulauskas, & Reid, 1986; Rovet & Ehrlich, 1988; Wertlieb, Hauser, & Jacobson, 1986). For example, Kovacs et al. (1986) followed school-aged children (8 to 13 years old) for the first year following diabetes onset. The psychological functioning of these children, as assessed by scores on standardized measures of anxiety, depression, and self-esteem, compared favorably to instrument norms. In fact, youngsters with diabetes typically had more positive scores than comparison youth. Considering the difficult and challenging nature of this chronic disease, the generally positive psychological adaptation of youngsters with IDDM and their families is especially noteworthy.

Within Group Research: Correlates of Metabolic Control

Given the limited support for a "diabetic personality" (Dunn & Turtle, 1981), in recent years psychosocial research has shifted away from between-group comparisons of diabetic and healthy youngsters to within-group investigations of behavioral, psychological, and family factors that are related to or predictive of disease-related outcomes for diabetic youth. In particular, metabolic control, as indexed by glycosylated hemoglobin levels, has been the most intensively investigated therapeutic outcome among youngsters with IDDM. Glycosylated hemoglobin is considered to be the gold standard for indexing metabolic control, as it evaluates integrated glucose control over a 6- to 8-week period (Bunn, 1981; Goldstein, Little, Wiedmeyer, England, & McKenzie, 1986). Moreover, high levels of glyco-hemoglobins have been associated with the development and progression of diabetes-related complications, such as retinopathy and renal disease (Skyler, 1987).

Research on psychological correlates of metabolic control has yielded a number of interesting findings. Youngsters with poor glycemic control have been found to be more depressed (Mazze, Lucide, & Shamoon, 1984), more anxious (Anderson, Miller, Auslander, & Santiago, 1981; Simonds, 1977), and less sociable (Lane et al., 1988) than those whose diabetes is well controlled. Similarly, family functioning has been linked with metabolic status. Youngsters from conflictual or dysfunctional families typically display difficulties with glycemic control (Anderson et al., 1981; Minuchin, Rosman, & Baker, 1978; White, Kolman, Wexler, Polin, & Winter, 1984). In contrast, positive family variables, such as support, cohesion, and organization, have been associated with better metabolic status (Anderson et al., 1981; Hanson, Henggeler, & Burghen, 1987a, 1987b; Klemp & La Greca, 1987).

Although such findings serve to highlight the role of psychological factors in glycemic control, the predominant research strategy has been to examine univariate relationships between psychological variables and youngsters' metabolic functioning. However, this research strategy presents serious limitations.

Perhaps the most notable concern is that it neglects other disease-specific factors that also contribute to therapeutic outcome. Therefore, it is not surprising that the magnitude of relationships obtained between psychosocial variables and metabolic control typically have been very modest. It is unlikely that substantial proportions of the variance in metabolic control could be accounted for by psychosocial factors alone, given the multitude of variables that potentially affect glycemic functioning. By assessing and/or controlling for the contributions of these other health status variables, the importance of the youngsters' and families' psychological functioning for glycemic control might be better appreciated.

Furthermore, univariate, correlational approaches do not specify the mechanisms or pathways for the observed relationships. Why is family support related to good metabolic control? Is it because supportive families have youngsters who are more adherent with their diabetes care than unsupportive families, and adherence, in turn, promotes better metabolic control? Or do such families create a secure, competent environment that buffers the potential adverse effects of stress, which could lead to metabolic disruptions? These issues must be considered in order for behavioral research in diabetes to foster the development of empirically based interventions for improving disease management and glycemic control.

MULTIVARIATE FRAMEWORK FOR PSYCHOSOCIAL RESEARCH IN CHILDHOOD DIABETES

In view of the concerns delineated here, we developed an initial framework for conceptualizing the role of psychosocial and family factors in childhood diabetes (La Greca, 1988). In addition to psychological variables, this initial model included behavioral, physiological, and diabetes-specific factors that were linked with metabolic control, either empirically or theoretically. However, based on findings from our own research, as well as those of other investigators, further refinement appeared indicated. A revised model is depicted in Fig. 14.1.

Each factor in the model should be viewed in the context of the other model components in a multivariate manner. Furthermore, each factor is complex and multifaceted. All diabetes-specific components might be considered to be necessary, but not sufficient conditions for good metabolic control. Psychosocial factors are viewed as affecting control primarily through these disease-specific variables.

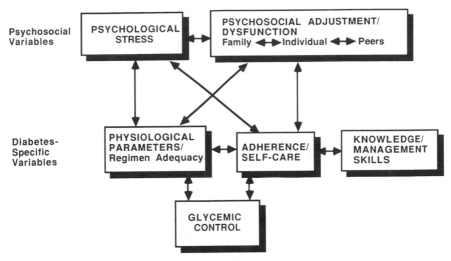

FIG. 14.1.   Model of psychosocial factors in relation to glycemic control.

The organization of the model implies that, in order to understand youngsters' metabolic functioning, assessment and intervention should begin at disease-specific levels (diabetes knowledge, self-care, regimen adequacy) before proceeding systematically to more complex psychological levels (stress and psychological adjustment). For instance, before attempting to improve metabolic control by altering family functioning, one should first determine whether the child and family know how to manage the disease and implement management tasks effectively. When gaps in knowledge exist, intervention should begin at an educational level.

This model also depicts likely pathways between psychosocial functioning and metabolic control. Two primary pathways — levels of self-care and physiological variables — are hypothesized as mediators between psychological variables and glycemic control. These are reviewed more carefully in the ensuing discussion. In order to adequately evaluate the mechanisms linking psychosocial variables with glycemic control, it would be desirable to assess these potential mediating variables in future psychosocial research.

Although this model was developed to examine factors that might affect metabolic control in the causal sense, with the idea that intervention in these areas should lead to improvements in metabolic functioning, most of the research supporting the model has been correlational. One assumption of the model is that the relationships depicted are likely to be complex and bidirectional in nature. For instance, poor self-care may lead to disruptions in metabolic control; however, it is also plausible that periods during which glycemic control is difficult to achieve may undermine self-care efforts.

Another caveat is that this model is cross-sectional; it examines one time point in the context of a longstanding chronic disease. Additional models are needed to appreciate the long-term and chronic aspects of diabetes. It is especially important to consider how periods of poor metabolic control, which inevitably occur with this chronic disease, might subsequently lead to problems with treatment adherence and general psychosocial adjustment.

Before describing the model, it should be emphasized that developmental parameters are important for each component of the model. Chronological age, for example, has been related to several aspects of diabetes care. Adolescents appear to know more about diabetes (Johnson et al., 1982; La Greca, Follansbee, & Skyler, 1990), but have poorer treatment adherence (Hamburg & Inoff, 1982; Hanson et al., 1987b; Johnson, Silverstein, Rosenbloom, Carter, & Cunningham, 1986), and worse metabolic control (Chase et al., 1989) than younger children.

Important developmental transitions also have been observed in the degree to which families are involved in diabetes care. Family members, especially mothers, assume considerable responsibility for diabetes management with young children, but are less involved in daily management tasks with older children and adolescents (Anderson, Auslander, Jung, Miller, & Santiago, 1990; Etzwiler & Sines, 1962; La Greca et al., 1990).

Factors Directly Affecting Metabolic Control: Physiological Pathways and Levels of Self-Care

Physiological Parameters

Metabolic control is determined by the balance between food intake, as a source of energy (calories and carbohydrates), and energy expenditure in daily activity. This balance is mediated by insulin availability. Consequently, physiological factors that affect insulin availability, such as the youngsters' degree of residual endogenous insulin secretion (Ludvigsson, Heding, Larsson, & Leander, 1977; Marner et al., 1985), or individual differences in insulin sensitivity or insulin resistance (Pedersen & Beck-Nielsen, 1987), will also influence metabolic control. For example, within the first 2 years after disease onset, endogenous insulin secretion (as measured by C-peptide concentrations) ceases in most youngsters with IDDM; however, some youngsters continue to secrete small amounts of insulin (Gonen et al., 1979; Grajwer, Pildes, Horowitz, & Rubenstein, 1977). The presence of residual endogenous insulin secretion has been associated with better glycemic control and a lower insulin dose requirement among children and adolescents with IDDM (Clarson, Daneman, Drash, Becker, & Ehrlich, 1987).

The attainment of metabolic control will also be easier in youngsters who have overcome the initial insulin resistance characteristically seen at disease onset or who have become insulin sensitive with decompensation (Yki-

Jarvinen & Kovisto, 1986). On the other hand, the increased insulin resistance that accompanies puberty (Bloch, Clemons, & Sperling, 1987) may contribute to problems with glycemic control among adolescents, and necessitate substantial adjustments in youngsters' insulin requirements to achieve acceptable levels of glycemia (Blethen, Sargeant, Whitlow, & Santiago, 1981; Daneman, Wolfson, Becker, & Drash, 1981; Mann & Johnston, 1984).

The complexities of achieving adequate levels of available insulin suggest that the prescribed insulin regimen will be an important factor contributing to youngsters' metabolic control. Yet, physicians' may differ markedly in their approach to insulin requirements and target glucose values. Marteau and colleagues (Marteau, Johnston, Baum, & Bloch, 1987) compared pediatricians and diabetologists with respect to the target glucose values they preferred to see in a child with diabetes. The two physician groups differed in that the pediatricians selected hyperglycemic profiles significantly more often than the diabetologists; the diabetologists were more likely to select profiles that reflected "tight" glucose control. To the extent that treatment goals are indicative of prescribed regimens, these findings suggest that physicians' treatment prescriptions for diabetes care must be considered in evaluating youngsters' glycemic control.

Finally, glycemic control will also be influenced by the glucose counter-regulatory hormones—the catecholamines (adrenaline and noradrenalin), glucagon, cortisol, and growth hormone (Cryer & Gerich, 1983, 1985). These hormones are secreted in increased amounts during times of physical stress (e.g., intercurrent illness), and/or extreme emotional distress. The physiological consequences of these hormones include the stimulation of glucose production, the production of free fatty acids (lipolysis and ketogenesis), and the inhibition of glucose uptake in tissue (see Goetsch, 1989). In nondiabetic individuals, increased insulin secretion offsets the effects of the counterregulatory hormones, so that normal levels of glycemia are achieved. However, insulin production is nearly or virtually absent in youngsters with IDDM, so that stress-related hormone release can result in ketonuria and disruptions in metabolic control (Baker, Barcai, Kay & Haque, 1969; Barglow, Hatcher, Edidin, & Sloan-Rossiter, 1984). This physiological pathway to metabolic control is discussed further in the section on psychological stress.

Treatment Adherence or Levels of Self-Care

Assuming that an adequate regimen has been prescribed, adherence to the treatment plan should be critical for good metabolic control. Rather than using the term *adherence* to reflect the degree to which a treatment plan is followed, perhaps *level of self-care* would be more appropriate. In fact, most investigators measure what the youngster or family actually does to manage diabetes, or their perceptions of self-care, rather than how closely they adhere to an actual prescription (La Greca, 1990a).

Maintaining adequate levels of self-care appears to be a significant problem among youngsters with IDDM, perhaps owing to the complex, demanding, and chronic nature of the treatment regimen. Problems with self-care appear soon after disease onset. Kovacs et al. (1986) followed school-aged children for 1 year after their initial diagnosis of IDDM. Youngsters reported "dietary compliance" to be the most difficult aspect of diabetes management by 5 to 8 months after disease onset, and again at 1-year follow-up. Increasing numbers of youngsters omitted their glucose tests over time (43% at study entry, 54% at 5–8 months; 70% at 1-year follow-up). Others have noted adherence to be problematic, particularly for adolescents (Johnson et al., 1986; La Greca, 1988).

Adherence is a very difficult construct to assess, given the numerous tasks that are involved in daily diabetes care. Measures must reflect the multi-component nature of the treatment regimen, and include assessments of such diverse tasks as insulin administration, glucose testing, content and timing of food consumption, and exercise. Assessment is further compli-cated by the fact that adherence to one aspect of the regimen may not be related to compliance with other aspects of diabetes care (Glasgow, McCaul, & Schafer, 1987; Johnson et al., 1986; Schafer, Glasgow, McCaul, & Dreher, 1983). (See Glasgow, Wilson, & McCaul, 1985, for a detailed discussion of problems in assessing adherence in diabetes.)

Furthermore, for any given management task, diverse barriers to self-care may be present that can inhibit or preclude adequate disease manage-ment (La Greca, 1988; La Greca & Hanna, 1983; Schafer et al., 1983). For example, youngsters have reported a variety of barriers to maintaining their prescribed meal plan, including social interference (e.g., skipping snacks or eating concentrated sweets when out with friends), planning and problem-solving difficulties (e.g., forgetting to shop for specific foods, difficulties in making substitutions for items on a prescribed meal plan), and appetite problems (e.g., not feeling hungry at the prescribed meal time, wanting to eat larger portions than the meal plan indicates; see La Greca, 1988).

Although the psychosocial model (Fig. 14.1) indicates a direct relation-ship between youngsters' self-care behaviors and metabolic control, empir-ical support for this relationship has been equivocal. Hanson et al. (1987a, 1987b) found adolescents' reports of adherence behaviors to be significantly associated with metabolic control. Using a variety of assessment methods, other recent investigations of adolescents with IDDM similarly support a relationship between several aspects of self-care and glycemic control (Kuttner, Delamater, & Santiago, 1990; La Greca et al., 1990; La Greca, Swales, Klemp, & Madigan, 1988; Schafer et al., 1983). On the other hand,

Johnson and colleagues (1986) developed a 24-hour recall interview measure to assess youngsters' adherence to diabetes care. This measure provides separate indices for various components of the diabetes regimen (e.g., exercise, insulin injections, etc.). In a sample of more than 200 youngsters with IDDM, glycemic control was not related to the various adherence factors derived from the 24-hour recall measure, with the exception of eating and testing frequency that were associated with better glycohemo- globin values (Johnson, 1989).

Although such findings appear puzzling at first, adequate self-care is not the only variable that is critical to successful therapeutic outcome. As suggested by the model (Fig. 14.1), high levels of treatment adherence do not guarantee acceptable metabolic functioning. Other model components will affect therapeutic outcome as well. For instance, a youngster could be prescribed an inadequate regimen; in this case, adherence may not have the desired therapeutic result. As another example, despite high levels of self-care, management tasks could be implemented incorrectly. Wing and associates (Wing et al., 1985; Wing, Koeske, New, Lamparski, & Becker, 1986) found children and adolescents to perform glucose testing tasks inaccurately; regimen adjustments based on incorrect test results may lead to poor management decisions.

In view of these findings, it becomes apparent that adherence-control relationships may be difficult to evaluate without also considering the adequacy of the treatment regimen, and the presence of stress or other emotional factors that could contribute to physiological disruptions in metabolic functioning. In other words, youngsters' self-care must be viewed within the context of the psychosocial, physiological, and diabetes-specific variables that can affect metabolic functioning, as delineated in the multivariate model.

Factors That May Affect Metabolic Control Indirectly: Knowledge, Psychological Stress, and Psychosocial Adjustment

Diabetes Knowledge and Management Skills

In the psychosocial model, diabetes knowledge and management skills are viewed as essential, but not sufficient, for good control. Given the complexities of daily diabetes care, youngsters and families must under- stand how to manage diabetes if good control is to be achieved. Active knowledge of diabetes care includes knowing how to execute daily manage- ment tasks correctly, how to plan for deviations in everyday routines, and how to adjust the regimen when problems arise. With the advent of intensified insulin regimens aimed at achieving near normal glycemic control (Schade, Santiago, Skyler, & Rizza, 1983), active diabetes knowledge might also include the youngster's ability to adjust insulin dosage or food intake based on target glucose values.

Marked developmental differences are apparent in youngsters' knowledge of diabetes and its management. Johnson et al. (1982) found that, on a measure of general knowledge about diabetes, 6- to 8-year-old children answered about 50% of the questions correctly, whereas older adolescents and mothers achieved scores of about 80% and 87%, respectively. Similar developmental trends were observed for diabetes problem-solving skills. Although most youngsters' and mothers' knowledge levels appeared to be adequate, some individuals displayed alarming gaps in their understanding of diabetes management.

Similar results were obtained with 7- to 15-year-olds and their mothers (La Greca et al., 1990). Consistent with previous findings, adolescents and mothers were more knowledgeable than preadolescent children. However, different patterns of relationships between knowledge and glycemic control were apparent for the children and adolescents. For preadolescents, mothers' knowledge of diabetes was associated with better treatment adherence and metabolic control. In contrast, adolescents' own understanding of diabetes, rather than their mothers', was significantly correlated with adherence and control. This developmental shift in the relative importance of parents' versus youngsters' diabetes knowledge is not surprising considering that adolescents typically assume greater responsibility for their diabetes care than younger children do (Anderson et al., 1990; Etzwiler & Sines, 1962; La Greca et al., 1990). As a result, adolescents' own knowledge and behavior should have a greater impact on diabetes management and control than their parents'.

Although support exists for a positive relationship between diabetes knowledge and glycemic control, some discrepant findings have been obtained. Hamburg and Inoff (1982) found youngsters' diabetes knowledge to be *negatively* related to metabolic functioning. These authors assessed a broad age range of youngsters (5 to 19 years of age), and did not evaluate parents' knowledge for the younger children in their sample. It is possible that poor metabolic control prompted reeducation efforts in these youngsters or promoted greater attention to their diabetes care, resulting in their higher knowledge levels. Equivocal results obtained across studies serve to highlight the difficulties of conducting correlational research in the context of an ongoing chronic disease.

With the advent of home blood glucose monitoring (HBGM), and intensified insulin therapy, comes the potential for youngsters to achieve near normal glucose control. However, recent findings indicate that HBGM alone has little impact on youngsters' glycemic control (Belmonte et al., 1988; Daneman et al., 1985; Wing et al., 1985; Wysocki, Green, & Huxtable, 1989). Unless glucose values are used to adjust the treatment regimen (e.g., altering insulin dose or food intake), HBGM will not likely effect metabolic functioning (Davidson, 1986a, 1986b; Skyler, Skyler, Seigler, & O'Sullivan, 1981). As with most aspects of diabetes knowledge, it may not be the information, per se, that is important, but the youngsters' and family's ability to use the information to adjust the diabetes regimen.

This contention is supported by recent work (Delamater et al., 1990) highlighting the value of teaching self-management skills to newly diagnosed children with IDDM and their parents. During the first 6 months after initial onset of diabetes, one group of children and parents were taught self-management skills and were compared with others receiving either standard care, or standard care plus a supportive intervention. The self-management intervention stressed the active use of glucose testing results to adjust the daily treatment regimen. Those who were taught self-management skills obtained consistently better levels of glycemic control over a 2-year follow-up than those who were provided standard diabetes instruction alone. This intervention study underscores the importance of active use of diabetes knowledge.

Most studies assessing diabetes knowledge and metabolic control have not considered the potential mediating effects of treatment adherence. One exception to this is the study by Hanson et al. (1987a). These investigators found that the family's overall level of diabetes knowledge was related to adolescents' treatment adherence, rather than directly to glycemic control.

It is possible that positive associations between knowledge and control obtained in some studies (e.g., La Greca et al., 1990), could be explained by the knowledgeable youngsters (and parents) also having higher levels of self-care. Consonant with this view, we propose that youngsters' and families' diabetes knowledge is related to glycemic control primarily through association with self-care (see Fig. 14.1). Youngsters who are knowledgeable about diabetes management, may be more adherent with recommendations for self-care. High levels of knowledge and self-care should lead to satisfactory metabolic functioning (assuming that other parameters in the model are favorable), whereas diabetes knowledge alone would be insufficient to produce adequate metabolic control.

Interactions between knowledge and self-care may also be of interest to investigate, but have not been studied to date. Good knowledge in the face of poor adherence should not have a positive impact on glucose control. Adequate levels of knowledge and adherence would appear to be necessary for satisfactory metabolic functioning. This hypothesis awaits further investigation.

Psychological Variables: Stress and Psychosocial Adaptation

Finally, psychological variables are essential aspects of the model, and include the individual's ability to cope with stress and his or her level of personal and family adjustment. These two major components are also interrelated. Even with satisfactory levels of knowledge and adherence, diabetes may be difficult to control when youngsters experience considerable stress or a high degree of personal or family conflict.

In the proposed multivariate model (Fig. 14.1), high levels of psychological stress and psychosocial dysfunction (depression, family conflict) are viewed as affecting metabolic control both through direct, physiologic pathways, as well as through relationships with treatment adherence. Similarly, positive psychosocial adaptation (e.g, family support, cohesion, and organization) may be associated with glycemic control either via better levels of self-care or through the stress-buffering effects of supportive family relations.

Stress and Diabetes. High levels of stress might affect metabolic functioning via several physiological pathways: (a) the pituitary-adrenal cortical system, through the release of cortisol, (b) the sympathetic-adrenal medullary system, through the effects of adrenaline and noradrenalin, or (c) increased secretion of glucagon, resulting from hepatic glucose production (Barglow et al., 1984; Hinkle & Wolf, 1952; Surwit, Scovern, & Feinglos, 1982). All of these counterregulatory hormones are secreted in greater quantities during times of intense emotional stress, and have the potential to destabilize glucose control. Furthermore, Barglow et al. (1984) point out that stress hormones may be elevated even before metabolic decompensation, suggesting that these hormones may play a role in initiating and exacerbating episodes of ketoacidosis in some individuals with IDDM.

Despite theoretical support for the destabilizing effects of psychological stress on individuals with IDDM, empirical investigations have been fraught with methodological difficulties, and findings have been equivocal, at best. Among adults with diabetes, reports of stressful life events have been associated with disruptions in metabolic control as evidenced by increased glycosuria, changes in insulin requirements, and increased frequency of clinic visits (Bradley, 1979; Grant, Kyle, Teichman, & Mendels, 1974). Adolescents' reports of negative, stressful life events also have been associated with higher levels of fasting serum glucose (Chase & Jackson, 1981; Hanson & Pichert, 1986), higher glycosylated hemoglobin levels (Chase & Jackson, 1981), and the presence of urine ketones among males (Brand, Johnson, & Johnson, 1986). In contrast, the frequency and intensity of daily stressors (Delamater, Kurtz, Bubb, White, & Santiago, 1987) and acute reactions to laboratory-induced stress (Delamater et al., 1988) have not differentiated adolescents in good versus poor glycemic control.

These discrepant reports may be a function of individual differences in physiological responses to acute stressors. Carter and colleagues (Carter, Gonder-Frederick, Cox, Clarke, & Scott, 1985) found that plasma glucose responses to laboratory stressors were idiosyncratic, but stable within individuals across time. Some individuals demonstrated a glucose rise, some a decline, and others no change in response to standardized "psychological" stressors (e.g., mental arithmetic). Summarizing their recent findings, Cox, Gonder-Frederick, and Carter (in press) noted that it is not reasonable to assume all types of stressors will produce a metabolic effect, nor that all individuals will respond similarly to the same stressor.

Following the notion of individual differences in stress responses, a recent investigation with children and adolescents identified the presence of a Type A behavior pattern as a possible discriminating personality variable (Stabler et al., 1987). Youngsters with IDDM, aged 8 to 16 years, who exhibited the Type A behavior pattern (aggressive, competitive, impatient behavior) demonstrated a plasma glucose rise in response to a challenging videogame stressor, whereas Type B youngsters (low on Type A characteristics) evidenced a plasma glucose decline. Although neurohormonal responses to stressors were not evaluated, they were presumed to underlie the stress-induced hyperglycemia observed in Type A youngsters. In apparent contrast to Stabler et al.'s findings, however, Cox et al. (in press) found Type A adults to demonstrate a plasma glucose decline, and Type B's to show a glucose rise in response to laboratory stressors. The reasons for these differences are not apparent, but a number of methodological differences across the two studies could be responsible. At this point, it is difficult to pinpoint reliable individual differences that predict youngsters' responses to stressors.

Although stress is thought to affect metabolic control primarily through physiological pathways, the adverse effects of psychological stressors could be mediated by levels of self-care. As Cox et al. (in press) noted, stress may affect self-care by promoting inappropriate behaviors (e.g., drinking or eating more than usual) or by interfering with routine aspects of diabetes care (e.g., not taking the time to test glucose). Anecdotal accounts of stress affecting diabetes care can be found. For instance, Simonds, Goldstein, Walker, and Rawlings (1981) noted that adolescent girls with IDDM reported that they were less likely to follow their diet when they were upset.

Additional support for this position can be derived from a recent investigation. Hanson and Pichert (1986) assessed stress, adherence, and glycemic control among adolescents (12 to 15 years old) for 3 days during a camp session for diabetic youth. Youngsters' stress levels were related to exercise adherence (more stress/less exercise), but were not consistently related to other adherence indices. Although negative cumulative stress (over 3 days) was related to higher levels of fasting blood glucose, the measures of adherence were not related to fasting glucose values. This study provides some limited support for stressful events affecting both daily diabetes management and glucose control.

In contrast to these results, Hanson et al. (1987b) did not find support for a stress-adherence relationship. These authors found that reports of stressful life events were associated with poorer metabolic control in adolescents with IDDM, but that this relationship could not be explained by a link between stress and adherence. In their sample, both stress and adherence were significantly and independently related to metabolic control; in fact, stress and adherence were unrelated. Although physiological pathways were presumed to underlie the relationships between stress and glycemic control, these pathways were not actually evaluated.

In view of these contradictory findings, further clarification of the effects of stress on metabolic functioning is needed. In particular, one cannot assume that stress affects control through physiological pathways when stress-adherence relationships are absent; given the problems inherent in measuring adherence to a complex diabetes regimen (Glasgow et al., 1987; La Greca, 1990a), methodological difficulties may account for such negative results. It is imperative to document physiological pathways between stress and glycemic control, rather than inferring them from the absence of support for adherence as a mediating variable. Finally, as Cox et al. (in press) noted, poor adherence and poor metabolic control might produce stress in some individuals with IDDM; the complex, bidirectional influences of stress, adherence, and glycemic control await further investigation.

Psychological Health of the Youngster and Family.　As discussed near the beginning of this chapter, considerable research has documented univariate relationships between glycemic control and the psychological health of youngsters with IDDM and their families (e.g., Anderson et al., 1981; Hanson et al., 1987a; Lane et al., 1988; Rovet & Ehrlich, 1988; Simonds, 1976–1977). As might be expected, family factors and child adjustment also are interrelated. For instance, behavioral and psychological adjustment problems in youngsters with diabetes have been associated with family conflict, and child adaptation has been linked with positive family factors, such as support and cohesion (Hauser, Jacobson, Wertlieb, Brink, & Wentworth, 1985; Wertlieb et al., 1986).

Individual Functioning.　On an individual level reports of anxiety, depression, and/or interpersonal conflict have been associated with problems in metabolic control among adolescents with diabetes (e.g., Anderson et al., 1981; Mazze et al., 1984; Simonds, 1977). Symptoms of anxiety and depression, and feelings of dysphoria about diabetes, have been noted among adolescent girls with IDDM (Simonds et al., 1981; Sullivan, 1978). Girls with IDDM have also been found to report more anxiety and greater concerns about physical appearance than boys with diabetes (Ryan &

Morrow, 1986). Although some of these studies suggest that greater psychological dysfunction is associated with poor diabetic control, even for poorly controlled youngsters mean levels of psychosocial distress are typically in the normal range of functioning.

Correlational analyses do not permit a determination of causal effects. It is quite likely that the link between psychosocial functioning and glycemic control is mutual and bidirectional, with each factor influencing the other. Improvements in glycemic control have been linked with positive changes in reports of anxiety, depression, and quality of life (Dupuis, Jones, & Peterson, 1980; Mazze et al., 1984; Seigler, La Greca, Citrin, Reeves, & Skyler, 1982; Shapiro, Wigg, Charles, & Perley, 1984). It is equally plausible that deterioration of glycemic control would lead to feelings of anxiety, depression, and emotional upset.

In a recent study, we examined whether relationships between anxiety, depression, and glucose control would be apparent when other diabetes-specific factors in the psychosocial model were considered (see La Greca & Skyler, 1991). Measures of depression (Beck Depression Inventory) and anxiety (State-Trait Anxiety Scale) were modified so that items that could be indicative of poor glycemic control (e.g., fatigue, irritability) were eliminated. Even with this precaution, adolescents who reported more symptoms of depression and anxiety displayed poorer glycemic control. However, reports of depressive symptoms were also associated with lower levels of self-care, diabetes knowledge, and problem solving; similarly, symptoms of anxiety were related to poorer levels of self-care and problem-solving skills. From these univariate analyses, it was not possible to determine whether depression and anxiety were related to metabolic control largely via associations with other health status variables, or whether other potential pathways should be considered as well.

Regression analyses revealed that age, disease duration, diabetes knowledge and problem solving, and self-care levels together accounted for almost 40% of the variance in glycohemoglobin. Depressive symptoms accounted for 9% unique variance beyond the other variables in the model. Although this represented significant incremental variance, this variance was considerably less than that obtained when depression was the only predictor for metabolic control. In contrast to these results, anxiety did not make a significant, unique contribution to the prediction of glycemic control above and beyond other variables in the model. These findings are consistent with literature on chronic illness, in that depression appears to be the most consistent psychological concomitant of chronic disease.

Our results further suggested that the relationship between depressive symptoms and metabolic control was at least partly mediated by other diabetes-specific factors in the psychosocial model. Moreover, the results were also consistent with the notion of depressive states being linked with glycemic control through physiological pathways, although no definitive conclusions can be drawn as physiological variables were not assessed.

On the other hand, symptoms of anxiety were related to glycemic control via poorer treatment adherence. Adolescents who reported more anxious symptomatology displayed less adequate self-care, which in turn was related to poor metabolic control. It is also possible that youngsters experienced anxiety as a result of poor diabetes management and problems with glycemic control. These analyses highlight the importance of examining diabetes-specific parameters as potential mediating variables in the relationship between psychological functioning and metabolic control.

Most investigations of youngsters with IDDM have examined levels of psychological distress; less attention has been devoted to investigations of coping strategies and positive psychological adaptation. One exception is a study by Hanson et al. (1987b) that evaluated the contributions of adolescents' social competence to adherence and metabolic control. These authors found that socially competent adolescents were more adherent with their prescribed diabetes regimen. Moreover, social competence appeared to buffer the relationship between stress and metabolic control. Specifically, for highly socially competent adolescents, high levels of stress were not associated with poor glycemic control, but for youngsters who were low in social competence, stress and metabolic control were strongly related. These data suggest that positive aspects of youngsters' psychosocial adjustment are linked with good glycemic control via better self-care, and fewer disruptions due to emotional stress.

In summary, youngsters' psychological adjustment and metabolic control appear to be interrelated. As with stress, potential pathways for such a relationship include adherence and physiological responses. It is also possible that youngsters' psychological dysfunction may be a sign of family dysfunction, which in turn, could be related to metabolic control via similar pathways. Most importantly, given the correlational nature of the studies in this area, it is not possible to determine whether symptoms of psychological distress lead to or result from poor metabolic control (or whether adaptation is a cause or a consequence of good control). Longitudinal research is necessary to evaluate potential causal pathways.

Family.   Parallel findings have been observed with respect to family functioning and diabetes. Family conflict and disruption have been associated with poor diabetic control, and family adaptation and cohesion with good control (Anderson et al., 1981; Baker et al., 1969; Hanson, Henggeler, Harris, Burghen, & Moore, 1989; Klemp & La Greca, 1987; Simonds, 1977; Swift, Seidman, & Stein, 1967).

According to the psychosocial model, we would anticipate family conflict to be associated with glycemic control largely through physiological pathways, but also through poor levels of treatment adherence. Supportive aspects of family functioning may be associated with control through better levels of self-care (Hanson et al., 1987a; Klemp & La Greca, 1987; Schafer et al., 1983), or through the stress-buffering effects of supportive interpersonal relationships.

In a recent investigation, we examined whether family variables were directly related to adolescents' glycemic control or were mediated by their relationship to treatment adherence, which in turn should be predictive of good control (Klemp & La Greca, 1987). Consistent with the psychosocial model, greater family cohesion and organization were associated with higher levels of self-care, whereas higher levels of family conflict were associated with poorer diabetes care. However, of these family variables, only perceived family conflict was associated with glycemic functioning, and it was linked with poorer control.

Path analyses provided support for a direct association (i.e., presumed physiological pathway) between metabolic control and family conflict. That is, the association between family conflict and poor adherence did not adequately account for the relationship between family conflict and adolescents' glycemic control. Given the correlational nature of the study, however, it is equally important to consider the possibility that poor metabolic functioning precipitates stress and conflict within families of adolescents with diabetes.

As an interesting counterpoint, positive family factors, such as cohesion and organization, were more closely aligned with youngsters' self-care than with their metabolic control (Klemp & La Greca, 1987). In turn, the adolescents' self-care was related to glycemic functioning. Similarly, using different measures of family functioning, Hanson et al. (1987b) found parental support to be related to adolescents' adherence, but not to their glycemic control. These data suggest that organized and supportive families may facilitate treatment adherence, and in this manner promote better glycemic control in their children.

The potential stress-buffering effects of supportive family relations have not been documented. To date, the one study that addressed this hypothesis (Hanson et al, 1987b) did not find family relations to moderate the negative relationship between adolescents' stress and their metabolic control. Further exploration of this issue would be desirable.

Peers.   A new addition to the psychosocial model is the inclusion of peer relations as an important aspect of psychosocial functioning to be considerered among youngsters with IDDM. Several investigators have observed social difficulties (e.g., introversion, social withdrawal, problems with dating) among youngsters whose diabetes was in poor control (e.g., Lane et al., 1988; Orr, Golden, Myers, & Marrero, 1983; Simonds, 1977), although for the most part, these studies were not designed to evaluate peer relations specifically. We might anticipate that children with good peer relationships and a supportive peer network would display more positive adaptation to diabetes and, conversely, that those with problematic social functioning would find diabetes management much more difficult to negotiate in social contexts, perhaps exacerbating preexisting social difficulties (see La Greca, 1990b).

Consistent with this perspective, Jacobson et al., (1986) evaluated the peer relations of newly diagnosed children and adolescents with IDDM. These investigators noted significant positive relationships between youngsters' perceptions of their social acceptance and their adjustment to diabetes. Although the youngsters' attitudes toward their diabetes were largely favorable, most of the children reported that they did not talk to their friends about their diabetes, and about one third of the sample reported thinking that their nondiabetic friends would like them better if they did not have diabetes.

During the adolescent years, peers become an increasingly important aspect of youngsters' daily life and social milieu. The presence of a chronic disease, such as IDDM, may further complicate youngsters' desires to fit in and be accepted by peers. For some adolescents, this might take the form of increased sensitivity about their diabetes. For example, Simonds et al. (1981) found that adolescent girls were more likely than boys to regard peers and siblings as treating them differently because of diabetes. Also, in a study of adolescents girls with diabetes and their mothers (Bobrow, AvRuskin, & Siller, 1985), most of the girls (50%) indicated that they would wait a long time before telling another girl they wanted to be friends with that they had diabetes, and 40% would wait very long before telling a boy they liked that they had diabetes.

Aside from increased sensitivity, peer social situations may also interfere with optimal diabetes care. In a study of barriers to diabetes care (La Greca & Hanna, 1983), children and adolescents with IDDM reported a large percentage of social barriers for several daily management tasks, most notably for dietary adherence and testing glucose (e.g., wanting to eat what friends are eating; not testing when out with peers). Youngsters who reported more barriers were less adherent with their diabetes regimen and were in worse metabolic control.

Kaplan, Chadwick, and Schimmel (1985) found that adolescents who were more satisfied with their social support were in worse glycemic control. And, in a study by Marrero (Marrero, Jacobs, & Orr, 1981), youngsters' metabolic control was related to reliance on parental, rather than peer, social support networks. It is possible that youngsters who are concerned about peer acceptance may compromise their diabetes care in order to fit in with their peer network. Additional research that explores the role of peer relations in diabetes management is both important and desirable.

DIRECTIONS FOR FUTURE PSYCHOSOCIAL RESEARCH

Although the psychosocial model presented herein may provide reasonable starting points for investigations of behavioral and psychosocial factors in diabetes care, several difficulties associated with this area of research may arise. First, testing the full psychosocial model is a challenge that requires large samples, and the availability of multiple, psychometrically sound measures to assess each model component. The requirement of large subject samples often means that only parts of the model can be tested at any one time. Alternatively, multicenter, collaborative research may be necessary to advance our understanding of psychosocial aspects of diabetes.

Second, there is a need for more illness-specific measures that assess youngsters' and families' behaviors and attitudes toward diabetes. Although several diabetes-specific measures exist (e.g., Grossman, Brink, & Hauser, 1987; Schafer, McCaul, & Glasgow, 1986; Sullivan, 1979), further refinement is indicated. Investigations that incorporate both diabetes-specific and generic psychosocial measures will have the advantage of promoting our understanding of the connections between global child and family constructs and specific diabetes outcomes, thereby providing an empirical base for developing relevant treatments (Jacobson, 1986). Retaining generic measures of psychosocial functioning is also advantageous in that it allows comparisons to be made between diabetic groups and other pediatric conditions.

Another consideration for future research is the need for longitudinal and prospective research designs. As mentioned throughout this chapter, such research designs are essential for appreciating complex, bidirectional relationships among emotional functioning, diabetes care, and therapeutic outcome. Coping with diabetes is a continual process that evolves and changes over time. This should be reflected in our research efforts.

Finally, it is important to consider developmental aspects of the disease. Factors that are important during the initial stages of the disease may not be as critical or relevant later on. Recent work by Kovacs and colleagues (Kovacs et al., 1985, 1986) indicates that family and individual adjustment improves significantly over the first year after the onset of diabetes. Moreover, family support may be most influential during the early years after diabetes onset. Among adolescents with a short duration of diabetes (2 years or less), Hanson et al. (1989) found family cohesion and flexibility to be strongly related to (better) glycemic functioning; yet, for adolescents with a longer disease duration, associations between family variables and control declined substantially. Studies that are sensitive to the developmental aspects of the child as well as the developmental aspects of the disease will be important for understanding the challenge of diabetes management for youngsters and families affected by this complex, demanding, chronic illness.

ACKNOWLEDGMENT

The preparation of this chapter was supported in part by grant HL 36588-04 from the National Heart, Lung and Blood Institute of NIH.

REFERENCES

Anderson, B. J., Auslander, W. F., Jung, K. C., Miller, J. P., & Santiago, J. (1990). Assessing family sharing of diabetes responsibilities. *Journal of Pediatric Psychology, 15,* 477–492.

Anderson, B. J., Miller, J. P., Auslander, W. F., & Santiago, J. (1981). Family characteristics of diabetic adolescents: Relations to metabolic control. *Diabetes Care, 4,* 586–594.

Baker, L., Barcai, A., Kay, R., & Haque, N. (1969). Beta adrenergic blockade and juvenile diabetes: Acute studies and long-term therapeutic trial. *Journal of Pediatrics, 75,* 19–29.

Barglow, P., Hatcher, R., Edidin, D. V., & Sloan-Rossiter, D. (1984). Stress and metabolic control in diabetes: Psychosomatic evidence and evaluation of methods. *Psychosomatic Medicine, 46,* 127–144.

Belmonte, M. M., Schiffrin, A., Dufresne, J., Suissa, S., Goldman, H., & Polychronakos, C. (1988). Impact of SMBG on control of diabetes as measured by Hb A1: A three year survey. *Diabetes Care, 11,* 484–488.

Blethen, S. L., Sargeant, D. T., Whitlow, M. G., & Santiago, J. V. (1981). Effect of pubertal stage and recent blood glucose control on plasma somatomedin C in children with insulin-dependent diabetes mellitus. *Diabetes, 30,* 868–872.

Bloch, C. A., Clemons, P., & Sperling, M. A. (1987). Puberty decreases insulin sensitivity. *Journal of Pediatrics, 110,* 481–487.

Bobrow, E. S., AvRuskin, T. W., & Siller, J. (1985). Mother-daughter interaction and adherence to diabetes regimens. *Diabetes Care, 8,* 146–151.

Bradley, C. (1979). Life events and the control of diabetes mellitus. *Journal of Psychosomatic Research, 23,* 159–162.

Brand, A. H., Johnson, J. H., & Johnson, S. B. (1986). Life stress and diabetic control in children and adolescents with insulin-dependent diabetes. *Journal of Pediatric Psychology, 11,* 481–495.

Bunn, H. F. (1981). Evaluation of glycosylated hemoglobin in diabetic patients. *Diabetes, 30,* 613–617.

Carter, W. R., Gonder-Frederick, L. A., Cox, D. J., Clarke, W. L., & Scott, D. (1985). Effect of stress on blood glucose control in IDDM. *Diabetes Care, 8,* 411–412.

Chase, H. P., & Jackson, G. G. (1981). Stress and sugar control in children with insulin-dependent diabetes mellitus. *Journal of Pediatrics, 98,* 1011–1013.

Chase, H. P., Jackson, W. E., & Hoops, S. L., Cockerham, R. S., Archer, P. G., & O'Brien, D. (1989). Glucose control and the renal and retinal complications of insulin-dependent diabetes. *Journal of the American Medical Association, 261,* 1155-1160.

Clarson, C., Daneman, D., Drash, A. L., Becker, D. J., & Ehrlich, R. M. (1987). Residual beta-cell function in children with IDDM: Reproducibility of testing and factors influencing insulin secretory reserve. *Diabetes Care, 10,* 33-38.

Cox, D. J., Gonder-Frederick, L. A., & Carter, W. R. (in press). The role of stress in diabetes mellitus. In D. J. Cox & L. A. Gonder-Frederick (Eds.), *Behavioral medicine handbook of diabetes mellitus.* Champaign-Urbana, IL: Research Press.

Cryer, P. E., & Gerich, J. E. (1983). Relevance of counterregulatory system to patients with diabetes: Critical roles of glucagon and epinephrine. *Diabetes Care, 6,* 95-99.

Cryer, P. E., & Gerich, J. E. (1985). Glucose counterregulation, hypoglycemia, and intensive insulin therapy in diabetes mellitus. *New England Journal of Medicine, 313,* 232-241.

Daneman, D., Siminerio, L., Transue, D., Betschart, J., Drash, A. & Becker, D. (1985). The role of self-monitoring of blood glucose in the routine management of children with insulin-dependent diabetes mellitus. *Diabetes Care, 8,* 1-4.

Daneman, D., Wolfson, D. H., Becker, D., & Drash, A. (1981). Factors affecting glycosylated hemoglobin values in children with insulin-dependent diabetes. *Journal of Pediatrics, 99,* 847-853.

Davidson, M. B. (1986a). *Diabetes mellitus: Diagnosis and treatment.* New York: Wiley.

Davidson, M. B. (1986b). Futility of self-monitoring of blood glucose without algorithms for adjusting insulin dose. *Diabetes Care, 9,* 209-210.

Delamater, A. M., Bubb, J., Davis, S., Smith, J., Schmidt, L., White, N., & Santiago, J. V. (1990). Randomized prospective study of self-management training with newly diagnosed diabetic children. *Diabetes Care, 13,* 492-498.

Delamater, A. M., Kurtz, S. M., Bubb, J., White, N., & Santiago, J. V. (1987). Stress and coping in relation to metabolic control of adolescents with Type I diabetes. *Developmental and Behavioral Pediatrics, 8,* 136-140.

Delamater, A. M., Kurtz, S. M., Kuntze, J., Smith, J. A., White, N. H., & Santiago, J. V. (1988). Physiologic responses to acute psychological stress in adolescents with Type I diabetes. *Journal of Pediatric Psychology, 13,* 69-86.

Dunn, S. M., & Turtle, J. R. (1981). The myth of the diabetic personality. *Diabetes Care, 4,* 640-646.

Dupuis, A., Jones, R. L., & Peterson, C. M. (1980). Psychological effects of blood glucose self-monitoring in diabetic patients. *Psychosomatics, 21,* 581-591.

Etzwiler, D. D., & Sines, L. K. (1962). Juvenile diabetes and its management: Family, social, and academic implications. *Journal of the American Medical Association, 181,* 304-308.

Fisher, E. B., Delamater, A., Bertelson, A., & Kirkley, B. (1982). Psychological factors in diabetes and its treatment. *Journal of Consulting and Clinical Psychology, 50,* 993-1003.

Glasgow, R. E., McCaul, K. D., & Schafer, L. C. (1987). Self-care behaviors and glycemic control in Type I diabetes. *Journal of Chronic Diseases, 40,* 399-412.

Glasgow, R. E., Wilson, W., & McCaul, K. D. (1985). Regimen adherence: A problematic construct in diabetes research. *Diabetes Care, 8,* 300-301.

Goetsch, V. L. (1989). Stress and blood glucose in diabetes mellitus: A review and methodological commentary. *Annals of Behavioral Medicine, 11,* 102-107.

Goldstein, D. E., Little, R. R., Wiedmeyer, H. M., England, J. D., & McKenzie, E. M. (1986). Glycated hemoglobin: Methodologies and clinical applications. *Clinical Chemistry, 32,* B64-B70.

Gonen, B., Goldman, J., Baldwin, D., Goldberg, R. B., Ryan, W. G., Blix, P. N., Schanzlin, D., Fritz, K. J., & Rubenstein, A. H. (1979). Metabolic control in diabetic patients: Effect of insulin-secretory reserve (measured by plasma C-peptide levels) and circulating insulin antibodies. *Diabetes, 28,* 749-753.

Grajwer, L. A., Pildes, R. S., Horowitz, D. L., & Rubenstein, A. H. (1977). Control of juvenile diabetes mellitus and its relationship to endogenous insulin secretion as measured by C-peptide and immunoreactivity. *Journal of Pediatrics, 90,* 41–48.

Grant, I., Kyle, G. C., Teichman, A., & Mendels, J. (1974). Recent life events and diabetes in adults. *Psychosomatic Medicine, 36,* 121–128.

Gross, A. M., Delcher, H. K., Snitzer, J., Bianchi, B., & Epstein, S. (1985). Personality variables and metabolic control in children with diabetes. *Journal of Genetic Psychology, 146,* 19–26.

Grossman, H. Y., Brink, S., & Hauser, S. T. (1987). Self-efficacy in adolescent girls and boys with insulin-dependent diabetes mellitus. *Diabetes Care, 10,* 324–329.

Hamburg, B. A., & Inoff, G. E. (1982). Relationships between behavioral factors and diabetic control in children and adolescents: A camp study. *Psychosomatic Medicine, 44,* 321–339.

Hamburg, B. A., Lipsett, L. F., Inoff, G. E., & Drash, A. L. (1979). *Behavioral and psychosocial issues in diabetes: Proceeding of the national conference* (Pub. No. 80–1993). Washington, DC: National Institute of Health.

Hanson, C. L., Henggeler, S. W., & Burghen, G. A. (1987a). Model of associations between psychosocial variables and health-outcome measures in adolescents with IDDM. *Diabetes Care, 10,* 752–763.

Hanson, C. L., Henggeler, S. W., & Burghen, G. A. (1987b). Social competence and parental support as mediators of the link between stress and metabolic control in adolescents with IDDM. *Journal of Consulting and Clinical Psychology, 55,* 529–533.

Hanson, C. L., Henggeler, S. W., Harris, M. A., Burghen, G. A., & Moore, M. (1989). Family system variables and the health status of adolescents with insulin-dependent diabetes mellitus. *Health Psychology, 8,* 239–254.

Hanson, S. L., & Pichert, J. W. (1986). Perceived stress and diabetes control in adolescents. *Health Psychology, 5,* 439–452.

Hauser, S., Jacobson, A., Wertlieb, D., Brink, S., & Wentworth, S. (1985). The contribution of family environment to perceived competence and illness adjustment in diabetic and acutely ill adolescents. *Family Relations, 34,* 99–108.

Hauser, S. T., & Pollets, D. (1979). Psychological aspects of diabetes mellitus: A critical review. *Diabetes Care, 2,* 227–232.

Hinkle, L. E., & Wolf, S. (1952). Importance of life stress in the course of management of diabetes mellitus. *Journal of the American Medical Association, 148,* 513–520.

Jacobson, A. M. (1986). Current status of psychosocial research in diabetes. *Diabetes Care, 9,* 546–547.

Jacobson, A. M., Hauser, S. T., Wertlieb, D., Wolfsdorf, J. I., Orleans, J., & Vieyra, M. (1986). Psychological adjustment of children with recently diagnosed diabetes mellitus. *Diabetes Care, 9,* 323–329.

Johnson, S. B. (1980). Psychological factors in juvenile diabetes. *Journal of Behavioral Medicine, 3,* 95–116.

Johnson, S. B. (1989, June). *Adherence and metabolic control in youngsters with IDDM.* Paper presented at the meeting of the Academy of Behavioral Medicine, Lake Mohonk, N.Y.

Johnson, S. B., Pollack, R. T., Silverstein, J. H., Rosenbloom, A. L., Spillar, R., McCallum, M., & Harkavy, J. (1982). Cognitive and behavioral knowledge about insulin-dependent diabetes among children and parents. *Pediatrics, 69,* 708–713.

Johnson, S. B., Silverstein, J. R., Rosenbloom, A., Carter, R., & Cunningham, W. (1986). Assessing daily management in childhood diabetes. *Health Psychology, 5,* 545–564.

Kaplan, R. M., Chadwick, M. W., & Schimmel, L. E. (1985). Social learning intervention to promote metabolic control in Type I diabetes mellitus: Pilot experimental results. *Diabetes Care, 8,* 152–155.

Keen, H. & Jarrett, J. (Eds.). (1982). *Complications of diabetes* (2nd ed.). London: Arnold.

Klein, R. (1988). Recent developments in the understanding and management of diabetic retinopathy. *Medical Clinics of North America, 72,* 1415–1437.

Klein, R., Klein, B., & Moss, S. E. (1985). A population-based study of diabetic retinopathy in insulin-using patients diagnosed before 30 years of age. *Diabetes Care, 8*(Suppl 1), 71–76.

Klemp, S. B., & La Greca, A. M. (1987). Adolescents with IDDM: The role of family cohesion and conflict. *Diabetes, 36*(Suppl 1), 18A.

Kovacs, M., Brent, D., Steinberg, T. F., Paulauskas, S., & Reid, J. (1986). Children's self-reports of psychologic adjustment and coping strategies during first year of insulin-dependent diabetes mellitus. *Diabetes Care, 9,* 472–479.

Kovacs, M., Feinberg, T. L., Paulauskas, S., Finkelstein, R., Pollock, M., & Crouse-Novack, M. (1985). Initial coping responses and psychosocial characteristics of children with insulin-dependent diabetes mellitus. *Journal of Pediatrics, 106,* 827–834.

Kuttner, M. J., Delamater, A. M., & Santiago, J. V. (1990). Learned helplessness in diabetic youth. *Journal of Pediatric Psychology, 15,* in press.

Krolewski, A. S., Warram, J. H., Rand, L. I., Christlieb, A. R., Busick, E. J., & Kahn, C. R. (1986). Risk of proliferative diabetic retinopathy in juvenile onset Type I diabetes: A 40-year follow-up study. *Diabetes Care, 9,* 443–452.

La Greca, A. M. (1988). Children with diabetes and their families: Coping and disease management. In T. M. Field, P. M. McCabe, & N. Schneiderman (Eds.), *Stress and coping across development* (pp. 139–159). Hillsdale, NJ: Lawrence Erlbaum Associates.

La Greca, A. M. (1989, June). *Psychosocial aspects of diabetes: A multivariate model.* Paper presented at the annual meeting of the Academy for Behavioral Medicine Research. Lake Mohonk, NY.

La Greca, A. M. (1990a). Issues in adherence with pediatric regimens. *Journal of Pediatric Psychology, 15,* 285–307.

La Greca, A. M. (1990b). Social consequences of pediatric conditions: Fertile area for future investigation and intervention? *Journal of Pediatric Psychology, 15,* 285–308.

La Greca, A. M., Follansbee, D., & Skyler, J. S. (1990). Developmental and behavioral aspects of diabetes management in children and adolescents. *Children's Health Care.*

La Greca, A. M., & Hanna, N. C. (1983). Health beliefs of children with diabetes and their mothers: Implications for treatment. *Diabetes, 32*(Supplement), 66.

La Greca, A. M., & Skyler, J. S. (1991). Psychosocial issues in IDDM: A multivariate framework. In P. M. McCabe, N. Schneiderman, T. M. Field, & J. S. Skyler (Eds.), *Stress, coping and disease* (pp. 169–190). Hillsdale, NJ: Lawrence Erlbaum Associates.

La Greca, A. M., Swales, T., Klemp, S., & Madigan, S. (1988). Self care behaviors among adolescents with diabetes. *Proceedings of the Ninth Annual Sessions of the Society of Behavioral Medicine,* Boston, A42.

Lane, J. D., Stabler, B., Ross, S. L., Morris, M. A., Litton, J. C., & Surwit, R. S. (1988). Psychological predictors of glucose control in patients with IDDM. *Diabetes Care, 11,* 798–800.

Ludvigsson, J., Heding, L. G., Larsson, Y., Leander, E. (1977). C-peptide in juvenile diabetics beyond the postinitial remission period. *Acta Pediatrica Scandinavia, 66,* 177–184.

Mann, N. P., Johnston, D. I. (1984). Improvement in metabolic control in diabetic adolescents by the use of increased insulin dose. *Diabetes Care, 7,* 460–464.

Marner, B., Agner, T., Binder, C., Lernmark, A., Nerup, J., Mandrup-Poulsen, T., & Walldorff, S. (1985). Increased reduction in fasting C-peptide is associated with islet cell antibodies in Type I (insulin-dependent) diabetic patients. *Diabetologia, 28,* 875–880.

Marteau, T. M., Johnston, M., Baum, J. D., & Bloch, S. (1987). Goals of treatment in diabetes: A comparison of doctors and parents of children with diabetes. *Journal of Behavioral Medicine, 10,* 33–48.

Marrero, D. G., Jacobs, S. V., & Orr, D. P. (1981). The influence of social support on adolescent diabetic metabolic control. *Diabetes* (Suppl), A 45.

Mazze, R. S., Lucide, D., & Shamoon, H. (1984). Psychological and social correlates of glycemic control. *Diabetes Care, 7,* 60–66.

Minuchin, S., Rosman, B., & Baker, L. (1978). *Psychosomatic families.* Cambridge, MA: Harvard University Press.

Orr, D. P., Golden, M. P., Myers, G., & Marrero, D. G. (1983). Characteristics of adolescents with poorly controlled diabetes referred to a tertiary care center. *Diabetes Care, 6,* 170–175.

Pedersen, O., & Beck-Nielsen, H. (1987). Insulin resistance and insulin-dependent diabetes mellitus. *Diabetes Care, 10,* 516–523.

Rovet, J. F., & Ehrlich, R. M. (1988). Effect of temperament on metabolic control in children with diabetes mellitus. *Diabetes Care, 11,* 77–82.

Ryan, C. M., & Morrow, L. A. (1986). Self-esteem in diabetic adolescents: Relationship between age at onset and gender. *Journal of Consulting and Clinical Psychology, 54,* 730–731.

Schade, D. S., Santiago, J. V., Skyler, J. S., & Rizza, R. A. (1983). *Intensive insulin therapy.* Princeton, NJ: Excerpta Medica.

Schafer, L. C., Glasgow, R. E., McCaul, K. D., & Dreher, M. (1983). Adherence to IDDM regimens: Relationship to psychosocial variables and metabolic control. *Diabetes Care, 6,* 493–498.

Schafer, L. C., McCaul, K. D., & Glasgow, R. E. (1986). Supportive and non-supportive family behaviors: Relationships to adherence and metabolic control in persons with Type I diabetes. *Diabetes Care, 9,* 179–185.

Schiffrin, A. (1987). Management of childhood diabetes. *Pediatric Annals, 16,* 694–710.

Seigler, D. E., La Greca, A. M., Citrin, W. S., Reeves, M. L., & Skyler, S. (1982). Psychological effects of intensification of diabetic control. *Diabetes Care, 5*(Suppl 1), 19–23.

Shapiro, J., Wigg, D., Charles, M. A., & Perley, M. (1984). Personality and family profiles of chronic insulin-dependent diabetic patients using portable insulin infusion pump therapy: A preliminary investigation. *Diabetes Care, 7,* 137–142.

Simonds, J. F. (1976–1977). Psychiatric status of diabetic youth in good and poor control. *International Journal of Psychiatry in Medicine, 7,* 133–151.

Simonds, J., Goldstein, D., Walker, B., & Rawlings, S. (1981). The relationship between psychological factors and blood glucose regulation in insulin-dependent diabetic adolescents. *Diabetes Care, 4,* 610–615.

Simonds, J. G. (1977). Psychiatric status of diabetic youth matched with a control group. *Diabetes, 26,* 921–925.

Skyler, J. S. (1987). Why control diabetes? Influence on chronic complications of diabetes. *Pediatric Annals, 16,* 713–724.

Skyler, J. S., Skyler, D. L., Seigler, D. E., & O'Sullivan, M. J. (1981). Algorithms for adjustment of insulin dosage by patients who monitor blood glucose. *Diabetes Care, 4,* 311–318.

Stabler, B., Surwit, R. S., Lane, J. D., Morris, M. A., Litton, J., & Feinglos, M. (1987). Type A behavior pattern and blood glucose control in diabetic children. *Psychosomatic Medicine, 49,* 313–316.

Sullivan, B. J. (1979). Adjustment in diabetic adolescent girls: Development of the diabetic adjustment scale. *Psychosomatic Medicine, 41,* 119–126.

Sullivan, B. J. (1978). Self-esteem and depression in adolescent diabetic girls. *Diabetes Care, 1,* 18–22.

Surwit, R. S., Scovern, A. W., & Feinglos, M. N. (1982). The role of behavior in diabetes care. *Diabetes Care, 5,* 337–342.

Swift, C. F., Seidman, F., & Stein, H. (1967). Adjustment problems in juvenile diabetics. *Psychosomatic Medicine, 29,* 555–571.

Wertlieb, D., Hauser, S. T., & Jacobson, A. M. (1986). Adaptation to diabetes: Behavior symptoms and family context. *Journal of Pediatric Psychology, 11,* 463–479.

White, K., Kolman, M. L., Wexler, P., Polin, G., & Winter, R. J. (1984). Unstable diabetes and unstable families: A psychosocial evaluation of diabetic children with recurrent ketoacidosis. *Pediatrics, 73,* 749–755.

Wing, R. R., Koeske, R., New, A., Lamparski, D., & Becker, D. (1986). Behavioral skills in self-monitoring of blood glucose: Relationship to accuracy. *Diabetes Care, 9,* 330 333.

Wing, R. R., Lamparski, D., Zaslow, S., Betschart, J., Siminerio, L., & Becker, D. (1985). Frequency and accuracy of self-monitoring of blood glucose in children: Relationship to glycemic control. *Diabetes Care, 8,* 214–218.

Wysocki, T., Green, L., & Huxtable, K. (1989). Blood glucose monitoring by diabetic adolescents: Compliance and metabolic control. *Health Psychology, 8,* 267–284.

Yki-Jarvinen, H., & Kovisto, V. A. (1986). Natural course of insulin resistance in Type I diabetes. *New England Journal of Medicine, 315,* 224–227.

15

Compliance and Control in Insulin-Dependent Diabetes: Does Behavior Really Make a Difference?

Suzanne Bennett Johnson
University of Florida Health Science Center

Pancreatic beta-cell destruction and the resultant inability of the pancreas to produce insulin is the pathological process underlying insulin-dependent diabetes mellitus (IDDM). Because insulin insufficiency is the underlying cause of this disease, treatment involves insulin replacement by injection once or twice a day. Exogenous insulin replacement prolongs life, but only crudely approximates normal pancreatic function. Although the goal of treatment is to maintain the patient's blood glucose within the normal range, blood glucose excursions readily occur in response to eating, exercise, illness, and stress. Consequently, the management of this disease requires a complex array of daily insulin injection, dietary, and exercise behaviors. In addition, the patient is taught to conduct multiple blood glucose tests to monitor current health status and to take appropriate action should significant blood glucose excursions occur.

IDDM is only one form of diabetes. Also known at Type I diabetes, onset typically occurs in childhood. Consequently, it is commonly referred to as juvenile or childhood diabetes. IDDM has no cure; children diagnosed with this disease remain diabetic throughout their lives. Hence, IDDM is a disease of both childhood and adulthood.

Most adult diabetics, however, suffer from noninsulin-dependent diabetes mellitus (NIDDM), also known as adult or Type II diabetes. When discussing the prevalence of IDDM, it is common to compare it with the prevalence of NIDDM. This comparison makes the problem of diabetes in children appear small because only 5% of all persons with diabetes in the United States have the juvenile form of the disorder. However, if one compares IDDM with other chronic diseases of childhood, a different picture emerges. In the United States, about 1 child in 600 (approximately 120,000 youngsters) has IDDM (LaPorte & Tajima, 1985). The risk of developing IDDM is higher than that for most other chronic diseases of childhood. It is equal to that of all childhood cancers combined and is much greater than that of other well-known diseases, such as cystic fibrosis, muscular dystrophy, and rheumatoid arthritis (La Porte & Cruickshanks, 1985).

As with other complex medical regimens, nonadherence is a major problem in IDDM populations. Watkins, Williams, Martin, Hogan, and Anderson (1967) published some of the first empirical data documenting the extent of this problem in adult patients. Over half were making insulin dosage errors, two thirds were testing incorrectly, and three quarters were judged "unacceptable" in terms of the quality, quantity, and timing of meals. More recent studies have documented similar problems among juveniles with this disease. We found that 40% of children studied were making insulin injection errors and 80% were making glucose testing errors (Johnson et al., 1982). Frequent errors in reading urine glucose tests were also reported by Epstein, Coburn, Becker, Drash, and Siminerio (1980), who noted that most of these errors were in one direction: The children tended to underestimate their urine–glucose concentrations.

In juveniles, nonadherence is far more common among adolescents. In a 1986 study, we compared four different age groups of children on 13 different diabetes adherence behaviors (Johnson, Silverstein, Rosenbloom, Carter, & Cunningham, 1986). Older youngsters were significantly less adherent on 8 of the 13 measures. They exercised less often, they administered their insulin injections at more irregular times and at less than ideal intervals, and they did not abide by the recommended injection time of 30 minutes before meal consumption. They also ate too much fat, too little carbohydrates, and ate and tested glucose less often. We have conducted a second study (Johnson, Freund, Silverstein, Hansen, & Malone, 1990), with a smaller sample, that essentially replicated these results: Significant age effects emerged for 7 of the 13 adherence behaviors, in all cases older youngsters were less adherent.

Although adherence is presumed to be related to diabetes control (i.e., how well blood glucose levels are maintained within the normal range), there have been surprisingly few empirical tests of this assumption. In fact, the literature documenting the prevalence of noncompliance in this population is larger than the literature documenting a link between compliance behaviors and diabetes control! Often, it is simply assumed that strict adherence leads to good control and poor adherence results in poor control. This assumption is so ingrained that most physicians assess adherence using measures of diabetes control! In 1985, Clarke, Snyder, and Nowacek conducted a survey of U.S. diabetologists. The diabetologists were asked how they assessed patient compliance in their clinics; 89% stated that they used glycosylated hemoglobin levels. Glycosylated hemoglobin is an index of the patient's average blood glucose level over the past 2 to 3 months and is the most widely accepted measure of diabetes control (Ziel & Davidson, 1987). It is a laboratory assay, not a measure of behavior. Yet, it is the measure of adherence used in the vast majority of pediatric clinics, highlighting the very ingrained assumption that adherence and diabetes control are so powerfully linked that one can be used as an index of the other.

The available literature contrasts sharply with this assumption as researchers have failed to document consistent, clinically significant relationships between compliance and diabetes control in IDDM samples. Using self-report data yielding a single adherence composite score, several researchers have reported low but statistically significant correlations between adherence and diabetes control (Brownlee-Duffeck et al., 1987; Hanson, Henggeler, & Burghen, 1987a). However, others using similar measures have failed to find significant relationships (Cox, Taylor, Nowacek, Holley-Wilcox, & Pohl, 1984; Hanson, Henggeler, & Burghen, 1987b; Simonds, Goldstein, Walker, & Rawlings, 1981). Kaplan, Chadwick, and Schimmel's (1985) report is noteworthy because of its high reported correlation between 19 IDDM adolescents' self-reported adherence behavior and their level of glycosylated hemoglobin ($r = -.78$). The authors reported a similar significant correlation between the adolescents' glycosylated hemoglobin levels and their scores on a Lie Scale, raising questions as to the validity of the adolescents' self-reported adherence data. Further, there is increasing evidence that adherence behaviors in diabetes are relatively independent of one another (Glasgow, McCaul, & Schafer, 1987; Johnson et al., 1986; Orme & Binik, 1989; Schafer, Glasgow, McCaul, & Dreher, 1983; Webb et al., 1984). Consequently, global ratings or composite scores of adherence may not adequately reflect the complexity of diabetes regimen behaviors.

Some investigators have studied particular diabetes adherence behaviors, such as dietary practices or blood glucose monitoring, and have attempted to link these specific behaviors to diabetes control. Again, inconsistent findings have emerged. Webb et al. (1984) reported that dietary compliance appeared to be related to diabetes control in a sample of IDDM adults. However, two intervention studies that improved patients' dietary adherence failed to produce concomitant changes in their diabetes control (Webb et al., 1982, 1984). Christensen, Terry, Wyatt, Pichert, and Lorenz (1983) reported that dietary compliance appeared to be associated with better diabetes control, but their statistical tests of this relationship only approached significance. Kaar, Akerblom, Huttunen, Knip, and Sakkinen (1984) reported that a nurse's rating of children's dietary compliance was related to the youngsters' diabetes control. However, this study can be criticized for measurement dependence. The nurse who made the dietary compliance ratings also knew the patient's current diabetes control status; this may have spuriously inflated the relationship between the two. An interesting study by Wing and her colleagues (Wing, Nowalk, Marcus, Koseke, & Finegold, 1986) did not assess daily dietary practices, but did find that unusual dietary behaviors, most notably bulemic behaviors, were associated with poorer diabetes control in IDDM adolescents.

Home blood glucose monitoring is the other specific regimen behavior that has attracted considerable empirical attention. Once again, highly compliant glucose testing behavior has not always been linked to good diabetes control. Gonder-Frederick, Julian, Cox, Clarke, and Carter (1988) reported that adult patients' self-reports of home blood glucose monitoring were linked to diabetes control but Wilson and Endres (1986) were unable to document such a relationship in a sample of IDDM adolescents. Some early intervention studies that used behavior therapy to improve patient adherence with glucose testing found concomitant changes in the patient's diabetes control (Carney, Schechter, & Davis, 1983; Schafer, Glasgow, & McCaul, 1982), but others did not (Epstein et al., 1981). More recent studies that have successfully increased the frequency and accuracy of home blood glucose monitoring in IDDM patients have been unable to document a link between increased home blood glucose monitoring and a subsequent improvement in diabetes control (Daneman et al., 1985; Mazze, Pasmantier, Murphy, & Shamoon, 1985; Wysocki, Green, & Huxtable, 1989).

Glasgow and his colleagues have published some of the most comprehensive studies of adherence/diabetes control relationships in IDDM populations. They treat insulin injection, dietary, exercise, and glucose testing behaviors as separate aspects of the diabetes regimen, instead of using a single compliance rating or composite score. Their early work documented some relationship between dietary, insulin injection, and glucose testing behaviors, and diabetes control in a small sample of IDDM adolescents (Schafer et al., 1983). However, their subsequent studies, conducted with larger samples and with greater methodological sophistication, failed to find any consistent relationship between patients' regimen behaviors and their diabetes control (Glasgow et al., 1987; Schafer, McCaul, & Glasgow, 1986).

Studies that have attempted to link adherence behaviors to health status in IDDM have varied in methodological rigor. Some studies have used global measures of adherence that may be insensitive to the complexities of the diabetes regimen. Most use self-report measures of adherence that are uncorroborated by another family member. None have repeatedly assessed multiple adherence behaviors across time to ensure that the temporal interval during which adherence is assessed is congruent with the temporal interval indexed by the diabetes control measure.

The typical intervention study has attempted to improve patients' metabolic status by improving regimen adherence. Ideally, intervention research should consider both behavioral and health status measures when evaluating outcome. Early studies focused solely on behavior although the goal of treatment was to improve health status by improving adherence (e.g., Gross, 1982; Gross, Johnson, Wildman, & Mullet, 1981; Lowe & Lutzker, 1979). More recent interventions have documented improved metabolic status as the result of a psychological intervention, but the mechanism of the treatment effect, improved adherence, was not carefully monitored (e.g., Anderson, Wolf, Burkhart, Cornell, & Bacon, 1989, Kaplan et al., 1985; Satin, La Greca, Zigo, & Skyler, 1989). A limited number of studies have provided data on both adherence behavior and health status (e.g., Carney et al., 1983; Epstein et al., 1981; Rubin, Peyrot, & Saudek, 1989; Schafer et al., 1982; Wysocki et al., 1989). Unfortunately, these studies fail to document a consistent association between improved adherence and improved metabolic status (e.g., Epstein et al., 1981; Wysocki et al., 1989). Further, despite data availability, the presumed relationship between changes in adherence and changes in diabetes control often remains untested (e.g., Rubin et al., 1989).

We have conducted a series of studies attempting to link adherence behaviors to diabetes control. However, before I describe these studies in more detail, more information about how we measure diabetes adherence should prove helpful.

MEASURING DIABETES ADHERENCE BEHAVIORS

Haynes (1979), probably the most cited author on the subject, defined *compliance* as "the extent to which a person's behavior (in terms of taking medication, following diets, or executing lifestyle changes) coincides with medical or health advice" (pp. 2–3). In diabetes, however, the medical advice is often very unclear. Physicians typically prescribe an insulin dose but documented prescriptions with regard to diet, exercise, and even timing of injections are usually unavailable. Instead, patients are given general prescriptions, such as "get some exercise" or "avoid sugar." These general prescriptions lack specificity and are usually undocumented. Consequently, the investigator is left with little in terms of a medical prescription except insulin type and dose. Glasgow, Wilson, and McCaul (1985) have recommended that "levels of self-care behaviors" be measured when there is no clear provider prescription available and that the terms *adherence* or *compliance* be avoided. However, because we were interested in adherence/diabetes control linkages, we decided to identify adherence standards that were either prescribed by the American Diabetes Association (ADA), stated in medical textbooks, or generally accepted within the medical community.

We identified 14 daily diabetes adherence behaviors to be monitored: 5 injection behaviors; 5 dietary behaviors; 3 exercise behaviors, and 1 glucose testing behavior. We ultimately dropped the first injection behavior, the percent of prescribed injections actually taken, because of uniformly high compliance; this measure exhibited so little variability that it was considered useless for research purposes. Glasgow et al. (1987) have also reported high compliance rates for this particular adherence measure. Table 15.1 provides a brief description of the remaining 13 adherence behaviors.

The advantages and disadvantages of various methods of measuring

TABLE 15.1
A Brief Description of 13 Adherence Measures Quantified From 24-Hour Recall Interview Data

Injection Behaviors

Injection Regularity: The degree to which injections are given at the same time every day.
Injection Interval: The degree to which the time between injections approaches ideal.
Injection-Meal Timing: The degree to which injections are given 30–60 minutes before eating.
Regularity of Injection-Meal Timing: The degree to which the time between injection and eating is consistent across days.

Exercise Behaviors

Exercise Frequency: How often a youngster exercises on a daily basis.
Exercise Duration: How long a youngster exercises on any exercise occasion.
Exercise Type: The strenuousness of the youngster's exercise.

Dietary Behaviors

% Calories: Carbohydrate: Percentage of total calories consumed consisting of carbohydrates in relationship to the 60% ideal recommended by the American Diabetes Association (Nuttal & Brunzall, 1979).
% Calories: Fat: Percentage of total calories consumed consisting of fats in relationship to the 25% ideal recommended by the American Diabetes Association (Nuttal & Brunzall, 1979).
Calories Consumed: The youngster's ideal total number of daily calories (based on age, sex, and height) subtracted from the youngster's reported daily calorie consumption.
Concentrated Sweets: The average number of concentrated sweet exchange units eaten on a daily basis (40 calories of any concentrated sweet equals one concentrated sweet exchange unit).
Eating Frequency: How often a youngster eats on a daily basis.

Glucose Testing

Testing Frequency: How often a youngster conducts a glucose test on a daily basis.

Note: For additional details concerning the definition and quantification of the 13 adherence measures, see Johnson, Silverstein, Rosenbloom, Carter, & Cunningham (1986).

adherence have been reviewed elsewhere (Johnson, 1990). Consequently, I restrict my comments to the particular method we selected: a modification of the 24-hour recall interview. The 24-hour recall interview has long been a standard dietary assessment technique and is considered the best of the available self-report methods (Marquis, Ware, & Relles, 1979). We expanded the interview to include all diabetes-relevant behaviors. Unlike the usual dietary assessment procedure in which one interview is conducted with a single informant, we conduct at least three interviews to ensure a more representative sample of daily diabetes management behavior. Instead of using a single informant, we conduct interviews with both the youngster and his or her mother. Each is interviewed separately about the youngster's behavior during the preceding 24 hours. The previous day's events are recalled in temporal sequence beginning with the child's awakening in the morning and ending with retiring to bed. To encourage honest reporting, all interviews are conducted by trained nonmedical personnel who are not associated with the clinic staff. Combining data obtained from both informants helps reduce memory errors associated with any recall procedure.

Obtaining adherence data from both mother and child permits estimates of parent-child agreement that have bearing on the reliability and validity of the procedure. Although perfect agreement cannot be expected because parents do not observe all of their children's activities, statistically significant correlations between child and parent reports have been documented in three separate samples (Freund, Johnson, Silverstein, & Thomas, 1991; Johnson, Silverstein, Rosenbloom, Carter, & Cunningham, 1986; Spevack, Johnson, & Riley, 1991; see Table 15.2); most are in the moderate to high range. Additional validity data have been obtained by comparing children's 24-hour recalls with observed behavior in a diabetes camp setting. For most diabetes management behaviors, the children's recalls exhibited good agreement with the observers' reports. However, the children tended to underestimate food consumption (Reynolds, Johnson, & Silverstein, 1990). Combining the data from both the child and parent recalls may help minimize this underestimation bias.

Although there are a myriad of diabetes regimen behaviors expected of the child, physicians and researchers have tended to treat adherence or compliance as a unitary trait or concept. Patients are described as "compliant" or "noncompliant" as if they exhibit a consistent pattern of disease management behavior. We addressed this issue by subjecting the 13 adherence behaviors, quantified from 24-hour recall data, to a principle component factor analysis (Johnson, Silverstein, Rosenbloom, Carter, & Cunningham, 1986). If a unitary conceptualization of adherence is correct, a single-factor solution should have emerged. Instead, a five-factor solution resulted accounting for over 70% of the variance. The first four of these factors were confirmed in a subsequent confirmatory factor analysis, but

TABLE 15.2
Parent–Child Agreement For 13 Diabetes Adherence Behaviors

Adherence Measures	Johnson et al. (1986) (n = 168) r (p<)	Freund et al. (1991) (n = 78) r (p<)	Spevack et al. (1991) (n = 64) r (p<)
Injection Behaviors			
Injection Regularity	.61 (.0001)	.62 (.0001)	.65 (.0001)
Injection Interval	.77 (.0001)	.74 (.0001)	.75 (.0001)
Injection-Meal Timing	.67 (.0001)	.64 (.0001)	.54 (.0001)
Regularity of Injection-Meal Timing	.42 (.0001)	.33 (.005)	.09 (ns)
Exercise Behaviors			
Exercise Frequency	.62 (.0001)	.75 (.0001)	.68 (.0001)
Exercise Duration	.59 (.0001)	.72 (.0001)	.29 (.02)
Exercise Type	.54 (.0001)	.76 (.0001)	.64 (.0001)
Dietary Behaviors			
Eating Frequency	.45 (.0001)	.65 (.0001)	.72 (.0001)
Calories Consumed	.77 (.0001)	.72 (.0001)	.73 (.0001)
% Calories: Carbohydrate	.64 (.0001)	.76 (.0001)	.72 (.0001)
% Calories: Fat	.64 (.0001)	.75 (.0001)	.78 (.0001)
Concentrated Sweets	.62 (.0001)	.67 (.0001)	.63 (.0001)
Glucose Testing Behavior			
Testing Frequency	.78 (.0001)	.94 (.0001)	.90 (.0001)

the fifth factor was not. It appeared that the two indicators of the fifth factor were better treated as separate constructs (Johnson, Tomer, Cunningham, & Henretta, 1990). Taken together, our factor-analytic studies suggest that adherence or compliance in diabetes is a multidimensional concept. There are at least six different adherence components that need to be assessed:

1. insulin injection, which is indexed by four different injection behaviors (i.e., regularity, interval, injection–meal timing, regularity of injection–meal timing);
2. exercise, which is indexed by three different exercise behaviors (i.e., duration, frequency, and strenuousness);
3. diet type, which is indexed by two measures (i.e., percent of total calories consumed consisting of carbohydrates, percent of total calories consumed consisting of fat);
4. testing/eating frequency, which is indexed by the frequency of meals and snacks and the frequency of glucose tests conducted;

5. calories consumed, a measure of the total calories consumed above or below an ideal based on the youngster's gender, age, and height; and

6. concentrated sweets, which consists of the amount of simple sugars consumed on a daily basis.

In all of our studies, we have considered compliance/control linkages between each of these six adherence constructs and glycosylated hemoglobin. This widely accepted index of diabetes control provides an index of average blood glucose levels over the past 2 to 3 months (Ziel & Davidson, 1987).

STUDY 1: A PRELIMINARY CROSS-SECTIONAL INVESTIGATION

Our first study (Johnson, Silverstein, Rosenbloom, Hansen, Carter, & Cunningham, 1986) was a cross-sectional analysis in which we attempted to link the adherence behaviors of 193 youngsters with their glycosylated hemoglobin levels. The data were collected during the years 1982 and 1983. The youngsters ranged in age from 6 to 19 years and had diabetes for at least 1 year. Blood was drawn for glycosylated hemoglobin (Hgb_{a1}) assay during a regularly scheduled clinic visit or upon arrival at diabetes summer camp. Adherence was measured by three 24-hour recall interviews, conducted with the child and parent, during the 2 weeks prior to or, for some of the clinic visits, immediately after the blood draw. The 24-hour recall interviews focused on two weekdays and one weekend day.

Data from the recall interviews were used to quantify the 13 adherence measures (see Table 15.1) which, in turn, were grouped into adherence constructs or factors. Each adherence measure was constructed so that scores close to zero indicated near perfect compliance and scores deviating from zero indicated increasing degrees of noncompliance (see Johnson, Silverstein, Rosenbloom, Carter, & Cunningham, 1986, for additional details). The 13 adherence measures were then standardized to the 1982 data set (on which the original factor analysis was based, see Johnson, Silverstein, Rosenbloom, Carter, & Cunningham, 1986) and grouped into adherence factors.

Hierarchical multiple regression (Cohen & Cohen, 1983) was used to test the relationship between the adherence factors and Hgb_{a1}. Cohort year, age, disease duration, and sex were entered first. Sex failed to offer predictive power and was dropped from subsequent analyses. The remaining variables were retained due to their significant association with Hgb_{a1}. Each adherence factor was added to the model singly or in combination; no significant increase in the R^2 occurred. Finally, interactions between each adherence factor and age and between each adherence factor and disease duration were considered. Only the injection factor offered predictive power, interacting with age.

This model is depicted in Table 15.3. Cohort year was a significant predictor of Hgb_{a1}; we attributed this to differences in laboratory assay technique that may have occurred between the 1982 and 1983 samples. Age was also a significant predictor. Older youngsters had higher Hgb_{a1} levels (i.e., worse diabetes control) which is consistent with clinical lore; deterioration in diabetes control is common during the adolescent years. Disease duration was a third significant predictor. As expected, longer diabetes duration was associated with poorer diabetes control (i.e., higher Hgb_{a1}). The interaction between injection and age was interpreted by calculating the nonstandardized beta weights for injection for varying ages from 6 to 19 using the regression equation depicted in Table 15.4 (as suggested by Cohen & Cohen, 1983). As is apparent from this table, injection behaviors in younger children (e.g., 6–9 years) were associated with Hgb_{a1} in the expected direction: Less compliant behavior (i.e., higher injection scores) was associated with higher Hgb_{a1} values (i.e., poorer diabetes control). In early adolescence, the relationship between injection behavior and Hgb_{a1} diminished to near zero. And in older adolescents (e.g., 16–19 years), the reverse trend was observed: Less compliant behavior (i.e., higher injection scores) was associated with lower Hgb_{a1} values (i.e., better diabetes control).

Table 15.5 depicts Hgb_{a1}, the injection factor scores, and the injection measures making up the injection factor by age group. Note that the adolescents were less adherent and were in worse diabetes control than their younger counterparts. Yet, the hierarchical multiple regression analyses failed to support a direct link between poorer injection adherence and poorer diabetes control. In fact, this relationship was more apparent in the younger as compared to the older youngsters.

Interpretation of these findings is difficult. It is possible that during early adolescence changes in sex and growth hormone production may be sufficiently powerful to diminish the effects of adherence seen in younger

TABLE 15.3
Study I: Hgb_{a1} Predicted by Cohort Year, Age, Disease Duration, Injection, and Injection × Age

Variable	Standardized B	p<	$R^2 = .212$
Cohort Year	−.16	.02	
Age	.25	.0003	
Disease Duration	.27	.0001	
Injection	.77	.03	
Injection × Age	−.83	.02	

TABLE 15.4
Study I: Nonstandardized Injection Beta
Weights at Varying Ages*

Age in years	Injection B weight
6	1.77
7	1.53
8	1.29
9	1.05
10	.81
11	.57
12	.33
13	.09
14	−.15
15	−.39
16	−.63
17	−.87
18	−1.11
19	−1.35

*$\hat{Y} = 8.32 - .91$ (Year) $+ .27$ (Age) $+ .23$ (Disease Duration) $+ 3.21$ (Injection) $- .24$ (Injection $\times$ Age).

TABLE 15.5
Study I: Hgb$_{a1}$[a] and Injection Measures[b] by Age Group

Age:	6–9	10–12	13–15	16–19
n =	40	89	49	15
Hgb$_{a1}$ %	10.99	11.98	13.20	13.32
Injection Factor Scores (standardized)	−.17	−.16	.21	.72
Injection Regularity (minutes)*	.48 (28.8)	.56 (33.6)	.85 (51.0)	1.13 (67.8)
Injection Interval (minutes)*	.69 (41.4)	.87 (52.2)	1.23 (73.8)	1.6 (96.6)
Injection-Meal Timing (minutes before meal)*	.76 (14.4)	.72 (16.8)	.86 (8.4)	.92 (4.8)
Regularity of Injection-Meal Timing (minutes)	25.56	18.60	21.91	43.36

[a]Lower scores indicate better diabetes control. [b]Lower scores indicate greater compliance.
*Numbers in parentheses provide an interpretation of the adherence measure using as more familiar measurement scale.

children. However, this does not explain the negative relationship between adherence and Hgb$_{a1}$ seen in older youngsters. Perhaps older adolescents who are in worse control are prodded by parents and physicians to become more adherent. Because efforts to become more adherent occur in response to the adolescent's poor diabetes control, the relationship between injection adherence and Hgb_{a1} is negative. Of course, such an interpretation is speculative at best. Longitudinal data would address this issue better by permitting changes in behavior to be associated with changes in health status over time.

Overall, the results of this initial study were disappointing. Only one of the adherence factors, injection, showed a significant association with Hgb_{a1}. The expected association between injection adherence and Hgb_{a1} occurred only for younger patients. In early adolescence there appeared to be no association and among older adolescents an inverse relationship occurred. Further, the addition of injection and its interaction with age to the model accounted for only 2% more variance than was predicted by patient demographics (i.e., age, disease duration, and cohort year). The full model accounted for only 21% of Hgb_{a1} variance. Clearly, our efforts to document a powerful link between adherence and diabetes control had met with failure.

However, this study, like all studies, had methodological shortcomings. We had two primary concerns. First, the study was cross-sectional; patients were studied at a single point in time. The absence of at least two repeated measures of Hgb_{a1} left us unable to detect whether change in Hgb_{a1} may be related to more or less adherent behavior. This is analogous to studying people's weight and eating habits. Although overall, there may be a relationship between weight and eating when weight and eating are measured only once, thin people who are eating a lot to gain weight and fat people who are dieting to lose weight are certainly going to diminish the relationship between weight and eating for the sample as a whole. A more sensitive method of studying weight (or Hgb_{a1}) and eating (or adherence) is to measure the health status indicator (e.g., weight or Hgb_{a1}) twice, and to measure adherence behavior (e.g., dietary habits) during the interval between the two health status measurements. Ideally, the two health status measurements should be taken at intervals during which a change in behavior could result in a change in health status.

This brings us to our second primary concern: the temporal congruity between the health status and the behavioral measures. Ideally, the temporal interval indexed by the health status and the behavioral measures should be the same. This did not occur in this initial investigation. Hgb_{a1} measures average blood glucose over a 2 to 4 month interval. For the behavioral measures to be temporally congruent with Hgb_{a1}, the 24-hour recall interviews should have been conducted for 2 to 3 months *before* the blood draw for the Hgb_{a1} assay. Instead, the interviews were conducted over 2 weeks and sometimes occurred after the blood draw for the laboratory assay. This lack of temporal congruity between Hgb_{a1} and the adherence measures may have further diminished the relationship between the two.

STUDY 2: A LONGITUDINAL ANALYSIS OF ADHERENCE/DIABETES CONTROL RELATIONSHIPS USING A 3-MONTH TEMPORAL INTERVAL

We set out to correct these methodological flaws in a second study of 78 youngsters with IDDM (Johnson, Freund, Silverstein, Hanson, & Malone, 1990). This study was labor intensive because we measured glycosylated hemoglobin levels at the beginning and the end of a 3-month study interval and we collected adherence data on nine separate occasions across the 3-month interval. Like Study 1, youngsters ranged in age from 6 to 19 yrs and had diabetes for a minimum of 1 year. Once again, adherence was measured using the 24-hour recall interview method; interviews were conducted with both parent and child. By the time this study was conducted, our laboratory had switched from a Hgb_{a1} to a Hgb_{a1c} assay. However, this had no substantive impact on the question we wished to address.

Despite our methodological improvements, we found little evidence that adherence behaviors were linked to glycosylated hemoglobin levels. Once again, the adolescents studied were less adherent and were in worse diabetes control than their younger counterparts. However, statistical tests failed to confirm a link between adherence behaviors and Hgb_{a1c}.

The best predictor of Hgb_{a1c} was prior Hgb_{a1c}, which accounted for some 47% of the variance. No adherence construct offered additional predictive power except for calories consumed. Nevertheless, calories consumed was a significant predictor only if it was permitted to interact with Hgb_{a1c} at study entry. Calories consumed showed the expected relationship to Hgb_{a1c} only for those youngsters who entered the study in relatively good control ($Hgb_{a1c} = 5\%-7\%$). Those entering in poor or very poor control ($Hgb_{a1c} = 8\%-15\%$) showed either no relationship between calories consumed and Hgb_{a1c} or an inverse relationship (i.e., lower calorie consumption was associated with higher Hgb_{a1c} levels). Further, the model that included calories consumed offered little predictive power above that offered by initial Hgb_{a1c} alone; only 4% additional variance was accounted for.

Because initial Hgb_{a1c} was such a powerful predictor of subsequent Hgb_{a1c}, one might argue that there was not enough variance left over to detect adherence/diabetes control linkages. It appeared that a longer temporal interval between glycosylated hemoglobin assessments might be more ideal. By this time, we had collected follow-up data on the youngsters we had initially studied cross-sectionally. The time between assessments was a lengthy 1.7 years. Hence, we could test our hypothesis using a longer temporal interval.

STUDY 3: A LONGITUDINAL ANALYSIS OF ADHERENCE/DIABETES CONTROL RELATIONSHIPS USING A 1.7-YEAR TEMPORAL INTERVAL

We managed to collect longitudinal data on almost 200 youngsters. As stated previously, the youngsters entering the study were 6–19 years old and had diabetes for at least 1 year. Obviously, 1.7 years later, the youngsters were older and had the disease longer. At both waves of data collection, adherence was measured via three 24-hour recall interviews, conducted with both parent and child. Although there was a change in glycosylated hemoglobin assay in our laboratory over the time course of the study (from Hgb_{a1} to Hgb_{a1c}), this did not substantively interfere with our analysis.

Because our sample size was relatively large and because we had multiple indicators of most of our adherence constructs, we elected to use linear structural equation modeling (LISREL VI-Joreskog & Sorbom, 1986) in hopes of detecting relationships between our adherence constructs and glycosylated hemoglobin levels (Johnson, Kelly, Henretta, Cunningham, Tomer, & Silverstein, in press). Once again, however, we were unable to detect consistent and significant associations between adherence and glycosylated hemoglobin.

Only testing/eating frequency exhibited any association to Hgb_{a1c}. This relationship is depicted in Fig. 15.1. To ease interpretation, all path coefficients were standardized. In this investigation, we were interested in lipid as well as glucose metabolism; hence, the inclusion of triglycerides in the model. Subscripts are used to depict the two time periods of data collection. As in all of our models, patient age and disease duration are included as predictor variables, as we are interested in whether adherence offers predictive power over and above these patient demographic characteristics.

Patient age was a significant predictor of patient adherence, triglyceride levels, and to a lesser extent glycosylated hemoglobin levels. All of these relationships are consistent with our earlier findings: older children are less adherent and are in worse diabetes control. Disease duration had a far less powerful effect, influencing triglyceride levels only at Evaluation 1, when some children may have been producing some insulin of their own. By Evaluation 2, all children had diabetes close to 3 years. Consequently, few or none were producing any endogenous insulin; at that time disease duration lost its predictive power.

The stability coefficients for both adherence and Hgb_{a1c} were significant and suggested moderate stability over the 1.7-year testing interval. In contrast, triglyceride levels evidenced no across-time stability. There was evidence that testing/eating frequency predicted Hgb_{a1c} at both Evaluation 1 and 2, although this relationship only approached significance at Evaluation 2. Further, the standardized path coefficients are decidedly small.

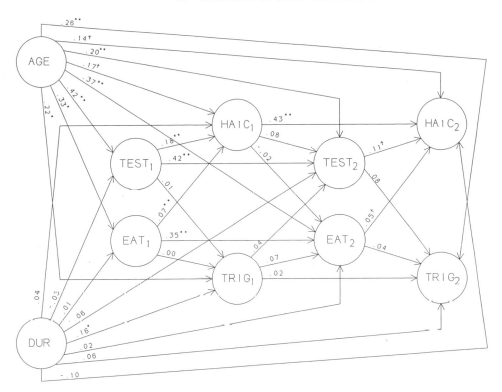

Note: For simplicity, observed variables and error terms are not depicted; *t > 1.96, $p < .05$; **t > 2.58, $p < .01$; + t > 1.65, $p < .10$. N = 193; $X^2(13) = 18.44$ ($p < .141$); $X^2/df = 1.42$; GFI = .982; AGFI = .923.

FIG. 15.1.   Longitudinal model for testing/eating frequency. Model Restrictions are (a) Eating Frequency and Testing Frequency are equally stable, (b) Eating Frequency and Testing Frequency have equal effects on HA1C, and (c) Eating Frequency and Testing Frequency have equal effects on TRIG.

Once again, the best predictor of Hgb_{a1c} was prior Hgb_{a1c}. However, only 28% of the variance of Hgb_{a1c} at Evaluation 2 could be accounted for by the model. There was no evidence supporting a strong link between adherence and diabetes control.

STUDY 4: THE IMPACT OF IMPROVED ADHERENCE ON DIABETES CONTROL

The first three studies I have described were all correlational efforts to detect an association between adherence and diabetes control. Although two of the studies were longitudinal, none attempted to manipulate adherence behaviors. We reasoned that if adherence behaviors are causally linked to diabetes control, a change in adherence should result in a change in diabetes control.

Diabetes camp provides a setting in which children's adherence behaviors are modified. By comparing children's adherence at home to the camp setting and monitoring diabetes control at the beginning and end of diabetes camp, we planned to test whether change in adherence was related to change in diabetes control.

Spevack et al. (1991) conducted this study with 64 7- to 12-year-old youngsters who had diabetes for at least 1 year. Using the 24-hour recall interview methodology the adherence behaviors of children were monitored before, during, and after attending diabetes summer camp. Because diabetes camp is only 2 weeks long, Hgb_{alc} would prove to be an insensitive test of change in diabetes control over such a short temporal interval. Consequently, we selected a glycosylated serum protein assay that provides an index of average blood glucose levels during the preceding 2 weeks. Blood was drawn at the beginning and at the end of the children's camp stay; a glycosylated serum protein assay was conducted on both samples.

As is depicted in Table 15.6, adherence behaviors did change during camp, although they reverted quickly to pre-camp levels once the children returned home. During camp, children took their injections more regularly, at more appropriate intervals, and closer to the 30-minute pre-meal ideal. They exercised more frequently, for longer periods, and more strenuously, and they tested their blood glucose more often. On the dietary measures, they ate more frequently and consumed more calories. However, the types of foods consumed did not change. Because food at camp was served family style, children could select as much of whatever types of foods they desired. Under these conditions, children did not change the types of foods consumed (compared to their home environment) but they did eat more. Although it appeared that children were actually less adherent during camp because they ate too many calories, their increased calorie consumption may have been appropriate in view of their increased exercise.

Despite the fact that change in adherence behaviors was clearly induced by the camp setting, we could find no evidence of a predictive relationship between any of our adherence constructs and glycosylated serum protein levels. The best predictor of glycosylated serum protein levels at the end of camp was glycosylated serum protein levels at the beginning of camp. Adherence behaviors during camp or change in adherence behaviors from home to camp offered no additional predictive power. Once again, there was no evidence for a strong link between adherence behaviors and diabetes control.

GENERAL DISCUSSION

In some respects, our studies confirm what many clinicians already know: Older youngsters are less adherent and older youngsters are in worse

TABLE 15.6
Adherence Behaviors Before, During, and After a Diabetes Summer Camp
(Spevack et al., 1991)

Adherence Measures*	2 Weeks Before Camp	2 Weeks During Camp	2 Weeks After Camp	6 Weeks After Camp	12 Weeks After Camp
Injection Behaviors					
**Injection Regularity	.47	.27	.50	.46	.68
(minutes)	(28.0)	(15.9)	(30.1)	(27.6)	(40.6)
**Injection Interval	.71	.59	.95	.87	.94
(minutes)	(42.5)	(35.1)	(56.9)	(52.2)	(56.2)
**Injection-Meal Timing	.70	.49	.68	.66	.71
(minutes before meal)	(17.6)	(30.3)	(19.2)	(20.5)	(17.3)
Regularity of Injection-Meal					
Timing (minutes)	18.7	18.1	19.5	12.0	18.2
Exercise Behaviors					
**Exercise Frequency	80.0	26.7	83.3	81.7	81.7
**Exercise Duration	.09	.03	.16	.17	.12
(minutes)	(20.0)	(42.4)	(14.4)	(15.4)	(14.1)
**Exercise Type	.97	.94	.98	.97	.97
(kcal/min.)	(.03)	(.06)	(.02)	(.03)	(.03)
Dietary Behaviors					
**Eating Frequency	15.4	2.6	15.3	17.3	16.3
(per day)	(5.1)	(5.8)	(5.1)	(5.0)	(5.0)
**Calories Consumed					
(above or below ideal)	−72	382	−35	−65	59
% Calories: Carbohydrate	24.3	23.3	25.4	24.8	23.3
(percent)	(35.7)	(36.7)	(34.6)	(35.2)	(36.7)
% Calories: Fat	23.7	22.0	24.5	23.9	22.7
(percent)	(48.7)	(47.0)	(49.5)	(48.9)	(47.7)
Concentrated Sweets					
(per day)	1.5	1.2	1.3	1.4	1.6
Glucose Testing Behaviors					
**Testing Frequency	51.2	45.8	54.1	59.2	60.8
(per day)	(2.0)	(2.2)	(1.8)	(1.6)	(1.6)

*Lower scores indicate greater adherence. In parentheses are interpretations of the adherence measures using more familiar measurement scales.
**Camp significantly different from before or after camp.

diabetes control. Given these associations, it is perhaps understandable that many, if not most, clinicians have come to believe that adolescents' poor control is caused by their poor compliance. However, our studies have failed to confirm such an association. We were able to identify few adherence/diabetes control linkages and those that were identified offered little in the way of predictive power. Our findings are consistent with the broader literature on this topic. Earlier studies have typically found a weak relationship between adherence and diabetes control, if a significant association emerged at all.

Where do we go from here? Some might argue that diabetes is simply too powerful a disease for behavior to make much difference. Although this may be true, there are several issues that need to be addressed before we can come to this conclusion.

First, there has been a tendency to reify glycosylated hemoglobin as the measure of diabetes control. Glycosylated hemoglobin is an index of average blood glucose. As such, it is insensitive to blood glucose variability. Two patients may differ greatly in terms of blood glucose variability and yet appear very much the same in terms of glycosylated hemoglobin levels. It is certainly possible that adherence behaviors influence blood glucose variability more than average blood glucose levels. Assessing glycosylated hemoglobin levels alone, will not permit us to assess such a relationship.

Glycosylated hemoglobin is a measure of glucose metabolism. Diabetes disrupts lipid metabolism as well. In fact, most children with diabetes ultimately die in adulthood of atherosclerotic heart disease (Barrett-Conner & Orchard, 1985). Yet, few studies have examined the effect of adherence behaviors on indices of lipid metabolism in IDDM individuals. Perhaps adherence behaviors exert a more powerful influence on lipid as compared to glucose metabolism in this population. Our own work suggests this is so (Johnson, Freund, Silverstein, Hanson, & Malone, 1990), although the relationship between adherence and measures of lipid metabolism is quite complex.

The consistent association between patient age and diabetes control found in many of our models suggests that biological changes associated with puberty may be exerting powerful effects on adolescents' diabetes control. A study by Amiel, Sherwin, Simonson, Lauritano, and Tamborlane (1986) offers some support for this hypothesis. These investigators examined insulin resistance in diabetic and nondiabetic adolescents, preadolescents, and adults. Insulin resistance was found to increase during adolescence for both the diabetic and nondiabetic groups, although the effect was most pronounced in the diabetic sample. The authors offered the following interpretation of their results: "it seems likely that physiologic factors, as well as psychosocial factors, have a role in the poor glycemic control often noted in teenage patients with diabetes. . . . Indeed, one can envision a vicious cycle in which the puberty-related reduction in insulin sensitivity leads to hyperglycemia, which leads in turn to further resistance and frustrates attempts to maintain compliance in these difficult cases" (p. 219). We agree. If biological factors associated with puberty were adequately assessed, true adherence/diabetes control linkages might be more readily discerned.

Insulin dose and insulin dose determination also need more careful consideration. We have not found insulin dose per se to offer predictive power in any of our causal models. However, it is also true that the strength of adherence/diabetes control relationships is ultimately dependent on the adequacy of a patient's prescribed insulin dose. Adherence should only make a difference if the medical treatment regimen prescribed is effective. No amount of adherence can make an ineffective regimen effective. If patients are over- or under-insulinized, this could have a profound effect on adherence/diabetes control associations. If adherence/diabetes control relationships differ when patients have too little as opposed to too much insulin, these relationships will be obscured when patients are combined into a single group for study. This is a knotty problem because there is no objective index of over- or under-insulinization (other than glycosylated hemoglobin level that is presumably affected by other variables in addition to insulin dose). Nevertheless, it is a problem with profound implications for any investigator attempting to delineate associations between patient behavior and diabetes control.

All of our studies to date assume that the influence of behavior on diabetes control is similar across individuals. This may not be the case. One person's diabetes may be influenced by the timing of injections whereas another person may be more sensitive to exercise. Yet another person may be effected by the timing or frequency of meals and still another person may be effected by the type of food consumed. Group analyses will never detect such individual patterns if they are truly idiosyncratic across individuals (although consistent within the individual). Although we know little about individual differences in adherence/diabetes control relationships, studies of patient hypo- or hyperglycemic experiences have confirmed individual symptom patterns that remain undetected when symptom/blood glucose relationships are examined using group data (Freund, Johnson, Rosenbloom, Alexander, & Hansen, 1986; Pennebaker et al., 1981). Assumptions about across-subject consistency may be obscuring true, but idiosyncratic, adherence/diabetes control relationships. We may need to turn to intrasubject designs to answer this important question.

Obviously, more research needs to be done before we can definitively answer the question: Does behavior really make a difference in the management of childhood diabetes? Nevertheless, it does seem clear that adherence does not have a simple and powerful link to diabetes control. Admittedly, failure to take insulin will have dire medical consequences. But, in our and others' (Glasgow et al., 1987) experience, most patients adhere to this aspect of the regimen. It is the impact of the myriad of remaining behaviors (which include multiple behaviors associated with insulin injections) that is open to question. Physicians generally believe that patients in poor control are nonadherent and those in good control are highly compliant. This belief is so ingrained that physicians commonly use glycosylated hemoglobin assay results as an indicator of patient adherence (Clarke et al., 1985). Yet, our and others' data do not support this assertion. Although we may not yet be able to definitively answer the question, "does behavior make a difference?", we certainly need to emphasize the importance of asking that question. Physician beliefs about powerful links between adherence behaviors and diabetes control have important implications for patient care. If poor control means poor adherence to the doctor, the patient may be blamed for his or her medical condition. The physician may do little to change the patient's medical prescription because the patient is seen as the source of the problem. In turn, the patient may develop feelings of discouragement and resentment, particularly if sincere efforts have been made to adhere to the medical regimen. It is probably best for all concerned if we emphasize the importance of the question rather than the definitiveness of its answer.

ACKNOWLEDGMENT

This chapter was supported by grants #R01 HD 13820 and K04 HD 00686 from the National Institute of Child Health and Human Development.

REFERENCES

Amiel, S. A., Sherwin, R. S., Simonson, D. C., Lauritano, A. A., & Tamborlane, W. V. (1986). Impaired insulin action in puberty: A contributing factor to poor glycemic control in adolescents with diabetes. *The New England Journal of Medicine, D1,* 215–219.

Anderson, B. J., Wolf, F. M., Burkhart, M. T., Cornell, R. G., & Bacon, G. E. (1989). Effects of peer-group intervention on metabolic control of adolescents with IDDM: Randomized outpatient study. *Diabetes Care 12,* 179–183.

Barrett-Conner, E., & Orchard, T. (1985). Diabetes and heart disease. In M. Harris & R. Hamman (Eds.). *Diabetes in America* (pp. XVI: 1–41). (NIH Publication No. 85–1468). Washington, DC: U.S. Department of Health and Human Services/Public Health Service.

Brownlee-Duffeck, M. Peterson, L., Simonds, J. F., Goldstein, D., Kilo, C., & Hoette, S. (1987). The role of health beliefs in the regimen adherence and metabolic control of adolescents and adults with diabetes mellitus. *Journal of Consulting and Clinical Psychology, 5,* 139–144.

Carney, R. M., Schechter, K., & Davis, T. (1983). Improving adherence to blood glucose testing in insulin-dependent diabetic children. *Behavior Therapy, 14,* 247–254.

Christensen, N. K., Terry, R. D., Wyatt, S., Pichert, J. W., & Lorenz, R. A. (1983). Quantitative assessment of dietary adherence in patients with insulin-dependent diabetes mellitus. *Diabetes Care, 6,* 245–250.

Clarke, W. L., Snyder, A. L., & Nowacek, G. (1985). Outpatient pediatric diabetes-I. Current practices. *Journal of Chronic Diseases, 38,* 85–90.

Cox, D. J., Taylor, A. G., Nowacek, G., Holley-Wilcox, P., & Pohl, S. L. (1984). The relationship between psychological stress and insulin-dependent diabetic blood glucose control: Preliminary investigations. *Health Psychology, 3,* 63–75.

Cohen, J., & Cohen, P. (1983). *Applied multiple regression/correlation analysis for the behavioral sciences* (2nd ed.). Hillsdale, NJ: Lawrence Erlbaum Associates.

Daneman, D., Siminerio, L., Transue, D., Betschart, J., Drash, A., & Becker, D. (1985). The role of self-monitoring of blood glucose in the routine management of children with insulin-dependent diabetes mellitus. *Diabetes Care, 8,* 1–4.

Epstein, L. H., Beck, S., Figueroa, J., Farkas, G., Kazdin, A. E., Daneman, D., & Becker, D. (1981). The effects of targeting improvements in urine glucose on metabolic control in children with insulin dependent diabetes. *Journal of Applied Behavior Analysis, 14,* 365–375.

Epstein, L. H., Coburn, P. C., Becker, D., Drash, A., & Siminerio, L. (1980). Measurement and modification of the accuracy of determinations of urine glucose concentration. *Diabetes Care, 3,* 535–536.

Freund, A., Johnson, S. B., Rosenbloom, A. L., Alexander, B., & Hansen, C. A. (1986). Subjective symptoms, blood glucose estimation, and blood glucose concentrations in adolescents with diabetes. *Diabetes Care, 9,* 236–243.

Freund, A., Johnson, S. B., Silverstein, J., & Thomas, J. (1991). Assessing daily management of childhood diabetes using 24-hr. recall interviews: Reliability and stability. *Health Psychology, 10,* 200–208.

Glasgow, R. E., McCaul, K. D., & Schafer, L. C. (1987). Self-care behaviors and glycemic control in type I diabetes. *Journal of Chronic Disease, 40,* 399–417.

Glasgow, R. E., Wilson, W., & McCaul, K. D. (1985). Regimen adherence: A problematic construct in diabetes research. *Diabetes Care, 8,* 300–301.

Gonder-Frederick, L. A., Julian, D. M., Cox, D. J., Clarke, W. L., & Carter, W. R. (1988). Self-measurement of blood glucose: Accuracy of self-reported data and adherence to recommended regimen. *Diabetes Care, 11,* 579–585.

Gross, A. M. (1982). Self-management training and medication compliance in children with diabetes. *Child and Family Behavior Therapy, 4,* 47–55.

Gross, A. M., Johnson, W. G., Wildman, H. E., & Mullett, J. (1981). Coping skills training with insulin-dependent preadolescent diabetics. *Child Behavior Therapy, 3,* 141–153.

Hanson, C. L., Henggeler, S. W., & Burghen, G. A. (1987a). Model of associations between psychosocial variables and health-outcome measures of adolescents with IDDM. *Diabetes Care, 10,* 752–758.

Hanson, C. L., Henggeler, S. W., & Burghen, G. A. (1987b). Race and sex differences in metabolic control of adolescents with IDDM: A function of psychosocial variables? *Diabetes Care, 10,* 313–318.

Haynes, R. B. (1979). Introduction. In R. B. Haynes, D. W. Taylor, & D. L. Sackett (Eds.), *Compliance in health care* (pp. 1–7). Baltimore, MD: Johns Hopkins Press.

Johnson, S. B. (1990). Adherence behaviors and health status in childhood diabetes. In C. Holmes (Ed.), *Neuropsychological and behavioral aspects of diabetes* (pp. 30–57). New York: Springer-Verlag.

Johnson, S. B., Freund, A., Silverstein, J., Hansen, C., & Malone, J. Adherence/health status relationships in childhood diabetes. *Health Psychology, 9,* 606–631.

Johnson, S. B., Kelly, M., Henretta, J. C., Cunningham, W. R., Tomer, A., & Silverstein, J. H. (in press). A longitudinal analysis of adherence and health status relationships in childhood diabetes. *Journal of Pediatric Psychology.*

Johnson, S. B., Pollak, T., Silverstein, J. H., Rosenbloom, A. L., Spillar, R., McCallum, M., & Harkavy, J. (1982). Cognitive and behavioral knowledge about insulin dependent diabetes among children and parents. *Pediatrics, 69,* 708–713.

Johnson, S. B., Silverstein, J., Rosenbloom, A., Carter, R., & Cunningham, W. (1986). Assessing daily management in childhood diabetes. *Health Psychology, 5,* 545–564.

Johnson, S. B., Silverstein, J., Rosenbloom, A., Hansen, C. A., Carter, R., & Cunningham, W. (1986). *Compliance and health status in childhood diabetes: A preliminary cross-sectional investigation.* Unpublished manuscript, University of Florida, Gainesville.

Johnson, S. B., Tomer, A., Cunningham, W. R., & Henretta, J. (1990). Adherence in childhood diabetes: Results of a confirmatory factor analysis. *Health Psychology, 9,* 493–501.

Joreskog, K. G., & Sorbom, D. (1986). *LISREL VI: Analysis of linear structural relationships by maximum likelihood, instrumental variables, and least square methods* (4th ed.). Uppsala, Sweden: University of Uppsala.

Kaplan, R. M., Chadwick, M. W., & Schimmel, L. E. (1985). Social learning intervention to promote metabolic control in type I diabetes mellitus: Pilot experiment results. *Diabetes Care, 8,* 107–206.

Kaar, M.-L., Akerblom, H. K., Huttunen, N.-P., Knip, M., & Sakkinen, K. (1984). Metabolic control in children and adolescents with insulin-dependent diabetes mellitus. *Acta Paediatrica Scandinavica, 73,* 102–108.

LaPorte, R. E., & Cruickshanks, K. J. (1985). Incidence and risk factors for insulin-dependent diabetes. In M. Harris & R. Hamman (Eds.), *Diabetes in America.* (pp. III:1–12). (NIH Publication No 85–1468.) Bethesda, MD: U.S. Department of Health and Human Services, National Institutes of Health.

LaPorte, R. E., & Tajima, N. (1985). Prevalence of insulin-dependent diabetes. In M. Harris & R. Hamman (Eds.), *Diabetes in America* (pp. V: 1–8). (NIH Publication No 85–1468.) Bethesda, MD: U.S. Department of Health and Human Services, National Institute of Health.

Lowe, K., & Lutzker, J. R. (1979). Increasing compliance to a medical regimen with a juvenile diabetic. *Behavior Therapy, 10,* 57–64.

Marquis, K. H., Ware, J. E., Jr., & Relles, D. A. (1979). *Measures of diabetic patient knowledge, attitudes and behavior regarding self-care: Summary Report* (NTIS No. PB83–134528). Atlanta, GA: Center for Disease Control.

Mazze, R. S., Pasmantier, R., Murphy, J., & Shamoon, H. (1985). Self-monitoring of capillary blood glucose: Changing the performance of individuals with diabetes. *Diabetes Care, 8,* 207–213.

Nuttall, F. Q., & Brunzall, J. D. (1979) Principles of nutrition and dietary recommendations for individuals with diabetes mellitus: 1979. *Journal of the American Dietary Association, 75,* 527–530.

Orme, C. M., & Binik, Y. M. (1989). Consistency of adherence across regimen demands. *Health Psychology, 8,* 27–43.

Pennebaker, J. W., Cox, D. J., Gonder-Frederick, L., Wunsch, M. G., Pohl, S., & Evans, W. (1981). Physical symptoms related to blood glucose in insulin-dependent diabetes mellitus. *Psychosomatic Medicine, 43,* 489–500.

Reynolds, L., Johnson, S. B., & Silverstein, J. (1990). Assessing daily diabetes management by 24-hr. recall interview: The validity of children's reports. *Journal of Pediatric Psychology, 15,* 493–509.

Rubin, R. R., Peyrot, M., & Saudek, C. D. (1989) Effect of diabetes education on self-care, metabolic control, and emotional well-being. *Diabetes Care, 12,* 673–679.

Satin, W., La Greca, A. M., Zigo, M. A., & Skyler, J. S. (1989). Diabetes in adolescence: Effects of multifamily group intervention and parent simulation of diabetes. *Journal of Pediatric Psychology, 14,* 259–275.

Schafer, L. C., Glasgow, R. E., & McCaul, K. D. (1982). Increasing the adherence of diabetic adolescents. *Journal of Behavioral Medicine, 5,* 353–362.

Schafer, L. C., Glasgow, R. E., McCaul, K. D., & Dreher, M. (1983). Adherence to IDDM regimens: Relationship to psychosocial variables and metabolic control. *Diabetes Care, 6,* 493–498.

Schafer, L. C., McCaul, K. D., & Glasgow, R. E. (1986). Supportive and nonsupportive family behaviors: Relationships to adherence and metabolic control in persons with Type I diabetes. *Diabetes Care, 9,* 179–185.

Simonds, J., Goldstein, D., Walker, B., & Rawlings, S. (1981). The relationship between psychological factors and blood glucose regulation in insulin-dependent diabetic adolescents. *Diabetes Care, 4,* 610–615.

Spevack, M., Johnson, S. B., & Riley, W. (1991) The effect of diabetes summer camp on adherence behaviors and glycemic control. In J. Johnson & S. B. Johnson (Eds.), *Advances in child health psychology,* (pp. 285–292). Gainesville, FL: University of Florida Press.

Watkins, J. D., Williams, R., Martin, D. A., Hogan, M. D., & Anderson, E. (1967). A study of diabetic patients at home. *American Journal of Public Health, 57,* 452–459.

Webb, K. L., Dobson, A. J., Tupling, H. E., Harris, G. W., O'Connell, D. L., Atkinson, J., Sulway, M. J., & Leeder, S. R. (1982). Evaluation of a diabetes education programme. *Australian/New Zealand Journal of Medicine, 12,* 153–160.

Webb, K. L., Dobson, A. J., O'Connell, D. L., Tupling, H. E., Harris, G. W., Moxon, J. A., Sulway, M. J., & Leeder, S. R. (1984). Dietary compliance among insulin-dependent diabetics. *Journal of Chronic Disease, 37,* 633–643.

Wilson, D. P., & Endres, R. K. (1986). Compliance with blood glucose monitoring in children with Type I diabetes mellitus. *The Journal of Pediatrics, 108,* 1022–1024.

Wing, R., Nowalk, M., Marcus, M., Koeske, R., & Finegold, D. (1986). Subclinical eating disorders and glycemic control in adolescents with Type I diabetes. *Diabetes Care, 9,* 162–167.

Wysocki, T., Green, L., & Huxtable, K. (1989). Blood glucose monitoring by diabetic adolescents: Compliance and metabolic control. *Health Psychology, 8,* 267–284.

Ziel, R. H., & Davidson, M. B. (1987). The role of glycosylated serum albumin in monitoring glycemic control in stable insulin-requiring diabetic out patients. *Journal of Clinical Endocrinology and Metabolism, 64,* 269–273.

Author Index

Subject Index